COMMUNITY HEALTH NURSING

An Alliance for Health

NOTICE

Medicine is an ever-changing science. As new research and clinical experience broaden our knowledge, changes in treatment and drug therapy are required. The authors and the publisher of this work have checked with sources believed to be reliable in their efforts to provide information that is complete and generally in accord with the standards accepted at the time of publication. However, in view of the possibility of human error or changes in medical sciences, neither the authors, nor the publisher nor any other party who has been involved in the preparation or publication of this work warrants that the information contained herein is in every respect accurate or complete, and they are not responsible for any errors or omissions or for the results obtained from use of such information. Readers are encouraged to confirm the information contained herein with other sources. For example and in particular, readers are advised to check the product information sheet included in the package of each drug they plan to administer to be certain that the information contained in this book is accurate and that changes have not been made in the recommended dose or in the contraindications for administration. This recommendation is of particular importance in connection with new or infrequently used drugs.

COMMUNITY HEALTH NURSING

An Alliance for Health

McGraw-Hill

Health Professions Division

McGRAW-HILL NURSING CORE SERIES

New York St. Louis San Francisco Auckland Bogotá Caracas Lisbon
London Madrid Mexico City Milan Montreal New Delhi San Juan
Singapore Sydney Tokyo Toronto

MARILYN B. KLAINBERG, R.N., Ed.D.

Assistant Professor
Adelphi University School of Nursing
Garden City, New York
Clinical Associate Professor and
    Director of Continuing Education
State University of New York
Health Science Center at Brooklyn
School of Nursing
Brooklyn, New York

STEPHEN P. HOLZEMER, Ph.D., R.N.

Dean and Professor
Long Island College Hospital
    School of Nursing
Brooklyn, New York
Consultant, Nursing Education
St. Francis College
Brooklyn, New York

MARGARET LEONARD, M.S., R.N.C., F.N.P.

Director of Quality Case Management
New York State Catholic Health Plan
Rego Park, New York
Adjunct Faculty
College of New Rochelle School of Nursing
New Rochelle, New York
Producer and Host, "Community Nurse—
    On Call"
WHPC–FM
Garden City, New York

JOAN ARNOLD, PH.D., R.N.

Associate Professor
College of New Rochelle School of Nursing
New Rochelle, New York

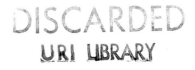

McGraw-Hill

A Division of The McGraw-Hill Companies

COMMUNITY HEALTH NURSING: An Alliance for Health

Copyright © 1998 by The McGraw-Hill Companies, Inc. All rights reserved. Printed in the United States of America. Except as permitted under the United States Copyright Act of 1976, no part of this publication may be reproduced or distributed in any form or by any means, or stored in a data base or retrieval system, without the prior written permission of the publisher.

1 2 3 4 5 6 7 8 9 0 DOW DOW 9 9 8 7

ISBN 0-07-105478-2

This book was set in Sabon by V&M Graphics, Inc.
The editors were John Dolan and Steven Melvin;
and the production supervisor was Richard Ruzycka;
the cover and text were designed by Patrice Sheridan.
The index was prepared by Patricia Perrier.
R.R. Donnelley and Sons was printer and binder.

This book is printed on acid-free paper.

Cataloging-in-Publication Data is on file for this title at the Library of Congress.

CONTENTS

CONTRIBUTORS

Lillian Anderson-Rafeldt, M.A., R.N., C.N.S. [15]
Instructor
Salve Regina College
Newport, Rhode Island
Consultant in Geriatric Nursing
Voluntown, Connecticut

Joan Arnold, Ph.D., R.N. [5, 6, 7, 8, 9, 10, 12]
Associate Professor
College of New Rochelle
    School of Nursing
New Rochelle, New York

Laurel Janssen Breen, M.A., R.N. [10]
Consultant in Health Care
Sea Cliff, New York
Senior Adjunct Faculty
Adelphi University
Garden City, New York

Susan Buchholtz, Ed.D., R.N. [2]
Instructor
Mt. Vernon Hospital
    School of Nursing
Mt. Vernon, New York

Carolyn A. Fish, M.P.H., R.N. [16]
Professor
University of New England
Westbrook Campus
Department of Nursing
Portland, Maine

Theresa M. Graf, C.I.J., Ed.D., R.N. [11]
Director of Health Services
Interfaith Nutrition Network
Hempstead, New York

**Carol Green-Hernandez, Ph.D., F.N.S.,
A.N.P./F.N.P.,C. [17]**
Associate Professor
Project Director, Primary Care Nurse
    Practitioner Program
University of Vermont
Burlington, Vermont

Numbers in brackets refer to chapters written or cowritten by the contributors.

Stephen Paul Holzemer, Ph.D., R.N. [5, 11, 13, 14, 15, 16, 17]
Dean and Professor
Long Island College Hospital
    School of Nursing
Brooklyn, New York
and
Consultant, Nursing Education
St. Francis College
Brooklyn, New York

Marilyn Klainberg, Ed.D., R.N. [1, 2, 3, 4, 11]
Assistant Professor
Adelphi University School of Nursing
Garden City, New York
and
Clinical Associate Professor and
    Director of Continuing Education
State University of New York
Health Science Center at Brooklyn
School of Nursing
Brooklyn, New York

Margaret Leonard, M.S., R.N.C., F.N.P. [11, 18, 19, 20, 21]
Director of Quality Case Management
New York State Catholic Health Plan
Rego Park, New York
and
Adjunct Faculty
College of New Rochelle
    School of Nursing
New Rochelle, New York
and
Producer and Host, "Community Nurse—On Call"
WHPC–FM
Garden City, New York

Maria E. Scaramuzzino, M.S.N., R.N., F.N.P. [13]
Instructor
The Long Island College Hospital
    School of Nursing
Brooklyn, New York

Joanne K. Singleton, Ph.D., R.N., C.S., F.N.P. [17]
Assistant Professor
Pace University
Leinhard School of Nursing
Pleasantville, New York

Numbers in brackets refer to chapters written or cowritten by the contributors.

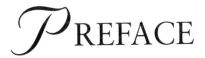

$\mathcal{P}$REFACE

Community Health Nursing: An Alliance for Health is intended as a basic text for the undergraduate student, serving as an introduction to community health nursing, and for the professional registered nurse practicing in community-based settings. This book presents community health nursing as part of a health alliance working collaboratively with members of the community and other health care professions to meet the health needs of clients. Whether the consumer of health care is viewed as an individual family, an aggregate, or the community, this book elucidates the need for providing seamless health care to the client. With an emphasis on care of the client in the community, this text serves as an important source and reference for nurses in this changing time of health care delivery.

Margin notes clarify and expand definitions and provide highlighted content areas that are emphasized for the reader. Annotated references are provided to direct readers toward more in-depth discussions of the concepts presented and toward further readings.

Part 1, Basic Principles of Community Health Nursing, serves as an introduction to the basic concepts of community health nursing, which are developed throughout this book. Chapter 1 provides an overview of community health and public health nursing; an introduction to changes in the health care system; an introduction to caring for families, groups, and communities; and a brief overview of the epidemiological process relative to community health. Chapter 2 provides a brief historic overview of community health nursing. Chapter 3 explores the impact of cultural diversity on how nurses provide health care to a community. Chapter 4 explores ethical issues related to community health nursing.

Part 2, The Community as Client, introduces the reader to the community as a system and client for care, using the Alliance for Health model. Chapter 5 details the Alliance Model, an interdisciplinary approach for community-based health care. The component parts of the model include community-based needs, systems of care management, and resource allocation decisions. This model is used to frame the application of the nursing process in the care of communities. Chapter 6 describes the community itself from a variety of perspectives. Chapter 7 identifies the community as a client system and provides the reader with ways in which to view the community and the importance of an interdisciplinary approach to care. Chapters 8, 9, and 10 apply the nursing process in caring for communities.

Part 3, Caring for People in Their Homes or Where They Live, provides information relevant to actual hands-on care of the client. Chapter 11 provides information relevant to making a home visit. Chapter 12 reviews the methodology for assessing the family, and Chapter 13 explores high-technology and home care. Chapter 14 looks at the challenges of working with a multitiered health care system. Chapter 15 provides an understanding of the infrastructure of the health care system and the role nurses play in it. Chapter 16 examines the effect of accreditation on certification and on continuity of care. Chapter 17 explores re-engineering of the nursing profession for survival in an ongoing care delivery system.

Part 5, The Business and Politics of Community Health Nursing, gives any student or registered nurse insight into the business and political aspects of community health nursing. Chapters 18 and 19 give the reader a basic understanding of the different types of businesses that are possible and the workings of the government. Chapter 20 covers managed care. Chapter 21 details the opportunities available to nurses in the changing health care industry and the important role professional organizations play in forging the nursing profession ahead.

$\mathcal{A}$CKNOWLEDGMENTS

It is with great appreciation that the authors thank the following persons for their contribution to this book: Laurel Janssen Breen, Jane Edwards, Janet Hand, Francine Medoff, and Linda Rubino.

A special thanks to our family and friends who have been most patient and supportive during this endeavor. For all your love, support, and encouragement, thank you to Ron Leonard; Denise and David McGraw; Billy Murphy; Cornelius, Virginia, Jack, Jennifer, P. J., and Jessica Brolly; Peter Suarez; Chris, Tom, Andrew, Eric, and Meaganne Hattorff; Elise, Lauren, and Erica Leonard; Kay and Dick Malenchek; Sally and Tim Boggan; John Shannon Keogh; Carolyn Fish; Rick, Michael, and Matthew Arnold; Bernard, Dennis, Dana, Greg, Jenny, Joshua, Max, Adam, Emma, and Sydney Klainberg; Danielle, Mark, and Sofia Rosenberg; Marcia Hammer; Anne Lupkin; Rose Ciampa; Nancy Giordano; and especially to the students who have been our teachers and have taught us so much.

COMMUNITY HEALTH NURSING

An Alliance for Health

BASIC PRINCIPLES OF COMMUNITY HEALTH NURSING

THE NATURE OF COMMUNITY HEALTH

CHANGE IN HEALTH CARE SYSTEM

Since 1990, the health care system in the United States has experienced and continues to experience tremendous change. During that time "the organizational, financial, and legal framework of much of the health care in the U. S. [has] been transformed" (Pew Health Professions Commission, 1995, p. 1). The greatest impact upon the American health care system has been the implementation of managed care and an increase in the number of clients who are cared for at home. The high cost of hospitalization has been drastically reduced by hospital closures and downsizing, resulting in a loss of hospital beds, thus decreasing hospital stays for clients. Because clients are sent home sooner, there is a critical need for increased as well as technologically sophisticated home care. By the year 2000, there will be an even greater focus on managed care with an emphasis on community and public health services.

COMMUNITY HEALTH NURSING

Community health nurses practice in a variety of settings with individuals, families, groups, and the community as a whole. The role of the community health nurse is dynamic and continues to change and grow as it meets the needs of society. As primary providers of health care, community health nurses maintain a variety of roles. Health care provided by the community health nurse to communities, groups, aggregates, families, and clients includes health education, health promotion, and screening and prevention programs through public health departments, ambulatory departments at hospitals, or voluntary community health-related organizations. Community health nurses may provide care to individual clients through voluntary agencies such as the visiting nurse service; proprietary, for-profit, home care agencies; hospital-based home care departments; and in ambulatory settings such as schools and places of work. The health care provided to individuals and families may involve direct client care services, including hands-on care for specific needs of the client (e.g., wound care or assessment of preexisting conditions). An in-depth look at these roles is discussed in Chap. 15.

Regardless of their focus, the community health nurse always provides health education and guidance to the client and the client's family. In addition, the community health nurse coordinates planning, case management, counseling, and referral of the client to other health care providers (e.g., physical therapists, nutrition counselors, occupational therapists). Together with the client and the community health nurse, these health care providers form a *health alliance*. By forming and encouraging alliances, community health nurses maintain a global approach to the health of individual clients and the community as a client. The notion of well communities fostering individual health is important as there is a reciprocal relationship between individual health, family health, and the health of communities. As the world "grows smaller" as a result of improved technology, extended global trade, increased recreational travel, and improved transportation systems, the opportunity to spread disease increases; thus, community health professionals must increasingly incorporate the concept of the well community into practice.

Community Health Nurse

Often the perception of the community health nurse is that of the visiting nurse who is concerned with the health of clients exclusively in their homes. Although this perception is somewhat true, the role of community health nurses as interpreted by the American Nurses Association (ANA) is to provide care to individuals, families, and aggregates within communities, using skills and knowledge relevant to both nursing and public health (ANA, 1986). They provide counseling services; conduct assessments; provide guidance and education; or implement research to improve client health care. In any of these roles, the community nurse always acts as the client advocate whether the client is an individual, family, group, or community. The ANA further defines community health nursing as a synthesis of nursing practice and public health practice concerned with the promotion and preservation of the health of populations. This is not limited to particular age groups or to a particular diagnosis. It is continual, not episodic, and while it is often directed at individuals, it contributes to the health of the total population. Thus, community health nursing practice is concerned with the promotion of the public's health (ANA, 1986).

Further confusion regarding the role of community health nurses has arisen from the fact that the terms "community health nurse" and "public health nurse" are often used interchangeably.

Public Health Nursing This term refers to the composite of nursing services and health promotion of populations. Its aim is to improve sanitation; control community epidemics; prevent the transmission of infection; provide education about the principles of personal hygiene; organize medical and nursing services for early diagnosis, prevention, and treatment of disease; and develop social mechanisms and standards of living that will ensure the health of individuals in the community and the world. The term public health nurse should be used to describe one who has been educationally prepared and supervised in clinical practice in public health nursing. At the basic level, the public health nurse holds a baccalaureate degree in nursing. A public health specialist is prepared at a graduate level with a focus in the public health sciences and holds a master's or doctoral degree [U.S. Department of Health and Human Services (DHHS), 1985].

Public health nursing synthesizes knowledge from public health science and professional nursing theories. It is used for the improvement of health for the entire community. Public health nursing embraces the goals of preventing illness and injury and promoting health (ANA, 1986).

Community Health Nursing This term is broader in that it incorporates public health nursing. It is defined as "...the synthesis of nursing theory and public health theory applied to promoting and preserving the health of populations. The focus of community health nursing practice is the community as a whole with nursing care of individuals, families, and groups being provided within the context of promoting and preserving the health of the community as a whole" (Association of Community Health Nursing Educators, 1990, p. 1). The term community health nurse refers to any nurse working within the community. This may be used to describe nurses at any level working within the community (e.g., occupational health nurses, school nurses, hospice nurses, home care nurses). A community health nursing specialist has a master's or doctoral degree in nursing (DHHS, 1985).

Community health nursing provides care and the insurance of high-level wellness to individuals, groups, and families within the scope of larger community needs.

Scope of Care

For many health care professionals unfamiliar with the principles and practice dimensions of community health nursing, the notion of providing care for a community or a population is a difficult concept to comprehend. Most nurses care exclusively for individuals in hospital settings. Community health nurses maintain a global approach to the health of a client be it an individual, a family, a group, or a community, regardless of the dimension. The notion of well communities fostering individual health is important to how community health nurses approach community health care.

Although primary care is an established role for the community health nurse, case management is a fairly new role. The community health nurse case manager manages the client's care and collaborates with other health care professionals. Case management has been defined as "a health care delivery process whose goals are to provide quality health care, decrease fragmentation, enhance clients' quality of life, and contain costs" (ANA Council on Community Health Nursing).

PUBLIC HEALTH SERVICES

"The mission of state and local health agencies is to protect and promote health, and prevent disease and injury" [National Association of County Health Officials (NACHO), 1993, p. 4]. To accomplish this, public health agency services include a multitude of activities, which can be grouped under one of three core functions: assessment, policy development, and assurance (NACHO, 1993). It is the responsibility of public health nurses working for a public health agency such as the DHHS to maintain the scope of these functions.

Assessment refers to the monitoring of the health status of communities or populations by public health agencies. It also includes the collection and analysis of statistics (e.g., morbidity and mortality data). Public health assessors view and measure the health resources, which meet or do not adequately meet the health needs of a community (NACHO, 1993).

Policy development is the formation of plans or actions developed to meet a community's assessed needs (NACHO, 1993).

Quality assurance refers to the method or process of establishing policies into services. Public health agencies assure that necessary services are available; it does not mean that the public health agencies actually provide the services.

Public Health Agencies

Public health agencies may be local, national, or international. International health agencies such as the World Health Organization (WHO) focus on global issues, set policy, develop standards, assess health conditions, and monitor health promotion programs. National agencies such as the U.S. Department of Health and Human Services (DHHS) provide funding and develop policy, but the states or local communities usually implement these policies. National agencies also develop and support programs for special groups (e.g., migrant workers, Native Americans, veterans, military personnel) and assess and monitor statewide health needs and services. The Centers for Disease Control (CDC) nationally monitor and report the occurrence of communicable diseases and publish a weekly report, the *Morbidity and Mortality Weekly Report (MMWR)*. Federal law requires that specific communicable diseases be reported to the CDC.

State and local government health agencies may vary considerably in how they implement programs and meet community needs, but federal or national standards ensure the maintenance of local standards. At the local level, city or county government may perform assessments (e.g., data collection), develop plans (e.g., inventory health resources, hold public forums, collect information, engage in research), and deliver health services.

Information is now readily available via the Internet, telephone, and fax. Air travel to distant destinations has not only made the swift transportation of vaccines, antibiotics, or rare blood possible, but it is also instrumental in spreading disease more rapidly.

COMMUNITY HEALTH STANDARDS OF PRACTICE

The community health standards of practice are based on the *Standards of Community Health Nursing Practice* (ANA, 1986) (See Table 1-1). These standards reflect two levels of practice: the generalist who is prepared at the baccalaureate level and the specialist who is prepared at the master's level (ANA, 1986). Nurses prepared at the baccalaureate level primarily provide care to individuals and families. They participate in the planning, implementation, and evaluation of quality assurance programs (ANA, 1995). The generalist nurse bases practice on the expertise of the specialist. The community health nurse generalist is a nurse prepared at a basic

---

TABLE 1-1

THE AMERICAN NURSES ASSOCIATION STANDARDS OF COMMUNITY HEALTH NURSING PRACTICE

Standard 1: *Theory.* The nurse applies theoretical concepts as a basis for decisions in practice.

Standard 2: *Data Collection.* The nurse systematically collects data that are comprehensive and accurate.

Standard 3: *Diagnosis.* The nurse analyzes data collected about the community, family, and individual to determine diagnosis.

Standard 4: *Planning.* At each level of prevention, the nurse develops plans that specify nursing actions unique to the client's needs.

Standard 5: *Intervention.* The nurse, guided by the plan, intervenes to promote, maintain, or restore health, to prevent illness, and to effect rehabilitation.

Standard 6: *Evaluation.* The nurse evaluates responses of the community, family, and individual to interventions to determine progress toward goal achievement and to revise the database, diagnoses, and plan.

Standard 7: *Quality Assurance and Professional Development.* The nurse participates in peer review and other means of evaluation to assure quality of nursing practice. The nurse assumes responsibility for professional development and contributes to the professional growth of others.

Standard 8: *Interdisciplinary Collaboration.* The nurse collaborates with other health care providers, professionals and community representatives in assessing, planning, implementing, and evaluating programs for community health.

Standard 9: *Research.* The nurse contributes to theory and practice in community health nursing through research.

NOTE: From *Standards of Community Health Nursing Practice*, by American Nurses Association, 1986, Washington, DC: American Nurses Publishing. Reprinted with permission.

level of nursing who works in a community setting. The community health nurse specialist is prepared with a master's or doctoral degree and demonstrates a depth and breadth of knowledge, competence, and skill in population-focused nursing practice (ANA, 1995). A specialist may perform all of the functions of a generalist. The nine standards of practice for the community health nurse are listed in Table 1-1.

CARING FOR INDIVIDUALS, FAMILIES, GROUPS, AND COMMUNITIES

Change in Community Health Care

Much has changed in the health care of communities. Until the 1990s, hospitals were the major provider of comprehensive care in most communities. Today, however, hospitals are considered only a part of the health care provided in the community. Now, in part because of economics and technology, many procedures formerly performed in the hospital setting are provided as outpatient services, through private practitioners or in managed care settings. Clients admitted to hospitals today are usually acutely ill and tend to be discharged from the hospital sooner—thus, the expression, "patients go home sicker and quicker." Accordingly, there is a greater emphasis given to discharge planning.

There is now a large client population at home in need of all levels of health care services such as acute care, long-term care, or hospice care—for example, clients on ventilators or with intravenous lines are now commonly receiving care at home. These clients require skilled professional nursing care, health education, and supervision. Families now are required to take a larger role in the care of these clients, often relying on the community health nurse as their main source of support.

The shift from hospital care to home-based care is due to the cost-saving methods embraced by managed care. Some clients may in fact do better and have less chance for infection in their own home; however, individuals should be assessed according to their individual needs, carefully considering the support that might be provided by the family or the community. Unfortunately, clients are often discharged too quickly to allow a thorough consideration of their needs. Furthermore, services offered often are based on insurance coverage not individual needs. For example, insurance coverage for women after childbirth allows only short hospital stays; thus, some new mothers go home without support systems in place. Additionally, short hospital stays may give the nurse little or no time to make an accurate assessment and to provide the necessary education or information to the new mother. New mothers are also often distracted by the birth of the child or too tired to concentrate on information that is conveyed by the nurse. Moreover, most insurance companies do not cover postpartum visits to newborns and mothers by the community health nurse. Lack of information concerning health norms can be dangerous for the mother and the newborn. The following case history is a case in point.

Ms. Stone, a community health nurse, visits Carol Hopewell, who was sent home from the hospital 1 day after the normal delivery of her first child. A 1-day postpartum stay was the policy of the hospital based on insurance reimbursement policies. The new mother was given instructions for the care of the newborn and herself by the hospital nurse, and it was agreed that her mother and her husband would help with the new infant. Ms. Stone called to make an appointment to visit the new mother and infant. She was told by Carol's mother that all was well and that the infant, who was being breast-fed, was the "best infant on earth," exactly the response one would expect from a new grandmother. The grandmother also said that the infant never cried and never woke for a feeding during the night. Ms. Stone asked her to elaborate her description of the infant because the situation sounded unusual. Because breast milk is digested more rapidly, breast-fed infants usually feed approximately every 2 h. The grandmother stated that the infant appeared to be more olive skinned than in the hospital. Ms. Stone asked if she could make a visit in the next hour. The nurse found the infant extremely jaundiced and dehydrated. She advised the family to call their pediatrician immediately. Upon examining the child, the physician determined that the infant's bilirubin was dangerously high; supplemental feedings of water or formula and special fluorescent lights at home were prescribed.

The outcome of this case was fine. In just 10 days, the infant was thriving on breast milk alone. However, sending the mother home early and without sufficient information might have caused significant danger to this infant. Not all infants who are jaundiced, which is common for neonates, need such dramatic attention, but most parents and grandparents lack the skill to make this distinction. The need for a follow-up home visit by the community health nurse in this situation is clear. However, because the decision to make postnatal visits is often driven by managed care and insurance coverage, home visits are often not made. This was an intact family with many support systems, including insurance coverage that included a home visit by a community health nurse. What about the new mother and infant who go home to a more compromised situation with little or no support or no professional nursing intervention at home?

One positive consequence of early discharge is that managed care groups have stressed improved client education and preventive education. Furthermore, shorter hospital stays limit exposure to nosocomial infections. One negative consequence of early discharge is that some patients go unnoticed, and they do not receive the care that they need until complications result in a full-blown crisis. This often leads to readmission of clients who are seriously ill and compromised.

Groups and Communities

Communities are comprised of the individuals, families, and groups that share the same environment. An *aggregate* is a group that not only shares common values and beliefs, but whose members interact with one another or take action on common issues. An example of an aggregate is a population aggregate that has age characteristics and health concerns in common, such as a senior citizen group [e.g., American Association of Retired Persons (AARP)]. Some communities may have different aggregates or groups with different characteristics that come together to deal with the health concerns of the larger community. Some aggregate populations develop their own communities (e.g., retirement communities). These are considered cluster communities within the larger community. When working with an aggregate, the community nurse works on the concerns of the aggregate not on individual problems.

Working with aggregate populations is in many way like working with other client groups or individuals. In the first stages, the nurse must develop an ongoing interaction with the aggregate group to determine its members' needs. In this assessment or data collection stage, the nurse uses many methods of data collection, including research, observation, and interviews. Of all the data collection methods, listening to the clients' needs is the most important. The information gathered by observation might include observing interactions among group members and observing people in their community environment. A "windshield survey" can be done by walking or driving through a community to see what it looks like. Nurses use many diverse methods to determine what services are available for the aggregate population, group, or community. Consider the following:

CASE HISTORY: ASSESSMENT OF AN AGGREGATE OF ELDERLY URBAN DWELLERS

By listening to a group and assessing the community, a community health nurse working with an elderly population in an inner city community determined that exercise and healthy food at reasonable prices were priority issues. As the nurse walked through the neighborhood, she noticed that all of the large food stores had moved away, leaving only small, high-priced, grocery stores. There was limited access to fresh fruits and vegetables. The streets were also poorly lit at night, and there had been several muggings of the elderly in the early evenings that past winter. The elderly in this community were afraid to go out for walks, and shopping had become difficult as a result.

With the help of a social service agency and the local public schools, the nurse arranged for school buses to take these senior citizens shopping weekly to a large supermarket. The nurse also worked with this group to organize walking teams, groups of two or three who walked together every morning for exercise. During the winter, additional buses were supplied to take these walking groups to a local shopping mall in the morning before the shops opened so that they could continue their exercise program in the cold weather. By using available resources and applying professional skills, the community health nurse helped community members help themselves.

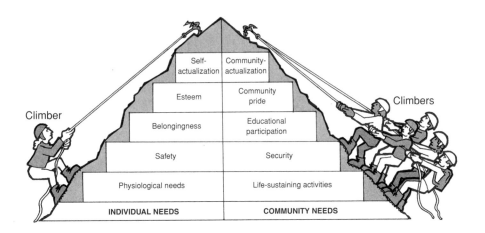

FIGURE 1-1

▧

A hierarchy based on Maslow's hierarchy of needs theory. Not unlike the healthy individual, the healthy community strives for actualization of needs. (Adapted from Higgs & Gustafson, with permission.)

Communities are often made up of persons with specific cultural, ethnic, racial, or religious beliefs in common, which may influence how the members view health. The economics of the community may also bias a community's view of its health needs. Health concerns and needs often exceed the community at hand. Thus, the expression, "think globally, act locally" has some truth. For example, environmental pollution may require local action but may also have a global effect.

The nursing process used in planning for community needs is the the same as the process used in planning for the needs of the individual client. First, the nurse does an assessment of the community, progressively compiling a database of vital statistics. Next, using the data, a diagnosis is made, and a plan is developed *with* the community. Finally, the plan is implemented and then evaluated by the community.

The method of viewing issues related to community needs is similar to Maslow's hierarchy of individual needs. To help a community move toward self-actualization, the nurse has to help the community meet its basic needs (Higgs & Gustafson, 1985). For a person to self-actualize, according to Maslow, they need to first meet their physiological needs, then safety needs, belongingness, love, and finally esteem. For a community to self-actualize, it must fulfill its needs for life-sustaining activities, security, protection, education, and community pride (Fig. 1-1).

*E*PIDEMIOLOGY

Epidemiology is concerned with phenomena related to health events in a population More specifically, epidemiology is the measurement of the distribution and determinants of states of health and illness in human populations (Harkness, 1995). Epidemiology is also concerned with patterns of health, disease, disability, and death in populations. In the past, epidemiology was concerned only with morbidity and mortality resulting from infectious disease; now it incorporates issues related to suicide, accidents, safety, violence, and chronic disease. Epidemiology, then, provides information about the type and size of the health problems with which a community must deal (Valanis, 1992). It also provides information that can act as a predictor for health planning. The inclusion of issues related to wellness in conjunction with improved technology for disease control and prevention have changed or shifted the paradigm of epidemiology.

The study of epidemiology can be traced to ancient times. Hippocrates, the father of modern medicine, was the first person to note the influence of environment upon humans. He encouraged those studying medicine to consider the effects of the four seasons, the wind, and water on the health of people. He was also concerned with how life styles influenced population wellness. In present times, the health effects of different life styles have become an increasingly important part of epidemiology.

In the 1800s, William Farr established the field of medical statistics, using the 17th century work of John Graunt. John Snow then used Farr's method for the collection of population data to investigate the cholera epidemic that took place from 1853 to 1854 (Harkness, 1995). With little sophisticated equipment or knowledge of bacteriology, Snow calculated the number of deaths from cholera by actually going door to door collecting data about the companies that provided water to the various districts of London. He found that the areas supplied by the Southwark and Vauxhall Water Company had 114 cholera deaths per 100,000 people, while those supplied by the Lambeth Company had no deaths from cholera. In areas supplied by both companies, there were 60 deaths per 100,000 people. Snow was convinced that the source of the epidemic was contaminated water. Accordingly, he removed the handles from the contaminated pumps that supplied the water, and thus stopped the outbreak of cholera. A plaque has been placed at the site of his discovery to commemorate this event (Fig. 1-2).

In 1909, Lilian Wald used an epidemiological approach to reduce high absence rates of schoolchildren with communicable diseases. Ms. Wald sent nurses to several New York City schools as a pilot project in school

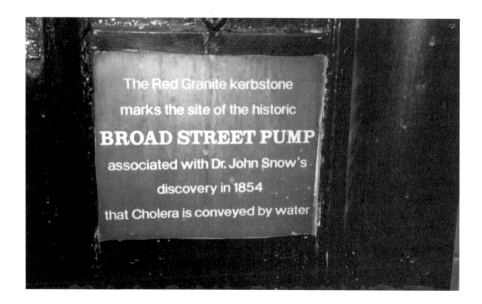

FIGURE 1-2

⬧

Plaque commemorating John Snow's discovery of the cause of the cholera outbreak in London in 1853–1854.

nursing. She believed that she could prevent the spread of communicable diseases and decrease absences among schoolchildren through health education. The outcome of her work was a decline of 90 percent in absences resulting from communicable illness. Since Lilian Wald, nurses such as Ann Nataro, R.N., M.S., in collaboration with community members and community agencies, have been instrumental in working with populations at risk to promote wellness. An excellent example of a community health nurse's effective response to the needs of the community follows.

CASE HISTORY: AN EFFECTIVE RESPONSE OF A COMMUNITY HEALTH NURSE

The director of a local day care center attended a national conference on infectious disease and day care. At the conference, the director heard several physicians speak about their concerns regarding the outbreak of diarrhea in day care centers. The director was concerned not only about the possibility of an outbreak in her center, the Happy Day Care Center, but also with the welfare of the children in the day care centers throughout Nassau County (New York).

The director conferred with Mrs. Anne Nataro, R.N., M.S., a community health nurse educator employed at a local school of nursing, who had done research on diarrhea outbreaks in day care centers. Mrs. Nataro was on the advisory board of the Day Care Council of Nassau County. Working with the director, other interested community members, the Day Care Council of Nassau County, the Health Department of Nassau County, and the Pediatric Association of Nassau County, Mrs. Nataro organized a health advisory committee to the Day Care Council. This committee formed an alliance to improve the health conditions in day care centers throughout Nassau County, and it organized workshops to educate day care workers about the health needs of children in day care.

The first such conference, held in Nassau County in 1986, dealt with the prevention of diarrhea outbreaks in day care centers. The solution was simple: proper diaper changing and hand-washing techniques were taught to day care workers, to children attending day care, and to their parents. Diaper changing locations were specified. Since 1986, conferences have been held each year on the health concerns of people working with children in day care. These are attended by day care workers and health care providers. Recently, Suffolk County formed a Day Care Advisory Committee, using the Nassau County Health Advisory Committee as a model.

In 1995, the *American Journal of Public Health* cited this study as being a significant factor in the prevention of diarrhea outbreaks in day care centers throughout Nassau County. The article stated that "an average of 20 centers have been visited each year over the past 9 years. Since the implementation of this program, there have been no reported outbreaks of fecally transmitted illness attributed to improper hygienic practices" (Esernio-Jenssen, 1995, p. 1710).

ℰPIDEMIOLOGICAL PROCESS

Like the nursing process, the epidemiological process is still evolving. Both processes are based upon methods of problem-solving, and both use methods of investigation as part of their process (Table 1-2).

Epidemiology has been compared to detective work because the epidemiologist must often determine the cause of or solution to a disease outbreak. Many interesting books have been written that explore the process of gathering information, such as *Anatomy of an Epidemic* by Gordon Thomas and Max Morgan-Witts and *Eleven Blue Men* by Barton Roueche. The discipline is based on a body of knowledge that includes population statistics and information developed about the natural history of disease.

Natural History of Disease

The goal of public health practice is to provide prevention at every phase of a disease process. Therefore, in addition to looking at prevention as a process that occurs before the onset of disease, community health nurses work toward prevention in the phases during and after the onset of the disease process.

The notion of the impact of the interaction of the epidemiologic triad—the agent, host, and environment—originated in the work of Leavell and

Agent is a causative factor that contributes to health problems. These may be chemical, physical, biological (e.g., virus, bacteria, fungi, worms, insects), or deficiencies (e.g., nutritional).

Host is a susceptible human (or animal) who harbors and supports a disease-causing agent. Host factors are often intrinsic such as age, race, genetic makeup, life style, exercise level, nutrition, health knowledge, and motivation for achieving wellness.

🔊

TABLE 1-2

COMPARISON OF THE NURSING AND EPIDEMIOLOGICAL PROCESS

Nursing Process	Epidemiological Process
Assessment: Establish database about client; gather related information from client and family; collect objective data	**Assessment**: Establish scope of problem; gather information from reliable sources; collect objective data related to problem (define problem)
Diagnosis: Interpret data; test subjective and objective hypotheses	**Develop hypothesis**: Analyze data
Planning: Develop plan to achieve level of wellness goals (clients included in development of plan)	**Planning**: Develop plan for prevention of condition or event (clients included in development of plan)
Implementation: Initiate plan with clients	**Implementation**: Implement plan with community or client
Evaluation: Determine achievement of goals with client and possibly redesign goals	**Evaluation**: Determine achievement of goals; reassess client; prepare report; conduct further research

Clark in 1965. Originally developed to examine the factors in infectious disease, this approach is now used to examine other health-related issues. The use of the epidemiologic triad in the analysis of health problems requires that all issues related to the interaction of each element of the triad must be considered. It is believed that all three components working in synchrony are necessary to influence one's health status.

When considering the triad—host, agent, and environment—it is helpful to think of a triangle balanced on a fulcrum (see Fig. 1-3). In order to become ill, the conditions of the agent, host, and environment become out of balance. In order to intervene, the nurse attempts to modify the characteristics of one of the components of the triad. An example of an intervention would be the immunization of a host; if the host is immunized against pertussis, this interferes with exposure to someone with pertussis. It is often not as easy to explain why one person becomes ill when several persons are subjected to the same pathogen. Host factors such as poor health or lack of immunization are simple explanations. Knowledge about the interaction among the host, agent, and environment often helps to clarify the forces and factors necessary for the development of an illness as the example below illustrates.

Environment is all external factors surrounding the host that might influence resistance to disease or injury. Environmental factors include biologic aspects of the environment (e.g., plants and animals needed for food, pathogenic microorganisms), physical aspects of the environment (e.g., heat, light, atmospheric pressure, radiation, air, water) as well as social, cultural, technological, educational, political, legal, demographic, sociological, and economic factors.

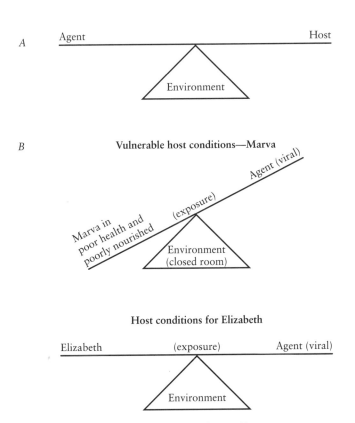

FIGURE 1-3. *A.* An example of conditions for wellness: Host, agent, and environment are perfectly balanced. *B.* An example of epidemiologic triad applied to Marva and Elizabeth. Marva's poor physical condition sets up a perfect condition for illness. Elizabeth's good physical condition helps protect her from illness. (Based on Leavell & Clark, 1965, with permission.)

CASE HISTORY: INTERACTION AMONG THE HOST, AGENT, AND
ENVIRONMENT

Elizabeth and a friend, Marva, visit a friend who is ill at home with a
viral infection. Lately, Marva has been under tremendous stress related
to her job. She has been working long hours, her diet has been poor,
and she has been complaining of fatigue. Following the visit Marva
becomes ill, but Elizabeth does not. In this example, both the environment and the agent are the same, but the host factors are not the same.
The stress due to overwork, fatigue, and a deficient diet have affected
the host, making the host vulnerable to disease (see Fig. 1-3).

The natural history of disease is the basis for intervention. The three levels
or stages upon which this is based are primary, secondary, and tertiary levels of prevention.

Primary Prevention Primary prevention is aimed at intervention before
disease—that is, the prepathogenic stage. Every disease process is divided
into two phases: the prepathogenic stage and the pathogenic stage.
Prepathogenesis is the period prior to illness. During this period, there are
factors within the host or the environment that have the ability to move
them either toward or away from the agent. The levels of prevention associated with the prepathogenic period are referred to as primary prevention
(Fig. 1-4). Primary prevention includes health promotion or specific protection. Examples of health promotion are education, housing, or good
nutrition. An example of health protection is immunization.

Secondary Prevention Secondary prevention occurs during early pathogenesis; this includes early diagnosis, prompt treatment, and the limitation of
disability. Examples of secondary prevention include case finding, screening, methods to prevent the spread of communicable disease, and adequate
therapies to treat the disease and prevent further complications (see Fig. 1-4).

Tertiary Prevention Tertiary prevention is also a period of pathogenesis.
This is the period of convalescence and rehabilitation. Examples of tertiary
prevention include re-education for the client (e.g., physical therapy, occupational therapy) and education of the public (e.g., to employ persons with
a disability) (see Fig. 1-4).

Descriptive Epidemiology

The aim of an epidemiologic investigation is to identify the client's health
goals and to develop ways of preventing illness. A descriptive epidemiologic study includes an investigation in order to collect information. Some
of the data may be collected by the community health nurse, while other
pieces of information may be collected by a variety of other agencies.

T H E   N A T U R A L   H I S T O R Y   o f   A N Y   D I S E A S E   o f   M A N

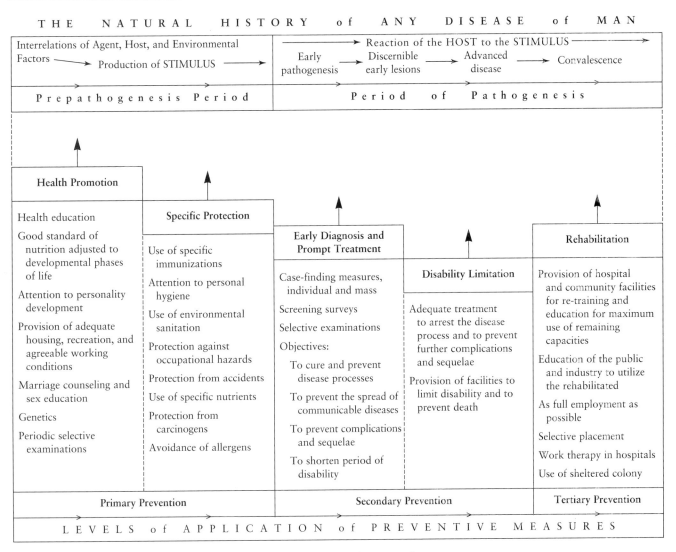

FIGURE 1-4. Levels of application of preventive measures in the natural history of disease. (NOTE: From *Preventive Medicine for the Doctor in His Community*, by H. R. Leavell & E. Clark, 1965, New York, McGraw-Hill. Reprinted with permission.)

A very basic way of collecting data is by actually counting the number of affected individuals. However, raw data (or numbers) can be misleading if they are taken at face value. For example, two cases of a disease in a population of 500,000 in a small town outside of Akron, Ohio, may not sound serious; however, if the disease in question is bubonic plague, these two cases are considered an epidemic. Conversely, 5000 cases of varicella in a New York City community in which there is a large population of children 10 years of age and under may not be unusual but may be considered *endemic* (Valanis, 1992). Endemic refers to "the habitual presence of disease or infectious agents in a defined geographical area or population" (Valanis, 1992, p. 428). Moreover, the same 5000 cases of varicella might be considered an epidemic on a college campus where there are

Census data are gathered about the population by the United States government every 10 years. These data provide information about populations. They include information by age, sex, race, socioeconomic status, housing, and employment. The census is used to compare trends in states and localities (census tract data). In the past few years, the accuracy of the census data regarding undocumented aliens and the homeless population has been questioned. Migrant workers may fall within these populations and so are also not accurately documented.

Endemic is a term used to describe the usual frequency of a disease in a community or area.

12,000 students. *Epidemics* are defined as rates of disease that are at a significantly higher level than the usual frequency (Valanis, 1992). The raw data, then, may be of little value.

Accordingly, ratios, proportions, and rates are used in epidemiology to provide a more accurate description of health situations. A *ratio* is the relationship between two numbers expressed as a fraction; the value is obtained by dividing the numerator of the fraction by the denominator. A *proportion* is a specific type of ratio in which the numerator is included in the denominator, and the resultant value is expressed as a percent (Valanis, 1992). A *rate* is a special form of a proportion that includes a specification of time. It is a statistical measure that can be used to measure and compare the health status in a community. A rate is the proportion of persons with a health problem among a population at risk. The total number of persons in this group then serve as the denominator. The numerator includes all of the events that are being measured. Rates are used to measure many things, including mortality and morbidity rates.

$$\text{Rate} = \frac{\text{Number of conditions or events that occur in a specific period of time}}{\text{Population at risk during the same time period}} \times \text{base multiple of 10}$$

Common morbidity rates measure the incidence and prevalence of disease risk among populations. *Crude rates* measure the entire population in a designated geographic area in relationship to a condition that is being investigated (Harkness, 1995).

$$\text{Crude death rate} = \frac{\text{Number of deaths in 1 year}}{\text{Average (midyear) population}} \times \text{per 100,000 population}$$

An *incidence rate* measures the number of new cases identified in a measure of time.

$$\text{Incidence rate} = \frac{\text{Number of new conditions or events that occur in a specific period of time}}{\text{Population at risk during the same period (usually midyear)}} \times \text{base multiple of 10}$$

A *prevalence rate* measures the existing number of cases in a population at a given time or over time.

$$\text{Prevalence rate} = \frac{\text{Number of existing conditions or events occurring within a specific period of time}}{\text{Population at risk during the same time period}} \times \text{base multiple of 10}$$

The *age-specific death rate* is another rate used to index health.

$$\text{Age-specific death rate} = \frac{\text{Number of deaths among persons in a given age group in 1 year}}{\text{Average (midyear) population in a specified age group}} \times \text{per 100,000 population}$$

The *infant mortality rate* is used to measure the health of a community or nation.

$$\text{Infant mortality rate} = \frac{\text{Number of deaths in children under 1 year of age during 1 year}}{\text{Number of live births in same year}} \times 1000$$

Summary

This chapter is an overview of the foundations of community health and public health nursing practice. Community health nursing is growing with the changes in health care being experienced by society. Based on standards of practice, community health and public health nurses use an epidemiological approach to care for individuals, families, groups, and communities. Community health nurses are concerned with prevention at the primary, secondary, and tertiary levels.

KEY WORDS

Agents
Census data
Community health nursing
Crude death rate
Endemic
Environmental factors
Host factors

Incidence rate
Prevalence rate
Proportion
Public health nursing
Rate
Ratio

QUESTIONS

DIRECTIONS: Choose the one *best* response to each of the following questions.

1. A group of persons who shares common values and beliefs and takes action on common issues is referred to as
   A. a community health action team.
   B. an aggregate.
   C. a neighborhood.
   D. a self-actualized community.

2. To determine if there is an epidemic, the community health nurse would
   A. examine the actual number of cases that occur.
   B. determine if the rate of a disease is significantly higher than the usual frequency of the disease.
   C. determine a relationship between the number of cases of a disease expressed by a fraction.
   D. measure the number of newly occurring cases.

3. During a blood pressure screening program provided by The State University College of Nursing, it is discovered that a client is hypertensive. This is an example of
   A. primary prevention.
   B. the good work done by nursing students.
   C. secondary prevention.
   D. the importance of blood pressure screening.

4. An incidence rate of a disease refers to
   A. the measurement of the existing number of cases in a population at a given time.
   B. the measurement of the number of new cases identified in a given period of time.
   C. how the community health nurse determines the risk factors of a disease.
   D. the measurement of the entire population at risk in a designated area.

5. The data gathered every 10 years by the United States government about the population are referred to as
   A. census tract data.
   B. primary data.
   C. host data.
   D. environmental data.

ANSWERS

1. *The answer is B.* An aggregate is a group of people who share common beliefs and values and who are concerned with similar issues.

2. *The answer is B.* Epidemics are defined as rates of disease that are at a significantly higher level than the usual frequency.

3. *The answer is C.* Discovering hypertension in a client in a blood pressure screening program is an example of secondary prevention.

4. *The answer is B.* An incidence rate of a disease refers to the measurement of the number of new cases identified in a given period of time.

5. *The answer is A.* The United State census is data collected every 10 years by the government about the population.

ANNOTATED REFERENCES

American Nurses Association. (1986). *Standards of community health nursing practice*. Washington, DC: American Nurses Publishing.

The standards of community health nursing practice are provided in this pamphlet along with the rationale and criteria for each standard. Additionally, this pamphlet defines community health nursing practice, presents ethical responsibilities, and provides guidelines for using the standards of community health practice. This document was developed to help nurses in practice to maintain and improve a high standard of client care.

American Nurses Association. (1995). *Scope of standards of population-focused nursing practice* (draft). Washington, DC: American Nurses Publishing.

This document was developed by the Quad Council (American Public Health Association, Public Health Nursing Section), the Association of State and Territorial Directors of Nursing, the Association of Community Health Nursing Educators, and the Council on Community, Primary, and Long-Term Care Nursing Practice, American Nurses Association. The scope and standards of care for public health, home health, and community health nursing practice are presented in this document.

Esernio-Jenssen, D. A. (1995). Teaching and reinforcing hygienic practices in child care centers (letter to the editor). *American Journal of Public Health 35* (12), 1710.

This letter to the editor refers to the outbreaks of diarrhea in the 1980s in Nassau County, New York. It reports on the collaboration of the Nassau County Department of Health, Adelphi University, and the Child Care Council of Nassau County in implementing a program that teaches and reinforces good hygienic practices in child care settings.

Harkness, G. A. (1995). *Epidemiology in nursing practice.* St. Louis, MO: C. V. Mosby.

Using nursing practice and research as its basis, this book presents the basic principles of epidemiology and helps nurses integrate these principles into practice. It includes the epidemiologic process from a historic perspective, and it presents various conceptual models, infectious and noninfectious processes, and the natural history of disease. Epidemiologic techniques are described, and there is a discussion of research methods, which include study designs.

Hickman, M. P. (Ed.). (1990). *Essentials of baccalaureate nursing education for entry level practice in community health nursing.* Lexington, KY: Association of Community Health Educators.

This document was prepared to delineate the essential education for entry level community health nursing practice and the scope and functions of community health nursing educators, researchers, and clinical practitioners.

Higgs, Z. R., & Gustafson, D. D. (1985). *Community as a client.* Philadelphia: F. A. Davis.

Using a variety of methods such as epidemiological, systems, and adaptation approaches, this book establishes an approach to community assessment and diagnosis. Application of theories such as Orem, Roy, and Rogers (Martha) are applied to community assessment and diagnosis.

Leavell, H. R., & Clark, E. (1965). *Preventive medicine for the doctor in his community.* New York: McGraw-Hill.

This book is the "grandfather" of preventive medicine. This landmark work is an epidemiological approach to preventive medicine. It explores the basic principles of preventive medicine, discusses in-depth levels of application of preventive medicine, and provides the natural history of disease. It addresses an approach to organized community action to achieve and plan for community health.

National Association of County Health Officials. (1993). *Core public health functions.* Olympia, WA: Washington State Association of Local Public Health Officials.

This report was initiated by the state and local public health leadership to develop an understanding and consensus with public health and in the public policy arena related to the cost of public health. This report defines core functions and population-based services. It develops roles of government in relationship to the health of the public.

Pew Health Professions Commission. (1995). *Critical challenges: Revitalizing the health professions for the twenty-first century* (Third Report of the Pew Professions Commission). San Francisco: Author.

This report indicates the future changes in the American health care system. It is an overview of health care in the 21st century. It reviews the impact on health care workers, managed care, and insurance, and develops a view of future health care.

Roueche, B. (1953). *Eleven blue men.* Boston: Little, Brown.

This book is a compilation of true epidemiological case studies. They are written in a narrative format about the epidemiologists who, through their investigative work, discover the causes of a variety of outbreaks in the New York metropolitan area.

Roueche, B. (1958). *The incurable wound and further narratives of medical detection.* Boston: Little, Brown.

This is a compilation of short stories based on actual epidemiological case studies.

Thomas, G., & Morgan-Witts, M. (1982). *Anatomy of an epidemic.* Garden City, NY: Doubleday.

This is true story of the outbreak of Legionnaires' disease that made headlines across the nation. It is the story of the medical detection team of epidemiologists 1who discovered the cause of this national outbreak.

U.S. Department of Health and Human Services. (1985). Consensus conference on the essentials of public health nursing practice and education (report of the conference September 5–7, 1984). Rockville, MD: Author.

This report includes the consensus definition of the roles of the community health nurse. It identifies basic educational requirements for the community health nurse as provider.

Valanis, B. (1992). *Epidemiology in nursing and health care* (2nd ed.). Norwalk, CT: Appleton & Lange.

Designed to furnish the reader with an introduction to the concepts and methodology as well as the application of epidemiology, this book addresses issues relevant to clinicians. It includes epidemiological measures, study design, and sources of data and critiques of epidemiological studies. The book addresses the natural history of disease and control of infectious and noninfectious disease.

AN HISTORICAL PERSPECTIVE OF COMMUNITY HEALTH NURSING

It has been said that "those who cannot remember the past are condemned to repeat it" (Santayana, 1953, p. 82). The efforts of those who have gone before then have a special meaning for our future, as our future is grounded in our past. Knowing how community health nursing has evolved into the profession it is today helps to give community health nurses the conviction to go forth and achieve greater things as well as the strength to meet the challenge of expected change and transformation.

Community health was the first form of nursing. Since the earliest days of civilization, wherever there was a "community," there were people who were in need of care because they were injured, ill, suffering the infirmities of old age, or giving birth to the next generation. The individuals who responded to those needs, using the skills and knowledge available to them in their particular time and place, were the first community health providers. Found in many guises over the course of history—medicine men, nuns, Knight's Hospitalers—community health nurses have provided care on battlefields, in cities afflicted by plagues, and in homes, both humble and affluent. That long tradition of community health care continues today to contribute to the emotional and physical well-being of people throughout the world.

Nursing is as old as humankind. The word nurse itself evolved from the Middle English *nurice* and the Old French *norice*, both of which found their roots in the Latin *nutricius* (nourishing). From the beginning of civilization, humankind has attempted to relieve the myriad of afflictions that brought pain, agony, suffering, and death.

The earliest people viewed illness and death as part of the natural phenomena of life and later as the work of the gods who were angry or displeased with them. The sickness and suffering that befell individuals were caused by wrathful gods and evil demons. Both death and recovery were looked upon as magic. These beliefs and practices gave rise to the custom of priests and religious orders serving as physicians and healers.

One of the earliest customs was to bring sick people to the marketplace so that others could inquire about their state of health. People somehow sensed that interest and attention paid to the sick had curative powers.

As awareness of the relationship between hygiene and sickness evolved, efforts turned towards the development of sanitariums, hot baths, and fresh air. Plagues were a major source of sickness, and when these scourges broke out, there was virtually no way to stop them other than to let them run their natural course. It was not until the 18th century that any formal health interventions toward community health were noted. Although the study of community health problems dates back to ancient Greece and Rome, the first indication of government interest in the recording or investigation of disease or issues relating to sanitation was during the 18th century.

Eighteenth Century

Although it was not until the 19th century that community health nursing was addressed explicitly, it was during the 18th century that the foundation was laid for community health nursing as we know it today.

The 18th century was notable for the beginning of the sanitary revolution that began to take hold in Europe, especially in England and then ultimately in colonial America. Furthermore, it was during this time that surveys, geographical mapping of diseases, and sanitation investigations and commissions were commonly done by regional governments (Swanson, 1993). Also during this time, as cities grew, slums also grew, as did the concomitant problems of the inner city environment. Birth rates and mortality rates were high. The average life span was no more than 30 years. In England, records indicate that over half of all children died before they were 5 years old, and abandonment of infants, especially in foundling hospitals, was not uncommon. The city hospitals, especially in London and Paris, could not keep up with the growing health needs; mortality rates were often well over 50 percent of the population.

In England, as a result of the Industrial Revolution, droves of people flocked into the cities, creating slums and spreading infectious diseases. The most significant health care discovery during that time was of inoculation in 1796 by Edward Jenner (1749–1823) (Swanson, 1993). At a time when almost 95 percent of the population was afflicted with small pox to some degree, Jenner realized that those people who worked with cattle had milder and fewer cases of small pox. His discovery led to an understanding of the idea of immunity, a concept previously unknown in science.

Thus, the 18th century was significant for the beginning of the sanitary revolution that spurred by the Industrial Revolution in England. With the migration of colonists, communicable disease then became an American health care problem. Although health care remained meager, the 18th century was significant to community health because it gave birth to the notion of creating and maintaining a database for the collection of health-related information.

COLONIAL AMERICA

Crossing the Atlantic Ocean did not improve the quality of available health care. Hospitals in America were either almshouses for the poor and indigent or pesthouses for those with contagious diseases. Most care of the ill as well as of births was provided at home by physicians or lay midwives. Institutions were often created to keep the impoverished away from the general public rather than to serve their needs. The medical profession, still without the benefit of antiseptics and antibiotics, could do little to help those afflicted. Treatment was still crude, as were methods for sanitation and hygiene. Physicians in America had no formal education, and skill and training were acquired in an apprentice system.

Hospital nurses were responsible for nothing more than general cleaning, scrubbing floors and pots, and doing the laundry. They were often from the lowest strata of society. Mostly illiterate, disinterested, and totally untrained, hospital nurses were often petty criminals who were used as labor instead of serving time in jail (Dolan, 1968).

Plagues were still the biggest health care problem, especially smallpox, which was estimated to affect one in five people, including our first President, George Washington. Later, it was yellow fever that brought terror to the colonies. The first hospital was in Philadelphia, established at the urging of Benjamin Franklin. It was his belief that the general public had a responsibility to the poor, sickly, and needy immigrant populations. He wrote a petition seeking the sanction to build what was to become the Pennsylvanian Hospital (1751). Later, the New York Hospital was built under a charter granted by George III in 1770 and opened in 1790. The purpose was to prevent the spread of infectious diseases that were brought into the port city by new immigrants and sailors. These hospitals were established along the format of those in England. Mainly used by individuals with no money or resources, these hospitals had no better success against the morbidity found in the slums in other parts of the world.

NINETEENTH CENTURY

Communicable diseases like typhoid and typhus ravaged Europe, killing more people than any of the wars. So desperate were the conditions that England passed the first sanitary legislation in 1837, establishing a National Vaccination Board (Swanson, 1993). Child mortality rates in industrial cities were still 50 percent before the age of 5. People who worked in the industrial plants lived an average of 16 years, tradesmen 22 years, and the upper class 36 years (Swanson, 1993).

Sir Edwin Chadwick (1800–1890), an English social reformer, was instrumental in amending the Poor Law in 1834. As an outcome of this, issues such as child welfare, care for the mentally ill, care of the elderly, standards for factory workers, and education were addressed. In 1842, Chadwick's publication, *The Sanitary Conditions of the Labouring Population*, increased the public's awareness to such an extent that the Public Health Act of 1848 was passed, which established a Board of Health.

An important discovery in England was made during this time by John Snow, a physician, anesthetist, and epidemiologist. During the major cholera epidemic of 1854 in London, Snow proved that water was the source of contamination and spread of cholera (Swanson, 1993). These discoveries helped to bring about an increase in civic understanding and moral commitment to the betterment of people's lives through economic, social, and environmental reform.

FLORENCE NIGHTINGALE

In freeing herself from the constraints of Victorian society, Florence Nightingale (1820–1910) irrevocably changed the profession of nursing for eternity. She came from the upper class at a time when it was considered unseemly for a well-bred lady to be involved in the unsightly and unsanitary care of the sick. Yet Nightingale was drawn to it, even before her famous trip to the Crimea. She was always attracted to philanthropic works, planning programs for the care and welfare of the needy. She wanted to study the care and treatment of diseases and afflictions and enrolled in a program for nursing under the direction of Pastor Fliedner at Kaiserswerth, Germany (Dolan, 1984). Fliedner established a training school in 1836 based upon a women's society for visiting and nursing care of sick persons at home started by his wife Frederika Fliedner. Upon graduating from the program, Florence Nightingale went to Paris to study with the Sisters of Charity.

With the outbreak of Crimean War between Russia and England in 1854 came the newspaper reports of the appalling health conditions of the wounded English solders. More lives were lost to contaminated wounds, infections, and an epidemic of cholera than were lost fighting the actual battles. During the famous battle of Balaklava, immortalized by the poem "Charge of the Light Brigade," thousands of soldiers were wounded with no hope of being cared for because of the staggeringly inefficient and obsolete British Army bureaucracy.

The upper strata of London society were stunned and horrified by the accounts they read. The stories of the plight of their young men were more than they could bear, and they let their political leaders know of their displeasure. The Secretary of State for War, Sir Sidney Herbert begged Nightingale for help. She and 14 nurses arrived at the military hospital at Scutari only to find that there were no beds, blankets, soap, or wash basins for the sick and wounded soldiers. Food was scarce and often inedible. The death rate among the wounded was almost 50 percent. Nightingale and her meager staff cleaned the barracks, washed clothes, cooked, and fed those too weak to feed themselves. At first they were resented by the medical and administrative staffs, but in short order, seeing the extraordinary changes that were made, Nightingale won their admiration. She also wrote to her family's wealthy friends and government officials to acquire much needed supplies and equipment. Reading the stories of her phenomenal work, the English responded overwhelmingly, and contributions for provisions poured forth.

Upon returning to London, Nightingale was asked to turn her efforts to the needs of England. In 1859, she published a 77-page text entitled *Notes on Nursing: What It Is and What It Is Not*. This text addressed issues of prevention and general good health. It was an immediate best seller. She stressed the need for hygiene, good food, sunlight, sanitation, sewerage, and attractive and comfortable surroundings. Nurses were to be sober, educated, well-trained, cleanly dressed, and above all kind and caring to their charges. Nightingale always stressed the importance of prevention as well as prompt and efficient care. Perhaps the most famous quote accorded her is the description of nursing that states that there are two major components of nursing, health nursing and sick nursing. Health nursing was "to keep or put the constitution of a healthy person in such a state as to have no disease," and sick nursing was "to help the person suffering from disease to live and regain a state of wellness" (Dolan, 1984, p. 164). Nightingale's work filtered across the Atlantic Ocean and became the basis for the modern nursing movement in the United States, a movement also generated by the horrors of war and the health care needs that war demands.

During this time, Florence Nightingale was prevailed upon to have nurses assigned to work in the community with physicians in a local dispensary. This has been referred to as the forerunner of community health nursing.

*C*IVIL WAR

Like the Crusades in Europe, the Civil War created the impetus for improvement of health care in the United States. The catastrophic number of wounded and mutilated soldiers that resulted from the Civil War created the need to provide health care for the troops wounded in battle. Over 2000 untrained nurses participated in the Civil War, and that number was not nearly enough. "Their (nurses') number was entirely inadequate . . . hygiene was atrocious . . . more victims resulted from disease than from bullets" (Rush, 1992, p. 409).

Seeing the inhumanity of the Civil War and outraged by its atrocities, Clara Barton, trained as a teacher and often referred to as the "American Florence Nightingale," became a national heroine as her reputation spread throughout the country. Founder of the American Red Cross, Barton began her one-woman crusade against the horrors of war after she witnessed the piles of corpses stacked in trenches and fields, rotting in 100°F heat. The sight of mangled bodies, crude amputations, rotting flesh, dysentery, and gangrene gave her the impetus to bring her wisdom and caring to the battlefields. She, like Nightingale, delivered lanterns so that surgeons could continue to treat and operate throughout the night. She brought food, clean bandages, blankets, and mostly, like Nightingale, she brought caring, kindness, and the knowledge that she could help save the lives of the young men in battle. Untrained but not unskilled, Barton, too, proved to the military leaders that her presence, and those she brought with her, would be a help and not a hindrance to the war effort (Oakes, 1994).

IMMIGRATION SURGES TO THE UNITED STATES

New York City has always been a major disembarkation point for immigrants who were seeking to start new lives. It is reflective of other cities that have served as ports of disembarkation, such as New Orleans and Miami. New York City has also been a place historically where economically deprived people live in large numbers, bringing their own unique set of health care needs. Historically, this has been a dilemma, as the city has often either insufficient resolution or resources to resolve these needs (Ravitch, 1974).

Government efforts to help the cities' poor and impoverished were minimal in the 19th century. City and governmental agencies often traded public assistance programs for party loyalty and promises of votes. Upper class reformers were not so altruistic as to be exclusively motivated to improve the lives of the poor. They were more concerned with honesty in government because ineptitude and wholesale theft led to high taxes (Ravitch, 1974). Upper class, well-born people were indifferent to the daily misery that surrounded the lives of the immigrant poor. Poverty was seen as a social problem that was to be alleviated almost exclusively by charity. At that time, there was a Commissioner of Public Charities and Corrections, which implied that poverty and punishment were related. New York City, like other cities of its size, had insane asylums, a poorhouse, a workhouse, and a few hospitals. Public institutions were chronically overcrowded, the largest of these being Bellevue Hospital with 768 beds (Ravitch, 1974).

The 1870s saw a shift in immigration patterns. Originally, most immigrants came from England, Ireland, and Germany, largely as a reaction to the economic and political conditions found in Europe at that time. As the influx from these countries decreased, the number of immigrants from the southern and eastern parts of Europe began to rise. This second wave accounted for more than half the number of all the immigrants in the United States (Ravitch, 1974).

Jewish and Italian immigrants moved into the slums previously occupied by the Germans and Irish. Little attention or consideration was given to light, air, or sanitation in the densely populated tenements. Garbage collection and sewage disposal were haphazard at best. Human value was minimal, where people worked long hours in horrible conditions for absurdly low wages, always living mired in poverty. By the end of the 1800s, those people who lived in comfort were becoming alarmed by the rising labor unrest and consistently increasing immigration. The city's rich began to sense a danger and potential for change to their way of life. Labor organizations and bold and unprecedented strikes with direct confrontation to the previously unchallenged law and order were occurring. The wealthy realized that the growth of the middle class and economically deprived could not be ignored. Eastern European immigrants, Russians, and Poles, created an environment of socialism, anarchism, militant unionism, and radical philosophies. The slum environment of discontent and unrest allowed these ideologies to flourish. It was the extremes of poverty, illiteracy, ignorance, misery, wretchedness, disease, filth, crime, corruption, depravity, and human degradation that allowed the political structure of the city to become so corrupt and crooked that the seeds for the social reform movement of the 19th century were activated. For some, it was the threat and spread of lawlessness into their own comfortable lives. For others, the motive was indeed compassion, stemming from deep religious principles and ideals of social justice, fairness, and equity. Many reformers were particularly concerned with improving the lives of the people who lived in tenements, eliminating sweatshops, and reforming child labor laws.

Trained nurses visiting at the homes of the sick first appeared in 1813 in the United States. The Ladies Benevolent Society was the first to organize women in Charleston, South Carolina to visit the sick poor. In 1819, the Hebrew Female Benevolent Society of Philadelphia organized a visiting nurse's organization of volunteer nurses who visited the sick. In 1839, the nurse's society of Philadelphia assigned women home visitors to care for the sick at home; in 1877, the first educated nurses were sent to care for the sick poor at home; and in 1885, the Visiting Nurse Association was established. The first settlement house in New York City was opened in 1893 (Ravitch, 1974). It was quickly followed by numerous other settlement houses, including one in Boston and one in Philadelphia, establishing several social service programs in the city slums (Tinkham, 1984). These houses were developed in the manner of William Rathbone, who formed the concept of district nursing in Liverpool, England in 1859. Each district or area of the city was assigned a nurse to provide some continuity of care and community recognition.

It could be argued that even more important and profound was the beginning social reform movement and the spirit of advocacy that the settlement workers brought to the consciousness of the city's wealthy. Most of these settlement workers themselves were from the privileged class, but they informed and ultimately interested their peers in the problems and plights of the poor. Social reformers were inspired with a sense of unrelenting mission to bring about change, and although working on several of the city's problems at the same time, the common belief was that the most important task was education. It was the conviction of the reformers that education held the fundamental promise to improve the future of humankind and society in general. The reformers' belief in the power of education to right the wrongs they saw in the cities was steadfast. As change agents, their faith and conviction in education as the means by which independence, power, affluence, health, and prosperity could be achieved for the masses became resolute over the following years.

Lillian Wald

Born in 1867, Lillian Wald, influenced by family relatives who were physicians, came to New York and entered the New York Hospital School of Nursing (Kalisch, 1978). Wald trained for the standard 3 years, graduating in 1891. She then went to work at the Juvenile Asylum for a year but left unhappy and frustrated by her lack of medical knowledge. This frustration brought her to the Woman's Medical College in New York. During her time there, she and another nurse, Mary Brewster, were asked to go to the Lower East Side of New York. Here they were to lecture to immigrant mothers about how to care for their sick children and family members. What Wald found there in 1893 shocked and horrified her. Wald and Brewster were from wealthy, upper class families. They were totally unprepared either emotionally or educationally for what was before them. One morning while teaching mothers how to properly make a bed, Wald was approached by a young child seeking help for his sick mother. Wald accompanied the child to a filthy, squalid tenement where she found nine people crammed into two rooms (Kalish, 1978). On the only bed lay a woman who had received no care for several days. She cleaned the woman, washed the bed linens, sent for a physician, and resolved to help people in the way they needed to be helped (Kalisch, 1978).

Inspired by this, Wald, accompanied by Brewster, began a district nursing service in New York City (Tinkham, 1984). Cleverly, they moved into the neighborhood that they were planning to serve because they felt that the community would view them as friends and be more willing to confide their problems. Their motive was simple, find the sick and nurse them. Their initial settlement house was on a Jefferson Street rooftop. Not aligned with any specific religious group or physician, the clinic was run on a "pay as you can" basis. They then let the community know that they were there to serve those in need. Within 2 years, the workload increased so much that they needed to find larger quarters. Thus, in 1895 with the help of the philanthropist, Jacob H. Schiff, Wald and Brewster opened the Nurses' Settlement at 265 Henry Street (Kalisch, 1978). Within a short time, nine other nurses were living at the Settlement, including the charismatic and progressive nursing educational leader, Lavinia Dock.

It was Wald who first used the term "public health nurse." She put a preface on Florence Nightingale's term "health nursing" because these nurses would be concerned directly with the needs of the public or society (Roberts, 1954).

By 1900, there were as many as 20 district nursing organizations with over 200 nurses, most of which existed in the large cities, although some did exist in small communities (Tinkham, 1984). So successful was the work of these nurses that Wald, working with the Board of Education in New York City, established a 1-month pilot program to have a nurse work directly in a school. Her impetus was the predicament of an intelligent 12-year-old boy who was unable to enter school because of an untreated skin condition (Roberts, 1954). During the 1-month program, the school's attendance went up. This positive outcome resulted in the hiring of the first school nurse in the United States in 1902 with 12 others to follow (Tinkham, 1984). School nursing rapidly became an integral and indispensable part of the health care of the young across the country.

At this time, the concept of occupational nursing also began. In 1895, at a Vermont marble company, a nursing service was established by the owner's "paternalistic and humanitarian interests in the welfare of his workers and their families" (Roberts, 1954, p. 85). An unabridged success, the service continued demonstrating the economic value of less time lost due to illness and accidents.

In 1913, the government provided for the establishment of the first state Division of Public Health Nursing in the New York State Department of Health, predating the Division of Nursing in the United States Public Health Service.

In 1910, the historic *Flexner Report* helped to formalize medical education, but with the enormous growth of communities, health care was unable to keep up the pace. Supplementing the cities' overused and exhausted resources were numerous private organizations that ran foundling homes, street baths, day care centers, orphan asylums, homes for destitute children, dispensaries, clinics, hospitals, homes for the aged, and lodging houses for vagrants (Ravitch, 1974). Despite these efforts and the reform trends, the slums of New York City grew in both numbers and in inherent misery, despondency, and depression. In a city where almost half the population was foreign born, turmoil and unrest saturated the air.

*T*WENTIETH CENTURY: ESTABLISHMENT OF COMMUNITY SERVICE

Nursing can and should be viewed as the earliest form of community service. It is related to the strong, perhaps instinctive, desire to preserve and protect the members of the group. As civilization grew, this notion extended to include other groups, tribes, clans, townspeople, and ultimately the stranger. It could be argued that the earliest form of nursing was that which took place in the community. When and how it all started is unknown. Dock writes "on nursing there is no record, save by military orderlies in the army, and an occasional old woman . . . it is possible that in the homes of the wealthy all nursing was done by slaves" (Dock, 1920, p. 38). It would be unfair to be critical of early societies for this behavior towards the sick and needy, says Dock, for it is "historically incorrect to assume that all neighborly kindness and charity began with the Christian era; it is also a temperamental error that narrows the mind by shutting out the view of the essential humanness of the whole race" (Dock, 1920 p. 38). Highborn Roman women were among the first in recorded history to recognize the value of nursing women in the recuperative process. Marcella turned her palace into the first free public hospital in about A.D. 390 (Dock, 1920). This was essentially the only way nursing women at that time could care for the needy other than to go out into the community with baskets of food, clean blankets, and bandages, practicing the most primitive and elementary form of community health.

It was during the beginning of the 20th century, with the enormous and persistent demands of immigration and infectious disease, that American nursing had the foresight, intuition, and historical experience to move into community-based care. Early memories of the original visiting nurses in long skirts, climbing over tenement rooftops, appear. Always aware that social context was important to the health care of its population, nurses fed the hungry in neighborhood soup kitchens, tended to the needs of schoolchildren with immunizations, growth scales, and hygiene classes. When the sickest of the sick could not get to the physician's office, the community health nurse came to the patient.

With the dawn of the new century, the reforms in nursing are perhaps no greater than in public health. In 1919, nearly 9000 trained nurses were devoting their careers to this type of care (Kalisch, 1978). At first their work was limited to the bedside, but gradually the awareness grew; if there was no food, heat, or sanitation, all the ministration in the world would be of no help. These nurses quickly discovered that their visits were often more psychosocial in nature due to the magnitude of the needs of the population. The knowledge and information they needed far outreached anything these caregivers had learned in nursing school. It was out of necessity that the specialty of the public health nurse emerged in thundering force. Historically, the term "public health" was used more often than "community health" although for a while they were thought to be interchangeable. Community health nursing is the result of the ever growing and changing needs of an exploding society. Community health, influenced by reforms in public health, education, and societal needs, is a direct reflection of the growth and change in the modern world. Today, the American Nurses Association (ANA) uses the term "community nursing" to encompass those that work in public health, schools, industry, and other community-based clinics, services, and organizations. The 20th century has seen many gains in the general health of the public, but as the 21st century nears, much of what has been attained in relationship to health care has begun to change and seems in some degree to have diminished. The high cost of health care has caused a reevaluation of how health care dollars are spent. There are threats of disbanding programs such as Medicare, hospital stays are shorter, and there is a possibility that a cap will be placed on health care to the elderly.

At the end of the 20th century, increased community health nursing services are again in great need. Although technologically advanced, it appears that the end of this century is not unlike the end of the 19th century inasmuch as the government at that time also assumed limited responsibility for health care. The economics of providing adequate health care has become a dilemma. The social environment that encouraged people like Lillian Wald to provide home health care service seems to be expanding the demand for increased community health nursing services (Chafey, 1996). In addition to decreased hospital stays, there are a growing number of people unable to pay for health care services and many with limited or no health insurance.

SUMMARY

The earliest functions of lay nurses were intuitive and geared toward the maintenance of health, comforting the morbid, and providing for the simplest needs of humankind. This included the provision of food, shelter, warmth, clothing, and care of the spirit. Persons referred to as nurses at that time were untrained but capable and concerned caretakers. These nurses used intuition, assessment, and common sense problem-solving to meet human needs.

Over time, as a body of knowledge developed, nurses were able to use intellectual, interpersonal, and psychomotor skills to meet human needs. Community health nurses, perhaps the oldest model of nursing, worked as health care extenders to achieve the purpose of a healthy citizenry. Their nurturing skills and achievements have been essential to the preservation of human life and to the improvement and cultivation of human welfare throughout civilization.

Historically, nurses have been seen in a variety of roles. Over the years nurses have been viewed as health preservationists, pharmacists, health educators, healers, and nurturers. Gradually, in response to social crises arising from wars, epidemics, and medical discoveries, nursing has assumed an essential role in the prevention, treatment, and education of the public. Despite objections from society, nurses fought for adequate education, preparation, and recognition of their position. Commitment to nursing care of those in need and education makes nursing unique and ensures our humanity as a civilized society.

QUESTIONS

DIRECTIONS: Choose the one *best* response to each of the following questions.

1. In the 19th century, the government's efforts to help the poor attain health were

   A. on the increase
   B. tied to political benefits
   C. well supported
   D. very limited

2. Lillian Wald and Mary Brewster began

   A. the visiting nurse service
   B. the first nursing program
   C. the Henry Street Settlement
   D. a women's health center

3. Florence Nightingale is affiliated with community health nursing because

    A. she fought in the Crimean War
    B. she assigned nurses to work in the community with the sick at home
    C. she sent nurses to assist soldiers during the Crimean War
    D. she was concerned with the need for good food, sunlight, and pleasant surroundings for her patients

4. Similar to the 19th century, at the end of the 20th century

    A. the government provides care for all citizens
    B. Americans are in need of improved sanitation and drinking water
    C. there is a need for improved and benevolent public policy concerning the provision of health care
    D. there are a multitude of health care programs that have emerged

5. Clara Barton has been referred to as the

    A. "American Florence Nightingale"
    B. the author of many home care nursing books
    C. the first nurse to provide home care
    D. the founder of the Henry Street Settlement

ANSWERS

1. *The answer is D.* Government efforts to help the impoverished attain health care was practically nonexistent in the 19th century.

2. *The answer is C.* Lilian Wald and Mary Brewster began the Henry Street Settlement House in 1895.

3. *The answer is B.* As Florence Nightingale was asked to assign nurses to work in the community with sick individuals, she became affiliated with community health nursing.

4. *The answer is C.* In the 20th century, as in the 19th century, there is a need for improved public policy and an increased role of the government in the provision of health care services.

5. *The answer is A.* Due to her work, Clara Barton has been referred to as the "American Florence Nightingale."

ANNOTATED REFERENCES

Kalisch, P. A., & Kalisch, B. J. (1978). *The advance of American nursing.* Boston: Little, Brown.

This book is an historical overview of nursing. It begins with ancient civilizations and ends with a portrayal of 20th century nursing. Florence Nightingale, Clara Barton, and Lillian Wald are among those highlighted in this well-written history of nursing.

Chafey, K. (1996). Caring is not enough. *Nursing and Home Care: Perspectives on Community, 17*(1), 10–15.

This article explores the ethical and moral dilemmas associated with health care provision. It provides an historical overview and presents the moral problems of the health care system in the United States today.

Dock, L. L. (1920). *A short history of nursing: From the earliest times to the present day.* New York: G. P. Putnam.

One of the first efforts to compile a history of the evolution of nursing by one of the profession's matriarchs. This work focuses on international influences and developments in health care.

Dolan, J. A. (1968). *History of nursing.* Philadelphia: W. B. Saunders.

This text is a short overview of the history of nursing. It is nicely organized and easy to read. This is a good introduction to the experience of nursing's past and its evolution.

Oakes, S. B. (1994). *A woman of valor: Clara Barton and the Civil War.* New York: Free Press.

A wonderfully written new novel about the founder of the American Red Cross. This story narrates the Civil War from the perspective of the women who followed the armies and tended the wounded and dying soldiers. It discloses Barton's personal relationships, reveals the political benefactors she cultivated, and portrays the influence and persuasion she developed in government.

Ravitch, D. (1974). *The great school wars: New York City: 1805–1973. A history of the public schools as a battlefield of social change.* New York: Basic Books.

A wonderfully written story of the growth of public education in New York City. Unfolding before the reader is the influence of each culture as its population reaches the shores of Ellis Island. Every wave of immigration had its own health care needs and changed the relationship between public education and its connection to health care education.

Roberts, M. M. (1954). *American nursing: History and interpretation.* New York: Macmillan.

A chronological compilation of the important developments in nursing and the author's perceived impact. Well written and easy to read, it provides the reader with an overview of a developing profession.

Santayana, G. (1953). *The life of reason.* New York: Charles Scribner's.

This is a revised edition written in collaboration with Daniel Cory. In one volume, it contains all five editions of the original work in 1907. The work itself is a view of mankind's attempts at explaining art, religion, and science in order to live a rational life.

Swanson, K. (1993). Nursing as informed caring for the well-being of others. *Image: The Journal of Nursing Scholarship, 25* (4), 352–357.

This article discusses the relationship of nursing practice to Jean Watson's theory of informed caring. Well written and organized, it helps the reader to understand the application of theory to practice and the needs of practice to the creation of theory.

❦

CULTURAL DIVERSITY WITHIN THE COMMUNITY

INFLUENCE OF HEALTH BELIEFS AND CULTURE

In the United States, many consider health care a right. Nonetheless, the responsibility for acquiring health care and maintaining one's personal health is largely placed upon the individual (Andrews & Boyle, 1995). This apportionment of the burden of responsibility upon the individual for maintaining one's own health suggests that there is a common standard of acceptable health; thus, self-care becomes an additional responsibility of one's health maintenance. In fact, the way people assess health is highly individual and often has a strong tie to culture. Differences in customs and values influence health care beliefs and practices among different cultures; regardless of how health care professionals evaluate a client's state of health, clients are inclined to measure their own sense of well-being. Naturally, then, a client's cultural beliefs or behaviors may conflict with the standards of the health care providers in a community.

The community health nurse may feel conflict when working with clients who, based on certain societal expectations, have not done all they could to maintain their health. Furthermore, the community health nurse's response to a client's health needs or demands is also influenced by the nurse's own cultural heritage and health beliefs. Health care providers must be sensitive to the enormous impact culture plays on clients' health and on providers' attitudes towards clients.

Culture is learned from a person's environment, and cultural learning is often likened to the way in which humans learn to speak (Spector, 1996). Accordingly, cultural norms are mostly implied and are often unexpressed by individuals. Most members of a family or cultural group have no need to discuss rules among themselves related to their culturally connected behaviors. Culture influences the foods we eat, how our children are reared, our reactions to pain, how we cope with stress, our response to health care, and the ways in which we deal with issues related to death. Cultural influences and organized support systems often set guidelines for living and provide foundations for client behaviors (Pender, 1996). In short, culture provides the underpinnings for a person's social development. The following case study is an example of how the community health nurse, using her knowledge about cultural diversity, makes an impact on the care of a client.

Diversity. Wherever things are not the same there is diversity. Diversity is not limited to culture, ethnicity, or race.

CASE STUDY: CULTURAL INFLUENCES ON RESPONSES TO HEALTH CARE

The community health nurse, making a routine postpartum home visit, found that the newborn had a serious breakdown of the skin in the area of the buttocks. The nurse referred the parents of the newborn to the local pediatric nurse practitioner who diagnosed this infant's condition as a bacterial infection and prescribed a topical antibacterial medication as treatment. The pediatric nurse practitioner recommended follow-up home visits by the community health nurse. After several home visits, the community health nurse realized that the parents, who were of Gypsy heritage, were not applying the prescribed medication as ordered, and there was evidence of increased infection. In all other respects, the infant was well cared for. Although this family seemed to trust the nurse, the parents remained noncompliant in the use of the cream. Furthermore, they seemed anxious about the prescribed treatment.

By inquiring about the culture of the Gypsy community, the nurse discovered that the community leader must approve all outside interventions, particularly medications. The community health nurse then asked the parents to accompany her on a visit to the community leader and matriarch, known as the "Queen." During this visit, the nurse discussed with the Queen the need for treatment of the infant. The Queen inspected the medication and the infant, then instructed the parents to comply with the treatment. The parents then began treating the infant. On the follow-up visit made by the community health nurse, the parents seemed relieved, and the infant's condition improved.

Clients' perceptions of health are based on the environment in which they live as well as the culture within which they have been socialized. Although ethnic, racial, and cultural differences are often key to the care of the client, environmentally derived health beliefs frequently determine how the client interprets health and seeks access to health care. For example, clients may believe that certain health problems are the norm for their age or condition and see no reason to seek health assistance. The following case study explores how an environmentally supported myth about women and aging could cause unnecessary health problems for a client.

CASE STUDY: MYTH AS A CAUSE OF HEALTH PROBLEMS

Mrs. Joel, a 46-year-old resident of a rural community, visited a mobile gynecology clinic managed by community health nurse practitioners. The clinic is funded by the state in which Mrs. Joel lives to provide outreach to rural women living in remote areas with few local services. Mrs. Joel came to the clinic for birth control education, breast cancer screening, and a Papanicolaou (Pap) screening test. Mrs. Joel reported that she had been experiencing a vaginal discharge and a fetid odor. After thoroughly examining the client, the nurse practitioner diagnosed an infection in the vaginal wall. In discussing the diagnosis with Mrs. Joel, the community health nurse discovered that Mrs. Joel believed the odor to be normal and had not considered seeking medical care. She told the nurse that all women in her family get an "odor" as they "reach the change" (menopause). Her experiences in a limited environment caused her to misinterpret her own symptoms of infection, believing them to be a normal part of aging. Had she not reached beyond the boundaries of her usual environment, Mrs. Joel's infection would have gone untreated and might have become more serious. As part of Mrs. Joel's treatment, the nurse educated her about women's health and the gynecological changes associated with aging and planned follow-up visits.

To create a health care plan competently with clients, the community health nurse must find ways of accommodating the client's perception of health and meeting his or her expectations of treatment (Spector, 1996). How this is achieved impacts on the state of health in our society. Clients who have the ability to improve their health conditions but refuse to do so because of health beliefs, religious restrictions, or cultural sway can be costly to the the health care system and compromise the client's health. For example, there are clients who refuse immunization against communicable diseases because of their beliefs, thereby increasing the possibility of the spread of disease. Such a client population can burden the health care system both because of the spread of the disease and because of the long-term effects to the clients themselves. Thus, to negotiate an effective health care plan, it is important to know how the client perceives health and illness and to understand the factors influencing the client's perceptions. Throughout this process, the community health nurse must respect the client's wishes. The nurse is then able to make predictive assumptions about behaviors of the client, based on a foundation of knowledge about the culture and the actions the client will take (Spector, 1996). As in the case study, some of our behaviors or expectations may occur from what we have experienced in our families or communities and what is considered the norm in our environment.

$\mathcal{P}$RACTITIONER'S BELIEFS

To meet the unique health needs of clients effectively, it is necessary for health professionals to be aware of their own health beliefs, their connections to their own cultures, and the influence the health care culture has had on them. It is important to note that the perception of health by a health provider is influenced simply by becoming a health care provider. Influenced by the health care system, health care providers incorporate a "health care provider culture" into their individual cultures as they become socialized into their professional roles (Spector, 1996). As health care providers become more aware of and sensitive to their own cultures and how they have arrived at their own belief systems, they can become more sensitive to the health needs and cultural norms of their clients. When community health nurses use information based on culture, health beliefs, and environment, they can help clients to make decisions supportive of a healthy life style.

$\mathcal{V}$ALUES CLARIFICATION

All societies and cultures have rules that identify appropriate and inappropriate behaviors. These are called **cultural norms**. Norms flow from cultural values, and provide directions for living up to and maintaining behaviors (Andrews & Boyle, 1995). Being in touch with one's values and the influence values have on the decisions one makes is essential to achieving and maintaining a high level of wellness. However, since cultures vary greatly, the values that guide a person's behavior also vary greatly. This is particularly true of how values influence health behaviors and health beliefs.

One way to help clients prioritize their health goals and behaviors is by using **values clarification** techniques. Values clarification is a process of self-evaluation and self-discovery that helps the client, whether the client is an individual, a family, or a community, to examine beliefs, behaviors, and assumptions. Values clarification has no set of rules nor are there any right or wrong choices implied when using values clarification techniques; it simply means that each person becomes aware of options for themselves. By understanding one's own values and their importance, as well as having the correct information related to these values, a person can make rational choices, not simply choices based on habit, cultural heritage, or social and environmental influences. By understanding one's values and their importance, a person, family, or a community can identify the best choices for themselves.

Most persons, however, do not notice the subtle influences that affect their values or beliefs and so may often make choices that are not in their own best interest. At certain ages, such as adolescence, external environmental pressures often exceed the values from one's culture. An example of this can be seen in inner city high schools where there is peer pressure

Cultural Norms. These norms are the cultural values of a group, which govern human behavior. Norms provide direction for the behavior that a person or group displays (Andrew & Boyle, 1995).

Values Clarification. This is a process by which individuals identify or express their personal preferences (i.e., likes and dislikes) relating to issues effecting their lives.

on adolescent girls to become pregnant. Pregnancy is often a symbol of maturity and love for many of these teenage girls. Despite the availability of sex education programs and birth control, many students in inner city high schools become pregnant each year.

Another example is concern about weight loss and its importance to health, which has been interpreted by some to mean excessively thin. The notion that "you cannot be too rich or too thin" has put tremendous pressure on members of our society. Extremely thin commercial models have become the standard by which many women and adolescent girls in our society judge themselves. Some young women and adolescents, attempting to be thin to fulfill this image, have developed eating disorders such as anorexia or bulimia. At times, people may base their belief system on poor information, which is believed to be true, or on a societal norm. The use of values clarification techniques could help clients beset by peer pressure to become more aware of the sometimes insidious interactions of their culture and their environment, opening the way to more beneficial behaviors.

A values clarification assessment concerning health beliefs might include the following questions:

1. What are the goals you would like to achieve in the next 5 years?
2. How do you spend your time?
3. How do you compare your health now with what you would expect your health to be?
4. Rank priorities concerning your health.

Question 1 will help the nurse to gain insight into the client's time orientation. Time orientation varies in different cultural groups. Some cultures tend to be future-oriented (Spector, 1996); they plan ahead and are concerned with long-range goals. Other groups are present-oriented and so do not plan for the future, concerning themselves only with events occurring now. As persons age, they often become oriented to the past, which may compromise their ability to function well in the present. For clients who are present- or past-oriented, this question may be difficult to answer as they will not have a plan for the future. Additionally, this question will give the community health nurse insight into the client's goal orientation.

Question 2 will give the nurse some insight into how clients are spending their time. Often clients do not stop to consider the amount of time they actually spend either at work or at play. It may help them to weigh the amount of time they spend on things or people they value.

Question 3 may give the nurse insight into what the client's image of health is. Clients often have a view of their health that is different from that of their health care provider.

Question 4 might help the clients to begin to assess and to develop their own health goals.

These questions may be asked by the community health nurse in interviews or may appear in the form of a written document or questionnaire. The responses to these questions will help the community health nurse gain insight and understanding of the client's goals.

Cultural Diversity

It was believed for a long time that the United States was a melting pot of cultures. More recently, the health care field has embraced the position that the United States is more like a salad bowl in which there is a mix of peoples, each group maintaining its own cultural identity and history. These are referred to as multicultural or diverse communities (Fig. 3-1). In the past, health care providers tended to deny or diminish the importance of cultural identity for individual and community health. Now, however, health care providers in the United States recognize that cultural forces have a significant impact on clients' conceptualization of and response to health and illness. Terms referring to the cultural heritage of people, such as African Americans, Italian Americans, and Asian Americans, are now more commonly used when describing and trying to understand the health needs and practices of clients. This affirmation of cultural diversity in the United States is a positive development that places several valuable assessment tools and perspectives in the hands of community health nurses.

Health beliefs or **mores** are not limited to cultural beliefs. They are often what clients have learned to expect from their social environment. Perceptions of health that clients have are also based upon the environment in which they live as well as the culture into which they have socialized. Although ethnic differences are often key to the care of the client, health beliefs frequently organize and manipulate how individuals interpret their own health and how they seek access to health care. Therefore, clients may believe that certain conditions are the norm for their age or condition and see no reason to seek out health assistance.

Cultural diversity is found in geographic environments in which a variety of culturally different persons or groups live together. Each group

Mores are habits and customs of society, usually those that come to be regarded as essential to the survival and well-being of the society.

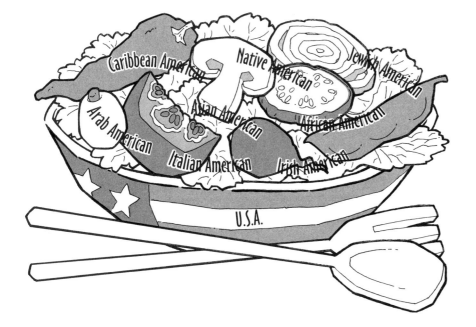

FIGURE 3-1

◙

The United States is like a salad bowl; that is, it is a mix of people with many groups maintaining their own cultural and religious identities and histories, making up one country.

brings its own expectations of health into the larger society. These expectations are influenced by a variety of forces, including changes in technology, advancements made in health care and the influence or pressures from the environment of the greater society.

Environmental press is the term used to refer to the effect or influence of the environment upon individuals or groups. Pressures from the environment in which clients live include both physical pressures (e.g., climate, available foods, altitude, size, location) and emotional pressures (e.g., religion, the need for formal education, the existence of more dominant cultures within the environment). These pressures may interfere with how persons experience or express their own culture. Much of this is based on theories of environmental press, which come from the landmark work of Kurt Lewin, a psychologist who practiced in the 1930s (Hall & Lindsay, 1970).

As the developer of an important environmental press theory, Lewin proposed that to study a person, scientists must look at the whole circumstances in which that person is placed (Lewin, 1936). For Lewin, individual functioning is a result of the complex relationship between the individual and the environment and is dependent on the state of the person as well as on the state of the environment (Lewin, 1936). In Lewin's cybernetic model, an individual's culture not only influences the environment but is influenced by the environment. Lewin's model provides a useful foundation for thinking about the interactions between individuals, their cultures, and the environment in which they live. Much of the work done by behaviorists uses Lewin's theories as a frame of reference (Klainberg, 1994).

ℰTHNOCENTRISM

Ethnocentrism is a belief in the superiority of one's culture or group.

Extreme devotion to one's own culture and the rejection or denial of other cultures is called **ethnocentrism**. This can lead to misunderstandings of other cultures as well as prejudice, racism, and discrimination. To provide effective care, the community health nurse must avoid ethnocentric behaviors. As one begins to respect cultural diversity, cultural sensitivity develops. "Cultural sensitivity is a prerequisite for personal, comprehensive nursing care" (Andrew & Boyle, 1995, p. 39).

𝒜SSIMILATION

Cultural assimilation is a process during which a person, family, or community adapts to a new cultural environment (Wadsworth, 1986). Most persons entering into new environments go through an assimilation process to some degree.

In most cases, assimilation involves the adaptation of a minority person or group to an established majority culture, usually referred to as the dominant culture. This is rarely an easy process, and persons undergoing it may feel both a need to become incorporated into the new environment and pulled by their inner sense of cultural ties. As culture is dynamic and individuals unique, there are usually differences in the ways in which each person incorporates the dominant culture into his or her cultural heritage. This may create cultural confusion or a cultural clash, sometimes between generations and more often within individuals. An example of the latter might be a sexually active adolescent male from a culture that frowns on sexual activity of adolescents and unmarried individuals in a dominant culture that encourages safe sex and the use of condoms; his inner conflicts about sexuality may interfere with his use of condoms and other safe sex practices, his incomplete assimilation denying him the protection of either his culture of origin or the dominant culture.

Although there are some minority cultures that assimilate eagerly to the dominant culture, other cultures attempt to maintain their cultural heritage intact despite external pressures. Examples of these are the Amish and the Hasidic Jewish communities. These communities make few compromises in an attempt to maintain their heritage. Despite the availability of technology, the Amish choose not to use many modern, labor-saving devices; contemporary medicine; or even electricity, and they continue to dress and live as they have for generations in an attempt to maintain their religion and culture. To maintain their religion, the Hasidic Jewish community has a dress code, dietary laws, limitations to the use of some technology, restrictions related to birth control, and restrictions that may have an impact on health practices. Community health nurses must respect and attempt to maintain the traditions of these and other groups when providing client care.

TIME, PERSONAL SPACE, AND FOLK HEALING

Culture influences how people express themselves in relationship to time and personal space and may affect how the community health nurse approaches clients in relationship to time and space.

In the United States, persons from the dominant culture tend to be very time dependent and, therefore, very concerned with the importance of time—that is, most Americans set appointments and are disturbed if the person with whom they have an appointment is late. Time is cut up into segments with work scheduled between the hours of 9 A.M. and 5 P.M., and entertainment similarly kept to a prescribed schedule. Television is divided into 30- or 60-min segments; theater or film begins at a specific time. Because Western culture tends to connote time with productivity, time is regarded as an important commodity. Accordingly, most Americans try never to waste time and try to be on time for appointments.

What has just been said about mainstream American culture is not true of all the diverse cultures within the United States. Some cultures view time as never ending, and they get to where they are going when they get there. If something does not get finished today, it is believed that it will get done tomorrow. Persons from such cultures have a different approach to keeping appointments and to what it means to be "on time." For persons from Ghana, for example, punctuality is of little importance. It is more important to continue a social interaction than being on time for another event (Geissler, 1994).

The physical distance people keep when interacting also differs from culture to culture. In the United States, people keep approximately 2 feet away from persons with whom they are conversing. In contrast to this practice, persons from many other cultures come either closer or further away to the person with whom they are speaking. Other practices, such as human touch, can also play an important part in how the community health nurse should approach a client. Additionally, eye contact has a significant meaning in most cultures. Many persons native to the Australian culture may combine direct eye contact with intermittent looking away, which they interpret as showing interest. Although direct eye contact may not be sustained by Australians, Argentines tend to maintain intense eye contact during conversation (Geissler, 1994). In short, cultural variation is the rule in the area of social interaction.

The degree to which physical touching is permitted is also dictated by cultural values and mores. While some degree of touching between persons of different sexes is generally acceptable to the dominant culture in the United States, Orthodox Jewish men are not permitted to be touched by women other than their wives. If hands-on care is to be delivered to an Orthodox Jewish male, the community health nurse delivering the care should also be a man whenever possible. If the community health nurse is a woman, she should instruct the wife or another man as to how to provide direct care to these male clients at home. The female nurse may oversee procedures to ensure that they are done correctly. South Korean clients also consider physical touching by members of the opposite sex inappropriate (Geissler, 1994).

In Singapore and Vietnam, the head is considered sacred; therefore, it is considered an affront to reach over someone's head and an offense to pat or touch a child on the head (Geissler, 1994). Strangers touching children is frankly frowned upon by many Hispanic parents (Andrew & Boyle, 1995). Mexican parents believe that this can cause illness. An example of this is Caida de la Mollera, which is a serious illness with a high mortality among infants and children 1 to 3 years of age. The cause is often related to diarrhea or vomiting; as a result of dehydration, the anterior fontanelle becomes depressed below the contour of the skull. Some poorly educated or rural Hispanic parents believe that this condition is caused by a non-family member touching the head of the infant. As it is common for the community health nurse to measure infants' skulls, this is easily mistaken for the cause of the problem (Spector, 1996). If Caida de la Mollera afflicts a child, a curandero, or folk healer, may be used to rid the child of Mal Ojo, or the evil eye, of the stranger. In an attempt to heal the child, the curandero may hold the infant upside down to help the fontanelle resume its placement; sadly, this practice may result in retinal hemorrhages

(Montelone, 1994). To prevent such tragedies, the parents must be encouraged to hydrate the infant. If they wish to use the curandero, this can be done in addition to hydration.

Regardless of education and assimilation into a more cosmopolitan health system, many Mexican Americans and other Hispanics may use the curandero for a variety of ailments and problems. Often these problems may be psychosocial. It is important for the community health nurse to understand the role and functions of the folk healers and work collaboratively with them. Without acceptance by the folk healer, Hispanic clients may not comply with the recommendations of the community health nurse.

Folk beliefs regarding illness and their cures can be found in all cultures. Nurses who wish to be optimally effective with the communities they serve should develop familiarity and appreciation of folk beliefs and other cultural differences, thus empowering themselves to help their clients toward wellness.

TRANSCULTURAL NURSING

Caring for clients from all cultures in a sensitive manner is referred to as *transcultural nursing* (Andrews & Boyle, 1995). Transcultural nursing was born from a synthesis of theories, concepts, and philosophies drawn from sociology, biology, and anthropology (Andrew & Boyle, 1995). The basis of transcultural nursing is that caring is a universal phenomenon that exists in all cultures (Leininger, 1978). Although caring occurs in all cultures, differences are evident in how each culture displays caring. Community health nurses must be sensitive to these differences in developing their plan of care. Because each culture displays caring in its own way, the health care plan should reflect both an acknowledgment and an understanding of how each client cares for others and wishes to be cared for.

Much of the literature written on transcultural nursing theory is based on the landmark work of Leininger in the 1970s. Leininger defines transcultural nursing theory as "as set of interrelated cross-cultural nursing concepts and hypotheses, which take into account individual and group caring behaviors, values, and beliefs based upon their cultural needs to provide effective and satisfying nursing care to people" (Leininger, 1978, p. 33). Leininger's work followed from her conviction that "if nursing practices fail to recognize [the cultural] aspects of human needs, there will be signs of less efficacious nursing care practices and some unfavorable consequences to those served" (Leininger, 1978, p. 33). Nursing, according to Leininger "is essentially a transcultural phenomenon in that the context and process of helping people involves at least two persons generally having different cultural orientations or intercultural lifestyles" (Leininger, 1978, p. 35).

Accordingly, she developed a Transcultural Health Model to study and analyze different health care systems and practices. Intended as a general guide for the health professional, this model provides a systematic method of identifying and analyzing major components of the health features of a culture (Leininger, 1978). Leininger's model is divided into four levels. Level one explores the relationship of health to the social structure of a culture, including the identification of dominant political, economic, familial, spiritual, technological, and educational systems with a demographic world view and environmental factors (Leininger, 1978). At level two, the nurse observes and listens to the people regarding their cultural values and health care. This is a vital part of the process as levels three and four are dependent on information gathered here. This information must be accurate and reflective of the client. Level three classifies the formal and informal health care systems of cultures, considering whether they are primarily preventive or restorative, ambulatory or nonambulatory, the age of the system, and who the providers are. Level four explores the roles and functions of the health care providers in the culture, analyzing their responsibilities, functions, and roles, as well as the contextual influences on roles and changes in roles (Leininger, 1978). Leininger believed that the development of cultural awareness is not an intuitive process but rather one that is achieved through a conscious effort (Leninger, 1978). This model is used as a guide for the community health nurse to explore the impact of the environment and culture upon the client and to facilitate the formation of a positive alliance between the client and the community health nurse.

CULTURAL ASSESSMENTS

Because clients have their own culturally defined ways of maintaining health, it is important for the community health nurse to include cultural information in the development plan for client care (Leininger, 1978). Such an assessment may use several strategies, including researching clients' cultural history and directly asking clients about their culture, religion, and individual health beliefs. Most clients are happy to answer questions if they are posed in a professional, nonthreatening manner. Throughout the assessment process, the community health nurse should keep in mind that although it is very important to understand the basic cultural differences that clients bring with them into the health care system, it is equally important not to stereotype clients. Instead, the community health nurse is encouraged to maintain an open mind and open communication concerning individual beliefs.

The community health nurse preparing to do a cultural assessment should be alert to the fact that there may be different degrees of assimilation by the clients. Some clients will have lived within the dominant culture for a long period of time, while others may be newcomers to the United States. Moreover, regardless of the length of stay, many clients will not have completely assimilated into the dominant culture, retaining traditional cultural beliefs and attitudes with respect to their health (Geissler, 1994). Language may further impede how one receives health care as well as health care information. Inability to communicate via the language of the dominant culture (if English is a second language) is of great importance and may impede the provision of health care. Also, translators may need to be utilized in the care of the hearing-impaired.

Below is an assessment instrument that can be used as a guide in conducting cultural assessments with individual clients. (To assess an entire community, please see the community assessment instrument in Chap. 5.)

Suggested Questions for the Cultural Assessment of an Individual

1. Where were you born?
2. Where were you raised? If not in the United State, how old were you when you came to this country?
3. Were you raised by your biological parents? (If adopted, do you have any information about your cultural history?)
4. Where were your parents/caregivers born? If first-generation inhabitants, when did they come to the United States?
5. Where were your grandparents born?
6. What language/languages do you speak? Can you read and write in your native language? Can you read and write in English?
7. What is your religion? What is your degree of involvement in your religion?
8. Is your spouse/partner the same religion as you?
9. Is your spouse/partner from your country of birth?
10. Are most of your friends from the neighborhood in which you live?
11. Do most of your friends come from the same background as you do?
12. Do you celebrate religious or ethnic holidays?
13. Where were you educated? Was your education religious or public?
14. What are the foods you like to eat on a regular basis? Are these foods unique to your culture?

Economics of culture

The degree of economic prosperity enjoyed or denied has a powerful impact on one's culture and degree of health. Poverty and low income are closely tied to poor health and poor health care services. On average, persons of low income have higher death rates than persons with incomes above the poverty level [U.S. Department of Health and Human Services (DHHS), 1992]. Violent and abusive behavior toward children and spouses, as well as homicide and assault in general, have been linked to poverty. Persons living in poverty live in a more violent environment, are sicker, and are more prone to health problems. Yet, despite this knowledge related to health threats, people living in poverty tend to have inadequate health systems. In fact, despite government health programs such as Medicaid and Medicare, 28.6 percent of the poor in 1990 did not have any type of medical insurance (DHHS, 1992). People living in poverty in our society—a group of nearly one out of eight Americans living below the poverty level—are, thus, identified as being at high risk for becoming ill (DHHS, 1992). Additionally, the elderly and persons with long-term health problems, such as acquired immunodeficiency syndrome (AIDS), multiple sclerosis (MS), and cancer are included in this high-risk group.

Efforts to identify people living in poverty in the United States have uncovered a disturbing correlation between poverty and culture. The official goals of the United States are articulated in the publication *Healthy People 2000: National Promotion and Disease Prevention Objectives* (1992). Prepared by the DHHS and the Public Health Service, *Healthy People 2000* identifies most minority populations as being at high risk for poor health (DHHS, 1992). This document provides a national strategy for improving the health of the nation over the next decade. It addresses issues of prevention of major chronic illness, injuries, and infectious disease. This report particularly addresses concern for high-risk groups and identifies most minority populations as being at high risk (DHHS, 1992). Minority populations include persons with low incomes, persons who are a member of either a racial or ethnic minority group, and persons with disabilities (DHHS, 1992). Predominant racial and ethnic minority populations identified in *Healthy People 2000* are African Americans, Hispanics, Asians, Pacific Islanders, Native Americans, and Native Alaskans (DHHS, 1992). Elderly clients and children constitute a large portion of the clients in these high-risk populations. High-risk factors that identify these populations are for the most part also identified with low income or at poverty levels. Poverty reduces a persons chances for a long life.

The link between culture, poverty, and ill health are especially evident in many of the statistics that describe African Americans living in the United States. According to the United States census in 1990, although poverty rates for whites and Hispanics have increased, the poverty rate for African Americans has remained the highest of these groups. African American infants have twice the average risk of having low birth weight (DHHS, 1992). Low birth weight is linked to neurological and developmental conditions, which include learning and behavioral problems. African Americans are prone to hypertension and sickle cell anemia. People with uncontrolled hypertension are also at great risk for developing other cardiovascular diseases, such as stroke or coronary artery disease. The life expectancy for African Americans is lower than that of whites.

In order to respond to the problems noted in this section, there must be improved access to health care services for all people, as well as more capable outreach to populations in ways that will address their community and cultural needs. It is important to note that most of the health issues mentioned above can be effectively addressed through preventive measures. Additionally, interventions through education, rehabilitative counseling, and direct medical attention can have a significant impact on primary, secondary, and tertiary levels of prevention for clients with hypertension, obesity, adolescent pregnancy, AIDS, diabetes, low birth weight infants, substance abuse, and violent behaviors. Clearly, issues of health belief and culture, not money alone, must be remembered when trying to meet the needs of a diverse population.

Gender, Age, and Health Care

Issues related to gender and age are included in this chapter because many of the ways that we treat and care for the elderly, women, and children are a reflection of our culture and its belief systems. The health of these aggregates is dependent on how society responds to them.

The Elderly

Older Americans make up the fastest growing members of our population with persons over 85 years of age constituting the faction with the greatest percentage of growth. Degrees of wellness among older Americans varies, but the majority of this aggregate are able to care for themselves (Abel & Nelson, 1996).

American society does not treat its elderly well. On the one hand, the technical environment that allows people to reach old age is provided; yet, on the other hand, a system that enhances or respects the lives of the elderly is not provided. Instead, our society reveres its youth. Many elderly live in poverty since they subsist on fixed incomes while the cost of living continually rises. Because of poverty, many older persons are without adequate health insurance for health care services, forcing them to assume out-of-pocket costs for medication and supplemental health insurance; unfortunately, these people cannot depend of their families or the community to provide them with adequate nourishment and care. Even those who are not economically deprived can become victims of a society that cares little about them. In addition to increased numbers of elder abuse cases reported in the media, there are reported cases of financial abuses directed at the elderly; these cases involve overcharging or cheating elderly persons on services that they may require for self-maintenance.

Furthermore, many inaccurate assumptions are made about the elderly. It is assumed that, as people age, they are no longer able to think or make practical decisions for themselves; instead, we tend to assume that they are impaired, slow, and unable to learn. These myths and others like them are called ageism. For many adults, their lives undergo less change as they age than many of us might imagine.

When changes do come with age, many elderly persons are able to respond to these changes effectively and resourcefully. Nurses frequently see older clients learning new self-care strategies as they relate to changes in the status of their health. These are often complex and difficult procedures for the lay person, such as the administration of a multitude of medications, diabetic care, or colostomy care. In providing health care services for the elderly, the community health nurse must remember that only a small percentage of the elderly fall into the category of *frail elderly* and that, for the most part, older clients remain well, active, and able to care for themselves. However, well and capable elderly are not without the need of support services to help to maintain themselves in a safe environment. It is the community health nurse who assesses these needs, using the data collection instruments, which evaluate the requirements of the client and how the community meets those needs. Misconceptions about the needs of the elderly can give rise to ageism. Ageism has no place in developing a plan of care with an elderly client, and it is important that the nurse is comfortable with the needs of the client and dispels negative personal experiences or myths.

Most frail elderly are not placed in nursing homes. Despite the myth that this is due to the high cost of institutional care, it is, in fact, primarily due to a desire of the older person to remain at home. Therefore, many elderly are cared for at home (Abel & Nelson, 1990). Although a spouse is often the main caregiver at home, adult children (primarily women) constitute the greatest number of caregivers (Abel & Nelson, 1990). The stress of long-term care can be emotionally, socially, and financially great. Middle-aged families are often referred to as "the sandwich generation," caring for both children and elderly parents simultaneously. Often aging themselves, many adult children are becoming the caregivers of their parents just as they come to the end of their duties as caregivers for their children.

All levels of prevention are practiced when caring for the elderly. Examples of *primary prevention* include acquiring security handrails for the tub or helping a senior citizen find a community support group for socialization and nutritional guidance. An example of *secondary prevention* is helping an arthritic client to obtain the assistance of a home health aide for several hours a day to shop and do household chores. Examples of *tertiary prevention* might include helping to access hospice services for the client and the client's family or assisting the family of a client in selecting either home care or nursing home care for a severely disabled client who has MS.

Women

The changing role of women in today's society impacts not only on their own health but the health needs of the entire community. Women are prominent in today's work force and are either equal economic heads or independent heads of households. As a result, women are now facing an increase in many of the stress-related health problems previously experienced only by men, including hypertension, cardiovascular disease, and lung cancer.

For the most part, middle-aged women, whether married or not, continue to maintain the home as a physical, social, and emotional environment despite major changes in their economic status. Although most American women are now among the work force, they still provide primary care for their aging parents and children. Adult children may also return home with children, and grandparents may find themselves caring for grandchildren as a result of illness, addiction, or death from accidents. This creates a variety of community health needs, including stress management for women, health services for children offered at times when women are available, day care services for children, and, in some cases, day care for elderly parents or sick children.

The stress-related health issues created for women by managing career and family are often addressed by the community health nurse. Planning for community health services to meet the requirements of these women is a tremendous community health need. By forming an alliance with women and other community members, the nurse can take preventive measures toward meeting these health needs.

Young Adult

Of growing interest to community health nurses is the newest aggregate in our society, the young adult population referred to as generation X (i.e., all persons born between 1961 and 1981; the "X" refers to extremes). In 1995, members of generation X accounted for 79.4 million people or approximately 30 percent of the United States population (Ritchie, 1995). In 1996, members of generation X in the United States ranged in age from 14 to 34 years of age. This generation has its own culture, which is very different from the cultures of previous generations. Meeting the health needs of these community members is a challenge.

As with all other generations, members of generation X are diverse, but they share many common values with which the community health nurse should become familiar. Most members of generation X are still living at home with their parents; some say these individuals have difficulty with transition to adulthood and that they have no reason to leave home except to marry, join the military, or go to college. For some, the cost of moving out is high, salaries are low, and jobs are scarce.

This is the television and fast food generation. Members of generation X relate to being at risk for crime, guns, and drugs in ways that former generations do not. Other generations have had to deal with violence, but it was viewed as organized in distant places, such as wars in foreign nations.

Generation X has also been decimated by acquired immunodeficiency syndrome (AIDS) even though it has had birth control measures, specifically condoms, available from an early age. This generation faces crime, guns, and drugs more locally.

As a group, members of generation X have not denied themselves personal luxury. They are well traveled, and many of them own new cars (Ritchie, 1995). They purchase more compact discs, disposable diapers, and electric can openers; eat more fast food; smoke more cigarettes; and are more likely to marry than members of the "baby boom" generation. They participate in aerobics; are concerned with a healthy diet; are likely to belong to an exercise club; and are major consumers of health and exercise equipment, sports equipment, and clothing.

Although reared in this culture, many members of generation X have a different view of how families and communities should operate. They are the children of "baby boomers" and women whose careers and education were significant. For older generation X children, there was little day care

Generation X includes all persons born between 1961 and 1981.

available; therefore, babysitters, private at-home care, and self-care (latch key) were called into service. These individuals learned to cook, shop, and help with housework. These are the children of the microwave oven and of fast food at home (Ritchie, 1995). Their experience has been to work in the household, and many worked outside the home while they were in high school (Ritchie, 1995). This is not a lazy generation, and they often undertake caregiving duties of siblings, the sick, and the elderly (Shellenbarger, 1996). Also, as children of divorced parents, they may belong to families with unique structures, including single-parent and multiple-parent families.

Partly as a result of their own early experiences, members of generation X have developed their own style of families. This relates not only to how families function as two-parent, single-parent, or heterosexual families, but also how they parent. There are now many single-parent and same-sex households. Many couples equally share parenting and work responsibilities outside as well as within the home. Most generation X families do not cling to roles that no longer fit their life style, including the roles associated with the traditional single-income household with the mother at home with the children and the father working. The economy is such that many couples have gone from being DINKS (double income no kids) to DIAKS (double income and kids). Although there have always been many varieties and types of families, there seems to be a greater latitude in today's world as families are more able to disclose their individuality and uniqueness. The community health nurse in working with generation X clients needs to be aware of their unique needs and life styles.

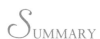

SUMMARY

Culture influences how people react and deal with health needs. Community health nurses working in the United States, particularly in urban environments, deal with a culturally diverse society. There is great need to be sensitive to the values and beliefs rooted in our clients' cultural, religious, and social heritages. Community health nurses must also understand their own beliefs and how these may impact their relationship with clients. To develop a health care plan competently, the community health nurse must consider all relevant facets of culture, gender, and health beliefs.

KEY WORDS

Cultural norms	Generation X
Diversity	Mores
Environmental press	Transcultural nursing
Ethnocentrism	Values clarification

QUESTIONS

DIRECTIONS: Choose the one *best* response to each of the following questions.

1. The term ethnocentrism refers to
   A. how serious a person is about being an American
   B. extreme devotion to one's own culture and rejection of others
   C. extreme caution in how an individual celebrates his or her culture
   D. how one accommodates becoming a citizen of a country

2. Correct statements concerning elderly individuals in this country include which of the following?
   A. They are well cared for in institutional settings
   B. They are the fastest growing segment of the population in the United States
   C. They are in need of tremendous care as they age
   D. They are mostly able to care for themselves with assistance

3. Middle-aged women are at high risk for
   A. surgical interventions
   B. stress-related diseases
   C. unwanted pregnancy
   D. economic instability

4. To provide quality care for clients, it is important for the community health nurse to first become
   A. a family nurse practitioner
   B. skilled in highly technological devices
   C. aware of their own beliefs and values
   D. skilled in using a values clarification instrument

5. Mrs. Jones attends a local screening for hypertension offered by the local health department. The community health nurse determines that Mrs. Jones has high blood pressure. Discovering hypertension at such a screening is considered
   A. primary prevention
   B. secondary prevention
   C. tertiary prevention
   D. assessment not prevention

ANSWERS

1. *The answer is B.* Ethnocentrism is a belief in the superiority of one's culture or ethnic group. There is a tendency to reject all other cultures.

2. *The answer is D.* Most elderly individuals in this country are able to take care of themselves, though often with some assistance.

3. *The answer is B.* Middle-aged women are at high risk for stress-related diseases.

4. *The answer is C.* It is important for the community health nurse to become aware of his or her own beliefs and values before being able to provide quality care to clients from many diverse backgrounds.

5. *The answer is B.* Hypertension screening programs are considered secondary prevention methods.

ANNOTATED REFERENCES

Abel E. K., & Nelson, M. K. (1990). *Circles of care, work, and identity in women's lives.* Albany: State University of New York Press.

This book examines the experiences of women who care for children, frail elderly, disabled persons, and the chronically ill. It looks at the unique experience of women as caregivers. It explores perceptions and feelings of the caregiver as well as the family and discusses the role of the caregiver in regard to the full scope of the duties and responsibilities of the provider from simple hands-on care to issues of total responsibility, including responsibilities related to home care and institutionalized care.

Andrews, M., & Boyle, J. S. (1995). *Transcultural concepts in nursing care* (2nd ed.). Philadelphia: J. B. Lippincott.

This book approaches the delivery of nursing care through the lens of transcultural issues. The three sections in this text—Theoretical Perspective, A Developmental Approach, and Clinical Topics and Issues—apply transcultural issues to the delivery of nursing care. This book uses natural and behavioral science as well as recent research as a foundation in its approach to the provision of care.

Geissler, E. M. (1994). *Pocket guide to cultural assessment.* St. Louis, MO: C. V. Mosby.

This pocket book provides information that is essential to assessing and caring for culturally diverse populations. This compact text contains cultural and ethical information for health care professionals on populations representing 166 countries. It explores concrete issues of childhood immunization and abstract matters like health care beliefs. Additionally, it identifies the language, religion, and location of each identified country.

Hall, C. S., & Lindzey, G. (1970). *Theories of personality.* New York: John Wiley.

This book is a compilation of selected theorists, including Freud, Jung, Murray, Lewin, Allport, Skinner, and others. Each theory is presented in a concise and positive manner.

Klainberg, M. (1994). *The impact of congruent-dissonant relationships between the nontraditional nursing student and the environment of an institution of higher education on the nontraditional nursing student's sense of mattering.* Doctoral dissertation, Columbia University Teachers College, New York (University of Michigan, Ann Arbor, Dissertation Services, order #9511051)

The research discussed in this dissertation explores the influence of educational practices and environments upon adult learners and culturally diverse populations. How people learn is influenced by the environment as well as their own belief systems. A sense of mattering enhances learning.

Leininger, M. (1978). *Transcultural nursing: Concepts, theories, and practices.* New York: John Wiley.

This book provides a comprehensive view of transcultural nursing to help nurses incorporate cultural concepts, theories, and research findings into their nursing practice. The book includes historical aspects, theories, and research development, transcultural nursing articles by nurse anthropologists, philosophical beliefs, and processes. Transcultural nursing and health care systems models are included as well as conceptual models to determine ways in which to weave cultural concepts into nursing.

Lewin, K. (1936). *Principles of topological psychology.* New York: McGraw-Hill.

Lewin's work is dedicated to the study of the person in the whole circumstance in which that person is placed. It explores how scientific psychology must take into account whole situations when working with clients. He believes that the environment of the individual serves to facilitate or inhibit a person's tendencies.

Monteleone, J. A. (1994). *Recognition of child abuse for the mandated reporter.* St. Louis, MO: C. V. Mosby.

This book is recommended for nurses, teachers, social workers, day care workers, and others who work with children. It contains information on recognizing abuse, including psychological, social, and physical abuse of children. There are identifying factors for concerned health care professionals who have reason to suspect abuse. It includes information on how to use the legal and social systems to protect children from abuse situations.

Pender, N. J. (1996). *Healthy promotion in nursing practice* (3rd ed.). Stamford, CT: Appleton & Lange.

This book offers an in-depth discussion of the nurse's role in prevention of disease through the promotion of healthy life styles. It provides an overview of major theoretical frameworks currently used in health promotion research and practice. It presents the utilization of nursing diagnosis and intervention classification systems, and it provides a framework for client assessment and health planning.

Ritchie, K. (1995). *Marketing to generation X.* New York: Lexington Books.

This book paints a picture of the population known as generation X. Aimed at advertisers, it compares generation X with the "baby boom" generation. It explores the roles of generation X, identifies family structure, and explores the development of members of generation X.

Shellenbarger, S. (1996). Caregiver duties make generation Xers anything but slackers. (Many people caring for a family member at home are under thirty.) *The Wall Street Journal*, May 22, 1996.

This article contain information about the post-baby boom generation. It views the social aspects of the generation Xers as well as the role of caregivers.

Spector, R. E. (1996). *Cultural diversity in health and illness* (4th ed.). Stamford, CT: Appleton & Lange.

This book discusses the dimensions involved in caring for people from diverse cultural backgrounds. It explores traditional and alternative health care beliefs and practices in a variety of ethnic perspectives. It shows how cultural heritage can affect health care delivery, and it articulates the need for sensitivity to clients' needs based upon culture and beliefs.

U.S. Department of Health and Human Services. (1992). *Healthy people 2000, National health promotion and disease prevention objectives.* Boston: Jones and Bartlett.

This text is a summary of a document that contains national strategies for improving the health of the nation over the coming decade. It addresses issues of prevention of major chronic illnesses, injuries, and infectious diseases. This work has been based upon the testimony of thousands of health care professionals from many different disciplines with an aim at producing measurable targets to be achieved by the year 2000.

U.S. Department of Health and Human Services. (1995). *Healthy people 2000: Midcourse review and 1995 revisions.* Boston: Jones and Bartlett.

This book is a report and mid-decade review of Healthy People 2000. It is a partnership among all levels of government and the private sector, attempting to make a positive difference in people's health. It a report in progress. It includes statistics related to physical activity and fitness, nutrition, tobacco, substance abuse, family planning, mental health, violent behavior, educational programs, occupational safety, oral health, cancer, maternal and infant health, sexually transmitted diseases, HIV, immunization, and prevention strategies.

Wadsworth, B. J. (1989). *Piaget's theory of cognitive and affective development* (4th ed.). New York: Longman.

This is an introduction to Piaget's theory of how children construct and acquire knowledge. There is an explanation of the central concepts in Piaget's theory of cognitive behavior, including the components of intelligence and the stages of cognitive and affective development.

Wywialowski, E. (1993). *Managing client care.* St. Louis, MO: C. V. Mosby.

This textbook addresses the management concepts and skills needed by entry level staff nurses and is primarily concerned with issues of nurse management and leadership. It is a book devoted to professional development issues.

☵
ℰTHICAL ISSUES

The community health nurse faces innumerable moral decisions and ethical dilemmas each day. Like other health care workers, community health nurses operate within a unique framework of ethical and moral decision-making. According to Davis and Aroskar, "health care ethics address four interrelated areas: (1) clinical; (2) allocation of scarce resources; (3) human experimentation; and (4) health policy" (Davis & Aroskar, 1983, p. 4). However, it may be argued that moral considerations related to health care and health sciences do not differ from other everyday moral considerations. Some believe that they both work with the same moral principles and use ethical reasoning in the decision-making process (Davis & Aroskar, 1983). Ethical and moral decisions are based on a standard of behavior developed within a culture or society (Ferrel & Gardiner, 1991).

ℰTHICS: WHAT IS IT?

The definition of ethics is complex. Although ethics are intensely personal, they are also a reflection of the society in which one lives (Mabie, 1993). Ethics are often referred to as a system of moral principles, or the rules or guidelines of a particular group, culture, or society. It is the branch of philosophy that deals with values and moral principles related to human conduct (Finn & Marshall, 1990). Whether or not one's actions are considered right or wrong or good or bad is often determined by the culture of a society. This was identified by Kurt Lewin as environmental press.

"An ethical act is one that leads to the greatest benefit for the most people (*utilitarianism*), or one that does not infringe on the basic inalienable human rights—such as life, freedom of speech, privacy, and due process—recognized by our society (*ethical formalism*). Second, an ethical act is one that increases the self-esteem and mental health of the person engaging in that act, particularly in the long run, but it may also expose the person to a great deal of short-term stress" (Ferrell & Gardiner, 1991, p. 3).

Environmental press refers to the pressure brought upon by a culture or society, which produces specific behaviors. Environmental pressures will facilitate or inhibit the person to behave in certain ways (Lewin, 1936). A person's behavior, according to Lewin's theory, is a function of the relationship between the person and the environment (Ijeoma, 1988). This is illustrated by the following example.

Since the late 1980s, as a result of economics and improved technology, providers of health care services in the United States have begun to debate the issue of rationing health care for severely disabled and elderly persons (Binstock & Post, 1991). Up until this time, it had been clearly the goal of health care providers to dispense equal care to all. Recently, however, cost factors and issues of quality of life related to health care have created fundamental questions about the aims and goals of health care (Binstock & Post, 1991). Despite this dialogue concerning cost containment, presently basic values of health care remain the same (Binstock & Post, 1991). However, it is an important matter, and with changes occurring in how health care is provided, it is an issue that must be deliberated.

Code of Ethics

Many professional groups have a code of ethics or principles that serve to act as a beacon for the way in which the profession is conducted. A *code of ethics* comprises the rules by which a profession is guided. The American Nurses Association (ANA) has its own code of ethics, which expresses the duties, values, and ethical responsibilities of the professional nurse. Nurses accept a moral and legal obligation to abide by this code (Table 4-1).

Autonomy   The term *autonomy* means independence or self-determination (Thompson, 1985). Autonomy is the right of individuals and society to decide for themselves how to mandate their own lives. The notion of autonomy implies respect for each person as unique and maintains each person's right to determine his or her own destiny (Mabie, 1993). Autonomy is an important part of American bioethics and means that adults have the right to make their own health care decisions (Powderly, 1996). When the community determines how persons should choose, even if the choice of the client is considered "bad" by society, the society is imposing its decisions on the rights of an individual. Although this imposition may seem to be in conflict with human rights, a society imposes its decisions when it believes that the decisions are for the betterment and safety of the larger community or in the best interest of the individual. Examples of this are mandated laws related to the use of seat belts and the deterrence of smoking in public places. These issues of prevention and safety are controversial; on the one hand, they seem to be aimed at increasing wellness, but on the other, they create are an ethical dilemma as they interfere with the autonomy of the individual. Autonomy means that people have the right to make their own health care decisions good or bad without interference from the society in which they live (Powderly, 1996)

◍

TABLE 4-1

CODE OF ETHICS OF THE AMERICAN NURSES ASSOCIATION

---

1. The nurse provides service with respect for human dignity and the uniqueness of the client unrestricted by consideration of social or economic status, personal attributes, or the nature of health problems.
2. The nurse safeguards the client's right to privacy by judiciously protecting information of a confidential nature.
3. The nurse acts to safeguard the client and the public when health care and safety are affected by the incompetent, unethical, or illegal practice of any persons.
4. The nurse assumes responsibility and accountability for individual nursing judgments and actions.
5. The nurse maintains competence in nursing.
6. The nurse exercises informed judgment and uses individual competence and qualifications as criteria in seeking consultation, accepting responsibilities, and delegating nursing activities to others.
7. The nurse participates in activities that contribute to the ongoing development of the profession's body of knowledge.
8. The nurse participates in the profession's efforts to implement and improve standards of nursing.
9. The nurse participates in the profession's efforts to establish and maintain conditions of employment conducive to high quality nursing care.
10. The nurse participates in the profession's effort to protect the pubic from misinformation and misrepresentation and to maintain the integrity of nursing.
11. The nurse collaborates with members of the health professions and other citizens in promoting community and national efforts to meet the health needs of the public

---

NOTE: Reprinted with permission. From the American Nurses Association.

Furthermore, the degree of participation and a striving toward autonomy by the individual or the community as a whole often indicate how well the community or an individual has succeeded in self-care or wellness. The degree of autonomy often predicts the degree of success toward a health goal. The extent to which individuals have control over their own lives affects their well-being (Robertson & Minkler, 1994). Therefore, empowering clients to take charge of health care decisions is a primary health promotion strategy.

CASE STUDY: CLIENT EMPOWERMENT

Mrs. King has had advanced multiple sclerosis (MS) and systemic lupus erythematosus (SLE) for 24 years. Although she had lost her

A DNR is a medical order to abstain from cardiopulmonary resuscitation (CPR) if a client's heart stops beating.

physical capabilities, her mind was sharp, and she was concerned with her loss of autonomy as her body deteriorated. At age 72, she wanted to die. She had been wheelchair-bound for more than 10 years. She needed the use of a Hoyer lift to get in and out of her wheelchair or bed, and the quality of her life had significantly deteriorated over the years. Over the last 15 years, she had been in and out of hospitals as a result of a multitude of medical crisis situations. This time she had been sent home from the intensive care unit (ICU) on a respirator. The ICU nurses were unable to wean her from the respirator in the hospital. She told her family and the discharge nurse that this was more than she could handle and did not want to use the respirator at home. She wanted to be taken off the respirator with full knowledge that this could end her life. She furthermore wanted a Do Not Resuscitate (**DNR**) order at home. Her physician refused to do this, as he believed Mrs. King was unable to make this decision on her own behalf. Although this was a difficult decision, Mrs. King's daughter, aware of her mother's feelings, felt that her mother must maintain her autonomy; thus, she consulted the community health nurse caring for Mrs. King and requested that her mother be seen by a psychiatrist to determine if in fact she was in sound mind to determine her own future concerning the DNR order. The community health nurse arranged a home visit by a psychiatrist. The psychiatrist determined that Mrs. King was in fact in sound mind and capable of acquiring a DNR order. The respirator was subsequently disconnected, and Mrs. King was able to breath on her own without the use of the respirator. It was believed by her daughter that taking charge of this part of her life gave her the will and ability to continue with her life at home. Mrs. King extended her DNR order to a Living Will/Health Care Proxy (pp. 66 and 67) to provide her with the autonomy she desired.

The right to receive or refuse treatment is a major ethical issue. The growth in the care of clients with long-term care needs or hospice care needs at home (either by family members or home health attendants) raises ethical questions of a different nature. In caring for a client at home, the principle of autonomy related to medical issues remains clear; however, unlike institutional settings, issues related to client care issues at home are complex (Dubler & Nimmons, 1992). Outside of the institution, there are other persons whose rights and interests are affected by the choices made by the client, and these must be included in how decisions are made. In these situations, autonomy may give way to accommodation (Dubler & Nimmons, 1992). Accommodations are made to include the needs of the family. If the main caregiver is unable to provide all the care necessary and desired by the client, the community health nurse helps the family adjust and accommodate to meet the needs of all parties concerned. The following situation is an example of accommodation.

CASE STUDY: FAMILY ACCOMMODATIONS

Mr. Peterson, an 89-year-old man, lives alone. He is visited by a community health nurse to monitor his physical condition. He has a history of Parkinson's disease but has been able to care for himself until the past 6 months when he needed assistance with shopping for groceries and to care for his home. Until recently, his 65-year-old daughter who has a full-time job drives 30 min to her father's house every other day to care for his shopping and other household needs. However, she has been diagnosed recently with breast cancer and needs to undergo chemotherapy; she is now unable to care for her father. Mr. Peterson refuses to live with another child who lives in a nearby state. The community health nurse intervenes and through accommodation helps this family face this dilemma. Mr. Peterson will stay at home with the assistance of a home attendant. His two children will call each week for socialization and support. His son will visit monthly as will his daughter as soon as she is able. His children will remain primarily responsible for his care, allowing Mr. Peterson his independence and personal freedom.

Beneficence Beneficence is a health care principle that mandates that the health care provider "does good for the client." This becomes a complicated issue when the health care provider also attempts to do that which the client wishes. If there is conflict between what is considered good by the profession and what the client wants, the nurse must abide by the client's wishes as long as it is within the professional scope of practice.

Nurses have the responsibility to inform and teach clients about their health care needs but should not attempt to impose their own or society's wishes upon the individual. For many religious groups, as a result of their beliefs and restrictions, this is an important issue. Hospitals in affiliation with such populations are developing outpatient as well as in-hospital settings to meet the needs of specific groups; for example, bloodless clinics have been established to care for Jehovah's Witnesses so that they may receive health care in a setting that is appropriate and supportive of their religious beliefs. Bloodless medical and surgical programs provide options for other individuals who do not wish to have a blood transfusion because of religious beliefs, personal choice, or other medical restrictions such as allergies, fever, or the fear of infection.

Confidentiality An important component of all health care professions, especially nursing within a community, is confidentiality. An obligation to uphold a client's privacy and maintain certain information in confidence has long been part of the nurses' code of ethics (Benjamin, 1991). Health information that an individual considers private must be kept confidential. The issue of privacy envelops the values of individual autonomy (Privacy and Technology Project of the Electronic Frontier Foundation, 1996).

Privacy provides the right of the individual to be left alone and free from unwanted publicity (Loeb, 1993). Confidentiality is merely the tool for privacy protection (Privacy and Technology Project of the Electronic Frontier Foundation, 1996).

In health care, the meaning of confidentiality goes beyond keeping information imparted to the health care provider secret. It goes to the core of the relationship between the client and the community nurse. It is an obligation of the nurse to preserve the confidentiality of the client (Benjamin, 1992). The code of ethics for nurses developed by the ANA embodies the concept of a client's right of privacy (see Table 4-1) so that the nurse has an obligation to protect the client's privacy and confidentiality. Without some protection, the client may not be completely honest with the nurse, which might inhibit other aspects of the client's care, as well as the well-being of the community.

In rare situations, there may be critical circumstances in which the nurse must break this confidentiality such as in a situation in which the failure to disclose information could cause serious harm to the client, the family, or others; in this case, disclosure may be legally binding upon the health care provider in some states (Loeb, 1992). For example, if a mentally ill client threatens the life of another, or if a client with acquired immunodeficiency syndrome (AIDS) confides that he or she is knowingly spreading the disease by unprotected sexual activity, the nurse would be required to break confidence with the client. In some states, health care providers have a "duty to warn," and in other states, disclosure of information remains prohibited by law (Benjamin, 1992).

Justice The most common perspectives of justice are distributive, egalitarian, and utilitarian. An important notion of utilitarian justice is that benefits should be first given to those who need them the most; thus, if there is a choice or a decision related to the provision of care, the best or most efficient choice would be made. An example of utilitarian justice is in a situation such as an accident in which there are limited resources and one victim can be saved and another cannot; care would be provided to the victim with the best chance of survival.

The concept of justice in providing care to a community is based on the notion that people are treated fairly and equally. The basis of this concept of justice is egalitarian justice. The notion of egalitarian justice or equal justice is that each person has access to the health services they need equally. The idea of fair and equal treatment is dependent, however, on issues that may be difficult to determine or may even be unmeasurable. Equal access to care may be dependent on many factors; for example, where one lives (i.e., an urban or rural location) may influence the actual delivery or access availability of services to a client or a community, thereby influencing the equity of care. Then the community health nurse may actually treat some clients unequally due to issues of equal access or availability.

Economics certainly has an effect on how health care is provided for a population or an individual client. If communities or nations have limited economic resources, the health care they provide, although equal among their members, may be less than services provided to other communities or nations. Although nurses are to provide care as needed to all clients regardless of financial status, there may be inequities based on financial realities.

In a health care system that uses distributive justice, health care services are distributed in the fairest way possible to all according to need (Davis, 1983). Although the principle of justice is the promotion of equity, using equity alone to measure justice is not sufficient. The needs of the community or an individual and availability of resources must be established to determine a just distribution of care.

ℰTHICAL ISSUES IN THE COMMUNITY

The need to explore ethical issues in relationship to community health is not new but has gained importance recently. The health care system in the United States is undergoing an enormous transformation due in part to factors such as the high cost of health care, improved technology, increased awareness by a concerned and informed population, and a large aging population. The influence of the insurance industry on how the health care system is used exemplifies the impact of business upon health care services, particularly home health care. The emergence of managed care reflects the sway of these changes (Fig. 4-1).

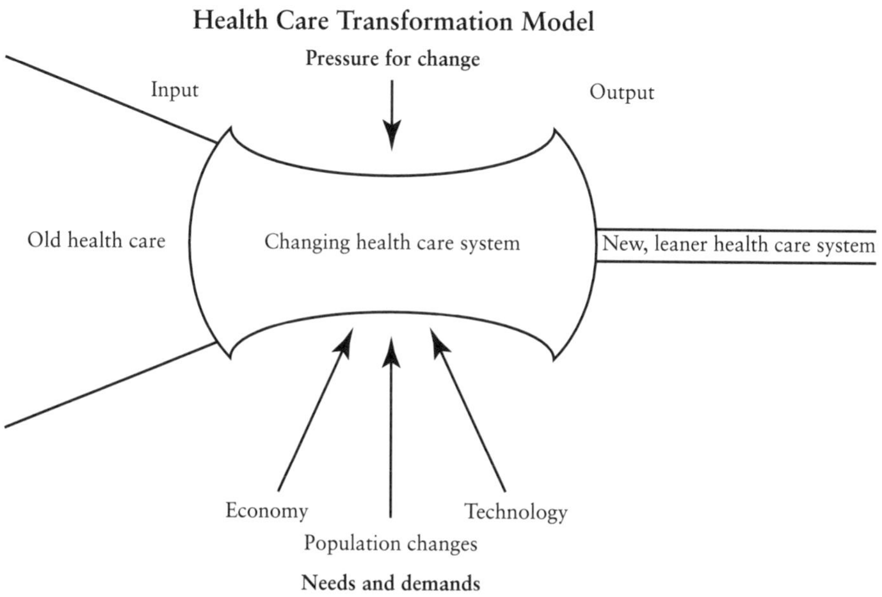

Health Care Transformation Model

FIGURE 4-1

◙

The Health Care Transformation Model represents pressure for change on a health care system caused by economics, population changes and shifts, or technological advances. The pressure for change creates a new health care system.

Changes in Health Insurance

Shortly after World War II, health insurance began to play a part in the culture of health care. The impact of health insurance has grown dramatically, particularly in the past decade.

Prior to the availability of health insurance, patients paid physicians directly for health care, a direct fee for service. The impact of a third-party payment system (health insurance) is significant as to how a client receives health care services and, thus, influences every aspect of health care. Third-party payment refers to how the health care provider is paid by the insurance companies for services rendered. The fees for care are paid by the insurance provider. Until recently, this meant the client would seek out the services of a physician and the insurer would pay a percentage of the cost of the service. The insurance company had guidelines as to what would or would not be covered by its policy and the amount it would pay for a specific service. The client and the physician had the most control over the selection of service. The physician could then order almost unlimited laboratory work, and the client could select any physician. This meant direct access to specialists without prior consultation with a family doctor. This grew to be very costly in terms of dollars and provided fragmented and, at times, expensive or unnecessary care for the client.

The high cost of health care and population age shifts to an older population, have created demands and pressure upon the health care system to change from the existing insurance system to a managed care system, with an emphasis on prevention, health promotion, and wellness (de Tornyay, 1992). As the system continues to change, health care, particularly care of the client at home and in the community, is significantly influenced by these changes in the insurance system. Payment by private insurers and government health insurance (i.e., Medicare and Medicaid) for health care services encourage and support as cost-effective health care services at home and in the community.

Advance Directives

Rapid advancements made in health care technology in addition to this changing economic climate has had an enormous influence on the home care system. Formerly limited to hospitals, highly technological care, requiring intravenous therapy or respirators, is now provided to clients at home. Some clients may be sent home on respirators or with intravenous lines with little or no support systems in place other than home care visits by the community health nurse; however, these visits are also limited by insurance coverage. Thus, advance directives, such as DNR orders and the Health Care Proxy, which are standard in hospitals, are now available to clients at home. Other advance directives include a Living Will or Durable Powers of Attorney for Health Care (Powderly, 1996). Advance directives are documents of empowerment, which extend the autonomy of clients beyond the point at which they lose their capacity to choose their own care (Powderly, 1996). Because this has become an issue of concern in the care of clients in the community, nurses must provide information to clients about advance directives that are available at home.

The Living Will and Health Care Proxy appoint a surrogate decision-maker to act on the client's behalf. DNR orders are only related to resuscitation. At home DNR orders tell emergency staff or attending personnel not to transfer the client to a hospital for cardiopulmonary resuscitation (CPR). Signing a Health Care Proxy allows clients to appoint someone they trust to make decisions about care in case they lose their ability to make decisions. Clients select someone they know as their health care agent; they can give that individual as little or as much authority as desired about health care or heath care treatments. As this is a legal document, clients need to discuss carefully with the health agent what they would or would not want the agent to do if a decision had to be made. This could include not providing CPR, artificial nutrition, hydration, transplant, and so on. The community health nurse provides information to a community about the availability of the Health Care Proxy to clients in the hospital as well as to individual clients at home (Fig. 4-2).

The ability to choose an assisted, at-home death is still a controversial issue and remains an ethical dilemma. It is presently being tested in the courts.

Cost vs. Care

Changes and shifts in the population further affect the health care system. An increase in the aging population and limited resources to meet the need for expanding services at home are an increasing burden for the community health care provider. Utilizing limited funds to provide programs to promote wellness by providing health care services and information has placed an economic strain on the health care system.

The high cost of health care has caused deep financial cuts, causing diminished health care services. Allocation of limited services to the community and individuals at home places a strain on the community health nurse. Ethical dilemmas concerning community health issues have grown as the general needs of society have changed and transformed how health care needs are met.

Like dominoes in a row, the effects on one component of health care affects another; for example, shorter hospital stays make increased home care necessary, which has had a major effect on home health care services. People are discharged from hospitals earlier than ever before following childbirth, surgery, and other medical treatment. Early discharge limits the time for predischarge health care education and may restrict the development of a thorough discharge assessment and plan for many clients.

Social concerns of a society may help to create a basis for meeting community needs. Health concerns of a society are often reflected in the development and implementation of health education programs. Examples of this are health promotion and educational programs within a community to provide addicts with clean needles and to instruct members about the use of condoms to prevent the spread of human immunodeficiency virus (HIV) or AIDS.

Health care concerns involving substance abuse, spousal abuse, child abuse, and AIDS are situations frequently approached by the community health nurse. With the economic burden related to the care of these clients, there has been a movement toward prevention and health education rather than a strictly curative approach. However, programs addressing prevention are at risk due to changes in the economy, and it is unknown how these programs will fare as economic resources diminish. It is unclear whether communities will continue to insist on economic support of preventable health problems as compared to those that cannot be prevented (e.g., MS). This is an example of an ethical dilemma based upon limited funds, which potentially affects the whole community.

Technological advances in health care and innovative research in recent years have increased longevity, but economic constraints make it difficult to provide safe environments for many aging or debilitated clients at home. Care of the client at home, using sophisticated equipment such as a respirator, is often offered with limited support to the family or the client. The burden of care sometimes is too great for families, and it is the family and the community health nurse who must deal with these dilemmas, often facing closed doors for the financial support from an overburdened insurance structure. Self-help or voluntary help programs are sometimes available to add support. Volunteer hospice workers who become friendly visitors to the dying and hospice professionals provide care at minimal cost; support groups for caregivers and respite programs are examples of

FIGURE 4-2

▧

A. Pocket-size Health Care Proxy. *B.* Advance Directive/ Health Care Proxy.

A

HEALTH CARE PROXY

I, _____ of

STREET   CITY   STATE

DAYTIME PHONE   EVENING PHONE

hereby appoint _____ of

STREET   CITY   STATE

DAYTIME PHONE   EVENING PHONE

as my health care agent to make all health care decisions for me if I become unable to decide for myself, including decisions about artificial nutrition and hydration.

SIGNATURE (PROXY INITIATOR)   DATE

This proxy was signed in my presence. The signer is known to me and appears to be of sound mind and to act of his/her own free will.

WITNESS   DATE

WITNESS   DATE

B THE ADVANCE DIRECTIVE / HEALTH CARE PROXY

(1) I, _____
    (please print your first, middle and last name)

hereby appoint _____
    (please print your proxy's first, middle and last name)

of _____
    (please print your proxy's home address and telephone number)
as my health care agent to make any and all health care decisions for me, except to the extent that I state otherwise. This proxy shall take effect when and if I become unable to make my own health care decisions.

(2) Optional instructions: I direct my proxy to make health care decisions in accord with my wishes and limitations as stated below, or as he or she otherwise knows. (Attach additional pages if necessary.)

_____

_____

Unless you state your wishes about artificial nutrition and hydration [feeding tubes], your agent will not be allowed to make decisions about artificial nutrition and hydration. See instructions on the back for samples of language you could use.

(3) Name of substitute or fill-in proxy if the person I appoint above is unable, unwilling or unavailable to act as my health care agent.

_____
    (please print your substitute proxy's first, middle and last name)

_____
    (please print your substitute proxy's home address and telephone number)

(4) Unless I revoke it, this proxy shall remain in effect indefinitely, or until the date or condition stated below. This proxy shall expire (specific date or conditions, if desired):

_____

_____

(5) Signature _____ Address _____ Date _____

(6) Statement by Witnesses (the person who is appointed agent or alternate agent cannot sign as witness, and must be 18 or older) *I declare that the person who signed this document is personally known to me and appears to be of sound mind and acting of his or her own free will. He or she signed (or asked another to sign for him or her) this document in my presence.*

Witness 1 _____ Address _____

Witness 2 _____ Address _____

communities negotiating these situations together in a positive manner. These services do not replace services lost to clients but indicate positive ways in which a community can begin to address its own health care needs (see Appendix I).

Many self-help groups exist for individuals with serious diseases such as Parkinson's disease, MS, SLE, and many others. Most local libraries have information about finding local self-help groups in the community. The *Source Book* provides a listing of self-help groups as well as social and health services in the greater New York City area.

Society may decide to withhold care from an elderly client because the cost to society is too great. Ceilings on surgical procedures exist in many communities simply because the economic burden upon the community is too great; thus, clients above a certain age may not be entitled to certain medical procedures. Financial issues are presently a concern, as the guidelines for health care are based on cost factors, which are changing how health care is provided. The alternative to limited health care based on economics is a society that provides care in spite of cost or because there are no limits; in this instance, a surgeon could collect insurance regardless of whether or not there was a legitimate basis for surgical intervention. For example, if a 90-year-old woman with end-stage Alzheimer's disease has a hysterectomy for fibroids, the surgeon is paid by the insurer despite the ludicrousness of the procedure for the client. Clients can be exploited when the benefit of treatment is not clear.

Financial issues are presently a concern in the United States, as the guidelines for health care are based on cost factors and are changing how health care is provided to clients. This has become a dilemma for the community health nurse manager who often must decide which community or person receives the limited health care services.

Community Participation

Sherry Arnstein, a social planner in the late 1960s, developed a method of measuring community participation. Arnstein called this the *ladder of participation*, which measures the participation of a community in eight steps, ranging from from nonparticipation to citizen control (Robertson & Minkler, 1994). The first step is manipulation, and the second step is therapy, both of which are considered areas of nonparticipation by a community. At these first two steps, the community health nurse can educate the community or client or provide services to the community. Steps three, four, and five are considered degrees of tokenism by the community. Step three is the informing step, step four is consultation, and step five is identified as placation. During this phase, clients may heed information and attempt to have a voice, but they are not considered in the community health care planning. The community health nurse must include clients during the planning stages of programs and provide for client input during this phase. Steps six, seven, and eight of the ladder are considered various stages of empowerment. Step six is partnership, stage seven is delegation of power, and stage eight is citizen control. During these stages, citizens engage in a partnership with health care providers, but it is not until stage eight when communities fully participate in an equal partnership with health professionals that clients take charge of their own health and that community members make a commitment to carry out a health care plan. The ladder of participation illustrates how a community embraces an issue (e.g., a health care issue) and takes charge of its own health decisions and improves its own health promotion activities.

The community health nurse has an important role in providing information by educating the community. How the members of a community decide to implement or participate in the community's health is impacted upon by a variety of issues.

Legal Issues

Providing health care to the community presents legal issues that concern the community nurse. All health care workers are responsible for practicing within a framework of laws. These laws reflect the mandates of local, state, and federal legislation. There are three types of laws under which community health nurses practice: constitutional law, legislative law, and common law. These are the legal guidelines that shape how community health workers practice. Private and community health care agencies under which nurses provide service are also bound by these laws. Therefore, nurses have legal standards, in addition to ethical standards, under which they practice.

The community nurse must know and follow closely the state laws and the Nurse Practice Act, which designates the scope of practice under which the nurse operates. The community health nurse may be a generalist, a clinical nurse specialist, a midwife, an occupational health nurse, a school nurse, or a nurse practitioner. It is important that the nurse operate in the appropriate scope of practice, according to the role designated by each state. This means the community nurse must know the legal limits of nursing practice within the community being served. Furthermore, scope of practice differentiates between the nurse's role in the care of the client and that of other health care professionals.

$\mathcal{E}$THICS, VALUES AND MORAL REASONING AS RELATED TO HEALTH CARE

Today, the community health nurse, as part of the health care team, must often deal with situations unlike those dealt with in the past. As technology has developed and enhanced our lives, it also brings with it many moral dilemmas. Community health care nurses must be concerned with a growing responsibility to confront these ethical and moral decisions in today's complex society.

Moral Reasoning

Moral attitudes and behaviors are developed through a combination of many factors. The environment in which one is raised, the family, the culture, or society all hold an important place in the development of one's morals.

Kohlberg's work suggests that moral development goes through stages of development that are characterized by different ways of understanding right or wrong. He believes that individuals pass through stages in an orderly fashion from a lower stage of moral development to a higher stage (Becker, 1982). He believes that all individuals in all cultures go through these stages in varying degrees. Kohlberg also claims that each successive stage is at a morally and cognitively higher level than the previous stage. Furthermore, his work indicates that at each higher stage of moral development, individuals are able to deal with issues of moral and ethical problems of greater complexity. The choices one makes then are dependent on one's moral and ethical development.

Gilligan's work on moral development elicits differences in the moral understandings between men and women (Becker, 1982). She believes that men and women interpret moral problems from distinct orientations. Gilligan believes that men's moral development is based on the ethic of rights and justice, and women's moral development is based on the ethic of care and responsibility. These theories are useful to the community health nurse in working with aggregate populations or individuals to create a positive and informed environment in which to help the client make health care decisions.

Moral Reasoning and Health Care

According to Emile Durkheim, to act morally is to act in such a way as to further the collective interest of society (Becker, 1982). Health care until recently claimed to be grounded in this theory. However, as our health care system previously functioned in a curative domain, there was little interest in prevention, and, therefore, there is a question if this was truly in the collective interest of society. The notion of collective interest may not have changed, but how we provide care to the society has been challenged.

Individual Good vs. Societal Good

There are times when the community health nurse in working with communities must consider the needs of an individual or an aggregate over the needs of the community. Health needs of one member or an aggregate population of a community may vary in terms of time, cultural differences, physical needs, technological levels, and economics from the community as a whole. At times, this may indicate a need for an individual approach to meeting some immediate or long-term goals. Accommodating the needs of individuals may cause an economic burden to the larger community, which may benefit only a few. Examples of this would be a community that provides sidewalk cuts to meet the demands of wheelchair users and a community that provides kneeling buses to meet the needs of persons who are otherwise unable to access public transportation.

Also, what may be good for society may be at the cost of endangering an individual. An example is the use of human subjects in research. Because many community health nurses are nurse researchers, they must be cognizant of the risks involved with human subjects in the research process. Ideally, by informing the client of the risks, there is a collaboration between the researcher and the subject. At the core of the research process is the informed consent procedure, which attempts to balance the risks to human subjects against the possible benefits to society (Davis & Aroskar, 1983). Community health nurses involved in research, as with any researcher working with human subjects, need to obtain informed consent from clients. Research involving human subjects should not be carried out unless the importance of the research is in proportion to the risk to the subject (Davis & Aroskar, 1983). It is a most important moral principle of informed consent that the client understand the terms and risks involved when agreeing to be involved in research.

Quality of Life vs. Quantity of Life

Issues such as equity in allocation of resources to individuals or society, the client's right to choose their quality of life, euthanasia for home-bound clients, or decisions on how one should live with an illness or potential illness are examples of ethical dilemmas regarding quality of life vs. quantity of life with which community health nurses are concerned. Choices regarding the rights of the client to the quality of life they desire vs. greater longevity is often driven by economics related to the health care system. Clients with large economic resources or with celebrity often stand a better chance of being a recipient of improved services. This has recently been a concern, particularly in situations related to organ transplantation.

A burden falls upon the resources of society when a client's behavior contributes to an illness or injury. Treating the client who drives without a seat belt and is injured is an economic burden to society. This is so even if the client can afford to pay for his medical expenses or has health insurance to pay for care. The actual care provided to one client requires time and energy to support that care despite the cost, and the time it takes to provide care reduces the time taken with another client. Is it not the responsibility of citizens to comply with laws to decrease this burden? Does this interfere with a person's rights?

The obese client who chooses not to lose weight may be in danger of ill health because of the choice not to lose weight. Obese clients are at higher risk for hypertension, adult onset diabetes, and heart disease. The need for treatment of health problems, which are directly or indirectly caused by the client's decisions, places an economic burden on the health care system. Being able to pay for care does not burden the system less. However, the wealthy obese person or the wealthy smoker or alcoholic has a better chance of receiving care or services than the person with fewer economic resources.

What about the issue of a client's right to self-determination? This is an ethical dilemma for the health care system. If clients choose not to follow the community health care provider's suggestions for care, are the clients noncompliant or using their own judgment or values to make independent decisions? Individuals have the right to make their own decisions. Clients may choose not to follow the suggestions or plan of the health care provider. Clients have a right to choose their own care and decide most issues related to their health as long as it does no harm to others. This does not include areas covered by laws, such as helmet laws for cyclists, wearing seat belts, or child safety seats in automobiles.

Personal and Social Responsibility

An individual's right to liberty is protected by the Constitution and can be impacted upon by disclosure by a health professional. In a situation where the client with an active case of tuberculosis refuses treatment yet continues living in close proximity to young children confronts the nurse with ethical, safety, as well as legal dilemmas. The nurse must choose between issues related to confidentiality and safety issues. This requires choosing the safety of one client over the confidentiality of another. The nurse faces an ethical dilemma when concerned with client confidentiality and an obligation to obey laws directed by society. This situation then imposes on the nurse to obey a law by reporting the situation to the health department and breaking confidentiality with the client to whom she is committed by the code of the profession.

Ethical Decisions of the Community Health Nurse

Using the ethical decision-making process, the nurse assists the client in developing a plan of care. A comparison of the nursing process and the ethical decision-making process is perhaps illustrative (Table 4-2). With the nursing process, nurses assess a client's needs, including both objective and subjective information; for example, an assessment could include blood work, a questionnaire, or verbal responses. Like the nursing process, in the ethical decision-making process nurses also initially gather relevant objective and subjective information. In the nursing process, nurses develop a nursing diagnosis, based on the North Atlantic Nursing Diagnosis

⌘

TABLE 4-2
COMPARISON OF THE NURSING PROCESS AND THE ETHICAL
DECISION-MAKING PROCESS

NURSING PROCESS	ETHICAL DECISION-MAKING PROCESS
1. Assessment	1. Assessment—gathering of relevant information
2. Diagnosis and analysis	2. Clarification of ethical component and social and legal implications
3. Plan	3. Identifying possible outcomes
4. Implementation	4. Implementation
5. Evaluation	5. Evaluation

Association (NANDA) guidelines. Use of the NANDA model in developing a community diagnosis is still fairly new. In the ethical decision-making process, nurses define the ethical, social, and legal implications with the client or the client's advocate. In the nursing process, nurses develop a plan of action based on the nursing diagnosis, and in ethical decision-making, nurses explore possible outcomes of a variety of decisions upon which a plan of action would be developed. Then in both the nursing process and the ethical decision-making process, the plan would be implemented and evaluated.

SUMMARY

The definition of ethics is complex. It is generally referred to as a system of moral principles that guide a society. As a society goes through changes, such as population changes or economic changes, the ethical framework of a society influences how we approach change. The health care system in the United States is in great flux, and how we approach that is guided by ethics already embedded within the system. This chapter explores our ethical values, discusses moral reasoning, and how the community health nurse makes decisions based on a code of ethics.

KEY WORDS

Autonomy
Beneficence
Code of ethics

Confidentiality
Ethical decisions
Moral reasoning

QUESTIONS

DIRECTIONS: Choose the one *best* response to each of the following questions.

1. The term beneficence is used correctly in which of the following statements?
   A. The client has the right to have a Do Not Resuscitate (DNR) order
   B. The community health nurse's responsibility is to see that the client is well cared for
   C. The first responsibility of the health care professional is "to do no wrong"
   D. The goal of the health care provider is "to do good" for the client

2. Having the right to decide how to direct one's own health care is an example of
   A. justice
   B. beneficence
   C. autonomy
   D. confidentiality

3. Providing equal access to needed health care, regardless of one's economic status is an example of
   A. utilitarian justice
   B. egalitarian justice
   C. an unattainable ideal of an ethical society
   D. an example of distributive justice

4. Providing drug addicts with clean needles is an example of a community health program that
   A. is striving toward health promotion
   B. is illegal and immoral in most states
   C. has limited community goals
   D. reflects a health prevention program

5. Technology has created the largest impact on how society meets the needs of
   A. the homeless
   B. schoolchildren
   C. caregivers
   D. the elderly

ANSWERS

1. *The answer is D.* Beneficence is described as the goal of the health care provider to "to do good" for the client.

2. *The answer is C.* An example of autonomy is having the right to decide how to direct one's own health care.

3. *The answer is B.* An example of egalitarian justice is providing equal access to needed health care, regardless of one's economic status.

4. *The answer is A.* Providing drug addicts with clean needles is an example of a community health program that is striving toward health promotion.

5. *The answer is D.* Technology has created the largest impact in how society meets the needs of the elderly.

ANNOTATED REFERENCES

Bandman, E. L., & Bandman, B. (1990). *Nursing ethics through the life span.* Norwalk, CT: Appleton & Lange.

This book approaches moral and ethical problems of everyday nursing practice, which appear throughout the life span of clients. It provides, in addition to many clinical cases, strategies and a foundation for ethical decision-making.

Becker, L. C., & Becker, C. B. (1992). *Encyclopedia of ethics.* New York: Garland.

This is an encyclopedia that contains anthologies, monographs, and bibliographies, including reports of legal cases and data from scholarly periodicals pertaining to ethics.

Benjamin, M., & Curtis, J. (1992). *Ethics in nursing.* New York: Oxford University Press.

This book provides nurses and student nurses with an introduction to an analysis of ethical issues. The book includes the nature of moral dilemmas, provides an introduction to basic ethical principles, and discusses issues related to ethics and public policy.

Binstock, R. H., & Post, S. G. (1991). *Too old for health care? Controversies in medicine, law, economics, and ethics.* Baltimore: Johns Hopkins University Press.

This book explores the rationing of health care for older people. It looks at alternative approaches to the problems of health care containment. A range of topics from economics of care, medical technology, legal issues, and religious views of rationing are explored in this book.

Bernard, P., & Chapman, C. M. (1993). *Professional and ethical issues in nursing.* London, Scutari Press.

Based upon the changes of the professional code in the United Kingdom, this book examines the code and explores the concepts and problems that relate to it. The goal of this book is to enable nurses to develop greater autonomy.

Curtin, L., & Flaherty, J. M. (1982). *Nursing ethics theories and pragmatics.* Bowie, MD: Prentice-Hall.

This scholarly book provides a theoretical basis and a philosophical approach for critical analysis of ethical problems. It provides direction for the nurse to develop an approach to ethical dilemmas in practice.

Davis, A. J., & Aroskar, M. A. (1983). *Ethical dilemmas and nursing practice*. Norwalk, CT: Appleton & Lange.

This book presents ethical dilemmas confronting health professionals through the lens of the nursing profession. Its aim is to make nurses more aware of the ethical dilemmas in health sciences and nursing practice.

de Tornyay, R. (1992). Reconsidering nursing education: The report of the Pew Health Professions Commission. Journal of Nursing Education, 31(7), 296–301.

This article explores the report of the Pew Commission for the year 2005 and its effects on nursing. It develops strategies for nurses in meeting the health needs for the future.

Dubler, N., & Nimmons, D. (1992). *Ethics on call*. New York: Harmony Books.

This book deals with everyday life and death decisions. It explains how patients can maintain their own autonomy in the throes of working within a large medical complex.

Ferrell, O. C., & Gardiner, G. (1991). *In pursuit of ethics, tough choices in the world of work*. Springfield, IL: Smith Collins.

This book explores the ethical choices one faces in the work world. Issues that include dilemmas faced by nurses and colleagues are discussed. A definition of ethics is presented. It examines how personal choices are made and the ethical choices and conflicts one faces in making decisions. The choices one faces are explored in the American work culture. The authors compare ethical decisions made in the United States with those made in Japan.

Finn, J., & Eliot L. M. (1990). *Medical ethics*. New York: Chelsea House.

This book explores the economics of health care. It questions the cost of providing these services and describes the nature of this issue. It includes issues such as abortion, euthanasia, drug testing, organ transplants, and maintenance of terminally ill patients. The book stresses the complex and conflicting moral principles on which health-related laws are based.

Ijeoma, M. E. (1988). *Relationships between educating environments and institutional goals in the institutions of higher education*. Unpublished doctoral thesis, University of Michigan, Ann Arbor.

This is a research thesis submitted to the faulty of the Graduate School of the University of Michigan. It includes work associated with Kurt Lewin's environmental theories.

Lewin, K. (1936). *Principles of topological psychology*. New York: McGraw-Hill.

This book explores the issues related to the theories of how the environment influences behavior.

Mabie, M. C. J. (1993). *Bioethics and the new medical technology*. New York: Atheneum.

This book examines the principles with which the advancement of science and technology has impacted on the provision of health care. Issues of life extension of the elderly, the ability to help otherwise unsuccessful couples in areas of fertility, sustaining life of the severely handicapped or comatose patients, and quality of life issues are explored.

Powderly, K. E. (1996). *Ethical issues for hospital-based risk managers.* Unpublished paper for the Department of Humanities in Medicine, State University of New York, Brooklyn.

This paper presents legal and ethical information and issues for health care providers. It presents issues of autonomy, and it includes information about advanced directives, HIV, human research, and clinical situations.

Privacy and Technology Project of the Electronic Frontier Foundation. (1996). *Primer of privacy.* E-mail: http://chmis.nwlink.com/effprivphtml.

This is a journal available on the Internet. It is intended for use by Community Health Management Information Systems and deals with ethical issues related to privacy.

Robertson, A., & Minkler, M. (1994). New health promotion movement: A critical examination. *Health Education Quarterly*, 21(3), 295–312

This article looks at the movement toward health promotion. It deals with the influence of health education upon health promotion and empowerment. In this article, Minkler links the notion of empowerment and community participation upon the health of the community and the individual.

Thompson, J. E., & Thompson, H. O. (1985). *Bioethical decision-making for nurses.* Norwalk, CT: Appleton & Lange.

This book provides guidance for nurses and other health care professionals in making practical bioethical decisions. It includes a discussion of the theoretical base for bioethics and presents a model for decision-making. Actual cases are provided for the reader.

United Way of NYC. (1995). *The source book.* New York: Oryx Press.

This book is an up-to-date directory of health and human service agencies of nearly 200 agencies at 5400 sites.

Veatch, R. M. (1987). *The patient as partner, a theory of human experimentation ethics.* Bloomington, IN: Indiana University Press.

This book explores the influence of the increasing sophistication of medical technology and the expanded perception of equal rights upon the research community, which the author calls a "revolution in medical ethics." This book presents a systematic approach to the risks faced by researchers and subjects in today's world. The author explores federal regulations, problems of research design and subject recruitment, ethical realities to experimentation, and other controversies.

APPENDIX I: SELF-HELP GROUPS

Self-Help Center
405 S. State Street
Champlain, IL 61820
217-352-0009
  This center has a listing of over 200 self-help groups.

Guided Tour to Self-Help on the Internet
http://odphp.osophs.dhhs.gov/eomfrnce/partnr96/ferg.htm
  Self-help groups available via the Internet are listed here.

Alanon/Alateen
1600 Corporate Landing Parkway
Virginia Beach, VA 23454
800-356-9996 (available 24 hours)
  This service is available for family and friends of alcoholics.

National Cancer Information Center
800-4-cancer

American Cancer Society
800-ACS-2345

Cancer Y-ME
800-221-2141
  These cancer organizations have access to many self-help groups. Cancer Y-ME has a list of over 200 self-help groups in the United States.

Share
19 West 44th Street
New York, NY 10036
212-719-0364
  This organization provides services for women with breast or ovarian cancers.

ALLIANCE FOR HEALTH: A MODEL FOR COMMUNITY HEALTH ASSESSMENT

Community health assessment is an ongoing process. Community health nurses and other health care providers in the community engage in ongoing assessments to keep their perception of the health of the community accurate. This process guides their interventions with the community so that their interventions are appropriate. Community assessment involves an investigation into three interrelated areas of concern: (1) **community-based needs**, (2) **systems of care management**, and (3) **influences affecting resource allocation decisions**. The accuracy of the assessment shapes the emerging plan of care with the additional influences that relate to the **validation of services by the client** and the **expertise of the nurse/interdisciplinary team**. Each of these components are discussed in this chapter.

The Alliance Model for Health, a model for community health assessment, is intended to serve as a template to inform nurses and other health care providers about forces that interact, making a composite picture of health and illness in the community. Figure 5-1 provides a schematic of the Alliance Model for Community Health Assessment. The reader should consider the three circles in this diagram, which represent a focus on community-based needs, the systems of care management, and influences on resource allocation decisions, as critical aspects of the overall community assessment.

Each circle includes an area of interaction with the other two circles as evidenced by the overlap of the three circles in the center of the diagram. These overlapping areas represent the degree of interaction of the three areas. The reader should note that there is minimal overlap of the three circles, suggesting minimal interaction among the spheres. Assessment of each area would identify parameters for potential intervention to expand these areas of interaction.

Community-based Needs are those identified by the nurse and other professionals with the input of the consumer or client.

Systems of Care Management are created to address community-based needs. These systems take into account the types of client problems, the public's expectations for care, the standard of accepted care, and the plans to meet client needs.

Influences Affecting Resource Allocation Decisions include the patterns of resource allocation, values and beliefs of the public, reliance on government funding, activities of special interest groups, and insurance coverage.

Client–Care Provider Alliance. Client–care provider alliance suggests that the interaction between the client and the nurse/interdisciplinary team is of mutual importance.

FIGURE 5-1.

◙

An alliance model for community health assessment.

The outer circle, encompassing the three inner circles, represents the mutual aspects of validation of services by the client and expertise of the nurse/interdisciplinary team. The placement of this circle suggests that the needs of the client and the ability of the nurse/interdisciplinary team to provide care are fundamental in concerns in every care delivery situation. *Arrows* suggest interaction and the mutual importance of care provider and care recipient concerns, hence the term *alliance*.

The most effective alliance or partnership is between the client and the interdisciplinary team, which includes the nurse as a team member. If a working interdisciplinary team is not in place, the nurse interacts with the client independently, until a team can be created. Teams have different members according to the needs of the client and the expertise of the team members. For example, a person recovering from diabetic ketoacidosis might have a team consisting of an endocrinologist, a nutritionist, a diabetic nurse specialist, and a clinical pharmacist. A family (client) in crisis due to a sudden infant death might receive care from a team consisting of a medical examiner or coroner, a community health nurse, a religious counselor, and a peer support provider (neighbor who recently experienced sudden infant death).

The working relationship between the client and the nurse/interdisciplinary team is the most significant aspect of the alliance model. A poor therapeutic or ineffective relationship between the client and the care provider negatively influences their alliance and, therefore, interferes with

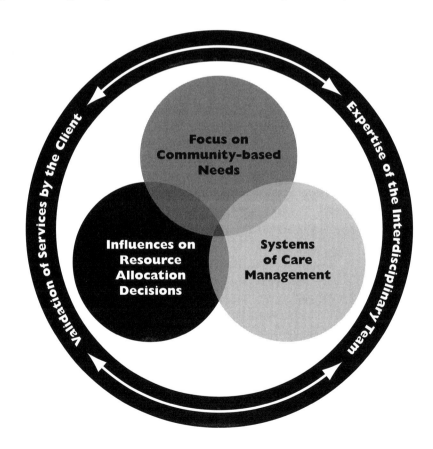

the interactions between the focus of care, the systems of care, and the influences on resource allocation decisions. Clients are increasingly viewed as partners in their care (Anderson & McFarlane, 1996). A well-developed alliance between the client and the care provider allows for full assessment of the strengths or problems in these spheres of interaction.

Clients are at times unable to participate fully in planning health care with providers. Children, people with mental and physical impairments, prisoners, or people with knowledge deficits are among the clients that may be unable to participate independently in planning for their health care. These clients can benefit from surrogates to assist with decision-making and to provide a voice to represent them. Novice nurses can seek mentors to improve their skills in relationship building so they can learn effective advocacy.

Nurses and other care providers will not always understand the community's needs, or how to work within the care systems in the community. Some providers are not able to interact fully with clients to plan their health care. Nurses in this situation need to refer immediate problems to more expert providers and resolve their skill and knowledge deficits through continuing or formal education. Nurses begin working in the community as novices and slowly master skills and knowledge at an expert level.

The Nurse Novice and Nurse Expert in the Community As community health nurses move from novice to expert care provider in the community, they use the referral process when they need assistance. Nurses can make referrals to other nurses or members of other disciplines. Nurses have the responsibility to remediate their knowledge and skill deficits through continuing and formal education, as they become expert providers.

$\mathcal{H}$EALTHY COMMUNITIES

Some communities are healthier than others; some work closely together to meet the needs of their members. Figure 5-2 suggests a more responsive and coordinated community compared to Figure 5-1 as represented by the increased overlap between the spheres of community-based needs, systems of care management, and influences on resource allocation decisions. This is a community where the expertise of the nurse/interdisciplinary team and the validation of services by the client are responsive to each other, well-developed, and interacting smoothly.

The community reflected in Figure 5-2 is not an ideal community in which there is a total absence of illness, where team members always make the best decision, or where resources are always available. Instead, it is a community where interaction and interrelatedness of the whole community are ongoing. In actuality, the level of interaction is always moving or changing, reflecting a living community.

In Figure 5-3, the sphere representing the focus on community-based needs is smaller than the other two circles. This signifies a community where the nurse, other team members, and the client need to direct more energy toward assessing, validating, and meeting community-based needs. For example, the diagram could represent a community experiencing a sudden influx of immigrants, a new emerging health problem, or the closing of a large health care facility.

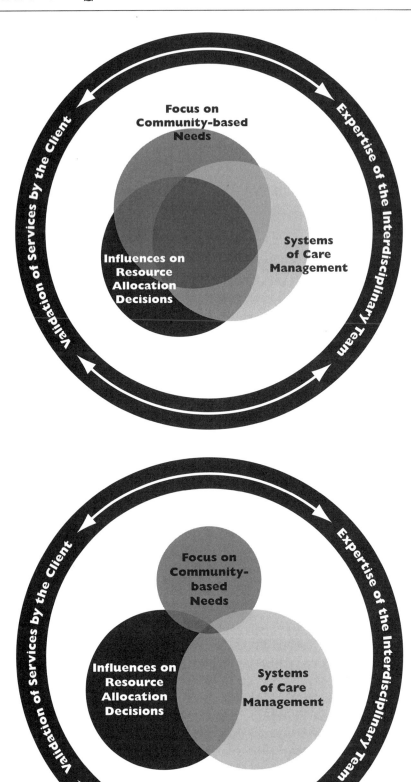

FIGURE 5-2. A reflection of a well-coordinated community.

FIGURE 5-3. A deficit in understanding community-based needs.

The major concern in the community represented in Figure 5-3 is the focus on community-based needs. After concerns with community-based needs are addressed, the circle would be the same size as the others, similar to Figure 5-2. The return of the circle to its original size represents stabilization of community-based needs. Examples of this stabilization would include: establishing services assimilate immigrants through cultural and English language support programs; identifying the cause of an emerging illness so treatment could begin; and establishing alternate care sites to meet people's needs. Community-based needs change on an ongoing basis and need continuous assessment.

Focus on Community-Based Needs

Community-based needs are those ever-changing needs that reflect the population of a particular area. For example, today's aging American population has requisite needs that are different from the baby-boom generation that followed the second World War. A community health nurse making an assessment in a large urban community would expect to find variations from an assessment made in a suburban or rural community. It is important for the nurse and other team members to assess each community on an ongoing basis to validate health-related concerns and account for changing health patterns to direct early and prompt intervention.

Community-based needs include but are not restricted to the measuring and analysis of the following sources of information: (1) patterns of morbidity and mortality, (2) demographics (e.g., age, gender, education level, income, housing), (3) environmental concerns, (4) public services (fire, police, sanitation, education, recreation, sports), (5) aesthetics (e.g., art, music, culture, religion), and (6) health-related facilities [e.g., hospitals, community-based organizations (CBOs), subacute and custodial care facilities, public health facilities, home care organizations]. Each of these data sources is explored below.

Patterns of Morbidity and Mortality

The patterns of morbidity (illness) and mortality (death) are significant variables in community health assessment. Knowledge of the causes of death and disability assists in the development of preventive health services as well as in the provision of early treatment and rehabilitation services. Patterns of morbidity and mortality change in communities. Epidemics, changes in immunization rates in children, and variations in how disease affects certain groups can all affect patterns of morbidity and mortality. Changes occur as communities develop, grow, or deteriorate.

Demographics

A community is known by the visible characteristics of the people such as age, race, gender, and location of housing and the invisible characteristics such as level of education, income, and religion. Demographics represent a way of describing a community statistically. Demographics can only describe the aspects of the community that can be measured. Some parts of the community demographics, like the homelessness rate, may be hard to measure because it is difficult to obtain an accurate count of the number of people in that category.

The complexity of measuring national demographics, usually through census counts every 10 years, results in problems with reporting findings. Some data take years to analyze and present to the public. The community may change while the old picture of a community (findings from the census) is still being developed. The massive task of measuring characteristics of the nation makes more frequent measurement unlikely.

International demographics are difficult to use because different variables are used to measure health statistics by different countries. Some countries do not record health-related information, which makes any comparison impossible. Also, exact definitions of what constitutes certain illnesses or syndromes vary from nation to nation.

Environmental Concerns

The environment is the context in which life is supported on earth. Concern about the global environment is necessary to protect the fragile ecosystem, a major determinant of health. It is important to advocate a healthy environment whether one is concerned about the loss of the atmospheric ozone layer and the resulting increase in harmful, carcinogenic rays from the sun, or a local chemical dump site, which threatens the drinking water of a community. People need to know about the health of the environment in which they live, work, and play. People need to act in a way that conserves resources for future generations.

Public Services

Public services include fire, police, sanitation, and education services as well as recreation and sports facilities. Every community provides protection from crime and disasters to its residents as well as activities that promote socialization and entertainment. A sign of a healthy community is one in which the public has adequate public services so that the members are safe to enjoy life. Large communities or those in certain hubs of the country may have more public services than other communities. In times of financial constraints, some communities limit access to public services that are not seen as essential.

Aesthetics—Art, Music, Culture, and Religion

Communities express the joys and pains of living through the creation of art and beauty. People may define art and beauty as a personal valuing of pottery, paintings, or music. Personal meaning of the aesthetic in a multiracial, multiethnic society like the United States is important to consider. People may have widely divergent views of what is artistic and beautiful.

A healthy community is one in which people can express what they find to be artistic and beautiful while tolerating the expressions of other groups different from themselves. The appreciation of diversity is key to the aesthetic component of a healthy community. Some of the ways communities appreciate the aesthetic are by building museums, funding public sculpture, remembering holy days and festivals, and holding ethnic celebrations.

Health-Related Facilities

Health-related facilities include ambulatory care clinics, hospitals, CBOs, subacute and custodial care facilities, public health departments, and home care and hospice organizations. These various health-related facilities are built by communities to meet the needs of the public. Contemporary trends are to decentralize health care services when possible and increase the use of CBOs. Rehabilitative services, for example, are moving into communities so that clients can receive services close to where they live.

Individuals and groups can also provide care out of private offices. Health maintenance organizations (HMOs) and preferred provider organizations (PPOs) also support health care by linking a number of facilities or practitioners together to provide health care with the intent of lowering costs.

Health Maintenance Organizations (HMO) A health maintenance organization (HMO) is an organized set of services usually provided at one site. Client's agree to join the HMO for a discount in the cost of services. A particular health insurance plan may have an HMO as one option that clients may choose to purchase. A guaranteed pool of clients makes cost control more possible. If clients wish to receive care from a different facility they will have a greater out-of-pocket expense.

Preferred Provider Organization (PPO) A preferred provider organization (PPO) is a group of care providers who see clients at a lower cost. Costs are lower because of the guaranteed client pool. As with the HMO, clients assume more financial risks if they visit a provider outside of the PPO structure.

CARE MANAGEMENT TECHNIQUES

The management of health care is a complex phenomenon. Variables include: (1) the mix of client problems, (2) the expectations of the public for care, (3) the competence of professionals, (4) the accepted standards of care, and (5) the use of interdisciplinary care plans (ICPs) or action plans. Care management techniques develop and change according to the changes in health care problems and how populations decide to allocate resources.

Mix of Client Problems

The mix of client problems may necessitate an ever-fluctuating level of intensity of needed services. Some individual clients in the community need total support while others need minimal intervention to maintain independence in living. Nurses in the community must make daily assessments of their case loads to decide which clients need a visit, which clients need a supportive phone call, and which clients need a different level of care, perhaps involving referral and coordination.

When the client mix includes families and groups of people as in a support group, care providers have a more diverse case load and confront a wider range of human problems. For example, the community health nurse caring for a family experiencing domestic disputes will likely be managing a complex plan of care. Clients with domestic dispute problems need special intervention services and psychosocial counseling.

The family unit needs a very different type of care from interventions focused on individuals. In domestic violence, the whole family needs care and support. Groups of people meeting for a common reason like a 12-step Alcoholic's Anonymous group have common needs, but the group needs various interventions so that all members can participate. Sometimes nursing groups of people is done for economy of time (giving similar instructions to many people at the same time), and sometimes it is done because people are better able to participate in their healing in the midst of group support. Some cancer support groups are founded on the idea that people with similar problems are best able to help cancer survivors cope with life.

Expectations of the Public for Care

The desire for health care services by the public is a major aspect of how care is managed. For example, prior to the advent of dialysis, people had fewer expectations about long-term care of clients with renal disease than they do today. Recent trends that support consumerism and make nutritional counseling and weight loss information a high priority encourage the public to expect this type of information from their care providers.

Advertising often teaches clients what they should expect from health care providers. Competing advertisements often present the idea that a special service is actually the normal service. This suggests that the organizations without the special service are actually substandard. Some deluxe maternity services are advertised as a service that a new family should expect, implying that hospitals without the service are not providing the basic service the new family needs.

Some people avoid the health care system because they fear providers, do not trust that the care they receive is adequate, or have had a poor experience with care in the past. The major problem with this situation is that the client avoids the care system until the illness or problem has so progressed that little or nothing can be done to correct it.

The challenge for health care providers is to assist the public to expect a reasonable level of care since unlimited care is no longer realistic. Even the reliance on the safety net of health care services for people who are uninsured or the underinsured, living in poverty, or with disabilities is now being called into question. In addition, American society has not yet defined *futile care*; many people receive care that will not help them become healthier. Some clients are kept on high-technology life support equipment long after it is useful.

Competence of Professionals

The competence of professionals affects how care is managed. Nurses need competence in theoretical as well as technical aspects of care. Care providers need to be skilled in issues related to capitated reimbursement, for example, to be fully able to manage care effectively from an economic perspective. Care providers need specific skills in negotiation, supervision, and collective bargaining to name a few.

Likewise, given the high level of acuity in home care services, nurses need the latest technical skills in areas such as intravenous home infusion therapy, use of respirators, administration of peritoneal dialysis, and managing complex medication regimens to be able to manage care in a safe way.

Each member of the interdisciplinary team brings various levels of skill in the physical, emotional, spiritual, and cultural care of clients; together the team is able to provide comprehensive care to the community. The smooth functioning of the interdisciplinary team suggests that the composite of the team, not necessarily each team member, has the skills and knowledge necessary to manage complex client situations.

Accepted Standards of Care

Each health care discipline performs its work using accepted standards of care. The American Nurses Association (ANA) sets general standards of care for the nursing profession, and the ANA together with specialty organizations, like the Association of Nurses in AIDS Care, set standards for specialized and advanced practice. Legally, the state nurse practice act sets the parameters of accepted nursing care for its jurisdiction.

Nurses are required to uphold standards for community-based care that are adapted for home care, school health, public health, and private practice. Nurses working in the community have the opportunity to share their concerns about care with their peers and professional associations so that the standards of care reflect contemporary practice. The National League for Nursing, Council for Community Health Services, and the Public Health Nursing section of the American Public Health Association are both involved in solving problems in community-based practice through discussions of their respective memberships.

Use of Interdisciplinary Care Plans (ICPs) or Action Plans

Interdisciplinary Care Plans
Interdisciplinary care plans
(ICPs) are guidelines for
providing interdisciplinary care
that will meet the needs of most
people having a procedure or
experiencing an illness. Clients
also have unique needs not
covered by ICPs. Professionals
must individualize care when
necessary.

ICPs or action plans influence care management by setting minimal expectations for client outcomes or responses to care interventions. These care plans are intended to capture the more general or typical response to interventions to accelerate discharge from a more acute level of care to a lesser level of care. For example, a client might be discharged from the hospital to home, or the home care nurse might discharge a client from a dependent care level of service to a level of greater self-care and independence.

Standardized ICPs are not useful for every client. People respond to care in unique or unexpected ways and may need a tailored, personal plan of care. It is important to remember that all clients together with the nurse need to evaluate continuously the plan of care for its fit with any predetermined ICP. Each provider has the legal responsibility to plan and provide care that meets the special needs of clients.

*I*NFLUENCES ON RESOURCE ALLOCATION DECISIONS

A number of variables influence how resource allocation decisions are made. They include: (1) patterns of resource allocation, (2) the values and beliefs of the population, (3) the reliance on local, regional, and federal government funding, (4) the influence of special interest groups on resource allocation, and (5) patterns of insurance coverage. In any community, one or more of these variables may influence resource allocation decisions at the same time.

The resurgence of tuberculosis (TB) in the United States points to the importance of various influences on resource allocation. In certain inner-city areas, there may no longer be an appropriate amount of funds allocated to the prevention and treatment of TB. The people controlling funds may judge the people living in poverty who have the disease, suggesting that they do not deserve costly treatments. There may be inequities in government funding because other diseases are competing for funding. Insurance companies may not pay for directly observed therapy (DOT) or watching people taking their medications because it is considered too expensive in certain settings.

Patterns of Resource Allocation

Every community has a pattern of how it allocates resources. Retirement communities allocate resources differently than aggregates of young families. One of the roles for nursing and other members of the interdisciplinary team relates to keeping a community informed about unmet needs of other parts of the community. For example, a community that does not value rehabilitative services may need to be educated about the importance of these services before it decides whether it wants or requires them.

Values and Beliefs of the Population

The values and beliefs of people dictate what types of health-related services they want developed. For example, a closed and isolated Amish community has different requirements for health services than a large metropolitan Hispanic community. Some populations with traditional religious beliefs could be expected to have different requisites for family planning services than groups who value various artificial birth control methods.

Populations are diverse and represent a variety of cultural values and beliefs. The community health nurse needs to uncover and learn various beliefs without supporting negative stereotypes. Nurses learn about beliefs different from their own by reading about other cultures as well as living and working with other groups of people. Diversity is found between cultural groups and within the groups themselves. Most groups have members who are conservative as well as liberal in how they interpret the values and beliefs of the overall group.

Reliance on Local, Regional, and Federal Government Funding

Communities that receive various levels of government funding for health-related programs allocate resources differently than communities that pay out-of-pocket for all health care services. Public hospitals subsidize approximately 70 percent of inpatient care and 50 percent of outpatient or ambulatory care (Rovner, 1996).

Changes in government funding could greatly change the services offered in certain communities that subsidize health care costs with public support. Each state varies in how it provides funds or services to the people who cannot pay for them. Local communities provide services after applying taxes on property and goods that are sold. The United States is different from other countries because it does not have an integrated national-state-local level of health services guaranteed to its citizens. The U.S. provides many health care services that are not always integrated (National Association of County Health Officers, 1993; U.S. Department of Health and Human Services, 1994).

Influence of Special Interest Groups

Special interest groups are those that use their influence to get the services that they want. For example, a certain political group may want more acute care cardiac services while limiting reproductive services for women. One of the concerns with special interest groups is that they may advocate for services for one group at the expense of another group's needs.

Health care planning can become inconsistent and chaotic when special interests are adopted without regard to the needs of the whole community. Clients from different age groups or with different diagnoses should not have to compete for care resources. Should resources go to the clients in the neonatal intensive care unit or the intermediate geriatric care unit? Does society want to focus on caring for people with acquired immune deficiency syndrome (AIDS) or Alzheimer's disease? There are no easy answers to these questions.

Advocates for the homeless, prisoners, and the physically and mentally challenged indicate that their needs are often not taken into account when health care choices are decided by the public. Advocacy groups, another type of special interest group, exist to assist less empowered groups to have a voice and get their needs met. The community health nurse advocates for different types of clients at different times in their experience of health and illness. Nurses advocate for other nurses by lobbying politicians to protect professional practice legislation.

Patterns of Insurance Coverage

The influence of third-party payment for health care as it relates to who has access to health care services is a complex issue. Increasingly, large segments of the population are uninsured or underinsured. Insurance coverage is not only a problem for people who do not work. Many people who work are not offered health care benefits or are paid per diem wages that do not include health care or other benefits. Some workers in the U.S. are undocumented non-residents who are impossible to cover with insurance.

The percent of people under age 65 with private health insurance decreased from 77 percent to 72 percent from 1986 to 1992. In this same time period, people without insurance rose from 15 percent to 17.2 percent (U.S. Department of Health and Human Services, 1995, pp. 9, 10). Since the insurance business is based on the economic rewards of keeping the pool of insurees healthy, and keeping risk of paying for benefits low, the number of uninsured could continue to rise.

$\mathcal{V}$ALIDATION OF SERVICES BY THE CLIENT

It is important to recognize that the measurement of health-related outcomes is dependent on the response of individuals to health-related interventions. The conceptual leap of viewing families, groups, and large aggregates as the clients of nursing care allows a more holistic view of nursing care, but measurement of these outcomes is difficult. Most assessment tools are related to the care of individuals (U.S. Department of Health and Human Services, 1994; Stanhope & Knollmueller, 1996).

Families, groups, and larger aggregates do receive nursing care, and the health of these aggregates may improve or stabilize. The techniques needed to measure aggregate wellness, however, are not always available to nurses or other care providers. For example, a family intervention to assist all members in coping with an unexpected death is intended to improve the functioning of the family unit. The nurse might expect to see improvements in communication as the family copes with the death experience. A tool to measure improvements in family coping, however, is not readily available to the community health nurse. Some of the limited areas where the measurement of aggregate health status is successful are immunization rates, communicable disease surveillance, and monitoring prenatal care.

One of the inherent problems with clients negotiating for their health care services is that they may not necessarily know what services they need. Clients may have unmet or unrecognized health care needs because they are unfamiliar with the services that are available. It is the responsibility of the health care provider to keep the consumer aware of their options in health care and to create linkages between providers and consumers of health care.

ℰXPERTISE OF THE NURSE/INTERDISCIPLINARY TEAM

It takes intervention from many health-related disciplines to improve the health of the community. Nursing, thus, as one discipline is a significant—but not isolated—contribution to the betterment of the public's health. Nursing needs to improve its ability to work with other team members continuously so care can be provided comprehensively. The skill of health care members in providing comprehensive care should be focused on care that is available, accessible, affordable, appropriate, adequate, and acceptable (Ferebee, 1994; Krout, 1994; Lillie-Blandon & Alfaro-Correa, 1995).

In the community, nurses' skills and knowledge, as well as the skills of other members of the interdisciplinary team, vary from novice to expert. The team is made up of newly licensed and experienced members, with a well-functioning team being one in which the members are able to work collaboratively to problem solve and meet client needs.

𝒾DENTIFYING PROBLEMS IN THE COMMUNITY HEALTH ASSESSMENT

In the ongoing community health assessment, deficits may be identified in various areas. Figure 5-4 represents an example of a problem in the integration of systems of care management. In Figure 5-4, the problem is not related to a deficit in the assessment of the issues affecting systems of care management, but rather to a deficit in the way this sphere is integrated with the other two areas.

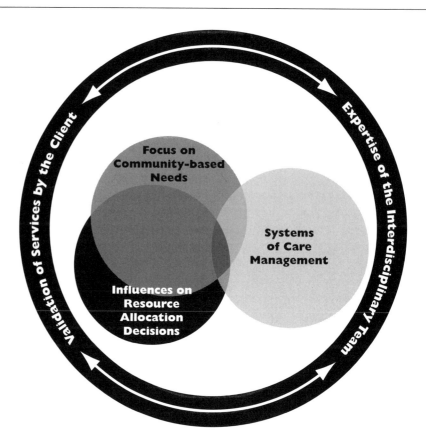

FIGURE 5-4. A problem in the integration of systems of care management.

The following scenario reflects a problem in the integration of systems of care management as reflected in Figure 5-4. In this fictitious situation, the change in one area of concern changes the entire system. The change in care management caused by a hospital closure affects the alliance between the clients who use the facility and the providers who care for them.

CASE STUDY: CLOSING PUBLIC HOSPITALS: A POLITICAL DECISION

Community health needs are carefully assessed on an ongoing basis by the community health department in a network of public hospitals in the Midwest. The political decision to close certain public hospitals came after a long and highly publicized period of public debate. Many people in the community believe that the medically indigent, who rely on public hospitals for care, were not considered in the decision to close these institutions.

The sudden closure of these hospitals made the system of care management completely unintegrated with the community-based needs as well as the influences on resource allocation. The remaining health-related facilities were unable to absorb requirements for care for people unable to pay for their health care.

Reintegration would be expected to occur when other systems of care management are developed or when the other health-related organizations adjust to the sudden closure of the hospitals by providing necessary care.

Summary

The focus on the Alliance Model of Community Health Assessment suggests that the process of community assessment is dynamic and never ending. The nurse or interdisciplinary team are always reevaluating their relationship with the client, as the client does with the nurse or interdisciplinary team. Their work together allows for continuous monitoring of community-based needs, the systems of care management, and influences on allocation decisions.

An Alliance Model for Community Health Assessment allows for full participation by professionals and the public in creating, using, and changing health care services. This comprehensive model promotes equal emphasis and attention on community-based needs, systems of care management, and influences affecting resource allocation decisions. None of these three areas of concern can be omitted in a comprehensive community health assessment. The area of overlap between these areas suggests the level of integration. A healthy community is represented by maximum overlap among these areas.

The outer circle in the model suggests the mutual importance of the validation of services by the client and the expertise of the nurse/interdisciplinary team. Clients with full knowledge of their health and ability to manage their care are more successful in negotiating with the nurse/interdisciplinary team. Although nurses sometimes work with clients alone, the best working relationship or alliance with clients is represented by an interdisciplinary team. (See the chapter appendix, for Alliance for Health: A Model Community Assessment Guidelines for Data Collection, which can be used in a community assessment.)

KEY WORDS

Client–care
   provider alliance

Health maintenance
   organization (HMO)

Prefered provider
   organization (PPO)

Interdisciplinary
   care plans (ICPs)

QUESTIONS

DIRECTIONS: Choose the one *best* response to each of the following questions.

1. When the newly employed community health nurse experiences a problem in the community, the best action is for this nurse is to
   A. work independently unless the problem increases.
   B. seek out other care providers to assist with problem solving as necessary.
   C. immediately refer the problem to a more experienced community health nurse.
   D. notify lay community leaders to get their opinions.

2. The needs and problems of a healthy community are
   A. continuously changing.
   B. usually fairly predictable.
   C. easily resolved.
   D. consistent over time.

3. Which source of information does **NOT** relate to measuring community-based needs?
   A. Environmental concerns
   B. Aesthetics
   C. Expectations for care
   D. Demographics

4. Which demographic variable would be the most difficult to measure?
   A. Household income
   B. Rate of premature births
   C. Causes of death
   D. Numbers of homeless people

5. The largest increase in the number of health-related facilities is occurring among
   A. community-based organizations (CBOs).
   B. hospitals.
   C. public health departments.
   D. nursing homes.

6. Interdisciplinary care plans (ICPs) would best be used with which of the following clients?
   A. A 12-year-old boy with an arm fracture and of normal weight
   B. An 87-year-old man with unstable angina and dementia
   C. A 45-year-old woman with chest trauma and poor health history
   D. A newborn with failure to thrive after a home delivery

7. A community health nurse working in a large Orthodox Jewish community would expect limitations in comprehensive
   A. coronary care services for men.
   B. services for older people.
   C. women's reproductive health services.
   D. services for infants and children.

ANSWERS

1. *The answer is B.* Seeking out other care providers begins the process of building a team of nurses and other professionals.

2. *The answer is A.* Problems are as fluid as the community and change with the community as it develops.

3. *The answer is C.* People's expectations for care relates to care management techniques in the Alliance Model for Community Health Assessment.

4. *The answer is D.* There has not been an organized effort to count the number of homeless people in the national census or other data collection activities.

5. *The answer is A.* Community-based organizations (CBOs) are rapidly expanding across the country.

6. *The answer is A.* An interdisciplinary care plan (ICP) is best used with situations that have more predictable outcomes.

7. *The answer is C.* The values and beliefs of the community might limit the services available for reproductive services such as abortion and artificial insemination.

ANNOTATED REFERENCES

Anderson, E. T., & McFarlane, J. M. (1996). *Community as partner: Theory and practice in nursing* (2nd. ed.). Philadelphia: Lippincott.

This textbook examines the potential relationships between nurses and clients as partners in creating solutions to health-related problems.

Ferebee, A. (1994). *Providing culturally appropriate services: Local health departments and community-based organizations working together.* Washington, DC: National Association of County Health Officials.

Culturally appropriate services are identified for the communities of Honolulu, HI; Howard County, MD; and San Luis Obispo County, CA. The use of leadership training, and interpersonal work with community leaders suggests improved health outcomes after projects are completed.

Krout, J. A. (Ed.). (1994). *Providing community-based services to the rural elderly.* Thousand Oaks, CA: Sage.

The needs of the elderly are reviewed in this text as they relate to the special needs in of this age group obtaining community-based care.

Lillie-Blandon, M. & Alfaro-Correa, A. (1995). *In the nation's interest: Equity in access to health care.* Washington, DC: Joint Center for Political and Economic Studies.

This summary report examines the health needs of Hispanics and African Americans. Multiple figures report health indicators by race and ethnicity as appropriate. Some of the topics of the figures are: numbers of physician visits, medical expenditures, percent uninsured, and usual sources of care.

National Association of County Health Officials. (1993). *Core public health functions.* Washington, DC: Author.

This document identifies the core functions of public health as: assessment of community health status and available resources; policy development resulting in proposals to support and encourage better health; and assurance that needed services are available.

Rovner, J. (1996). The safety net: What's happening to health care of last resort? *Advances* (supplement), (1), 1, 4.

This report of The Robert Wood Johnson Foundation identifies problems in the concept of a health care safety net. It explores the potential problems with a growing group of people without health insurance coverage.

Stanhope, M., & Knollmueller, R. N. (1996). *Handbook of community and home health nursing* (2nd. ed.). Mosby: New York.

This comprehensive text provides assessment tools for the assessment of individuals, families, and communities. The assessment tools focus on various ages and diagnoses. Extensive guides relate to nutrition, first aid, and emergency procedures as well as procedures completed in the home.

U.S. Department of Health and Human Services. (1994). *Prevention '93/'94: Federal programs and progress.* Washington, DC: Author.

This document explains the national effort: Healthy People 2000. Existing services and proposed solutions to problems are identified for all units of the Public Health Service, Administration on Aging, Administration for Children and Families, and the Health Care Financing Administration.

U.S. Department of Health and Human Services. (1994). *Clinician's handbook of preventive services.* Washington, DC: Author.

This book identifies screening, immunization/prophylaxis, and counseling concerns for children, adolescents, adults, and older adults.

U. S. Department of Health and Human Services. (1995). *Healthy people 2000: Midcourse review and 1995 revisions.* Hyattsville, MD: Author.

Healthy people 2000 identifies the health goals of the U.S. Department of Health and Human Services.

ALLIANCE FOR HEALTH: A MODEL COMMUNITY ASSESSMENT
GUIDELINES FOR DATA COLLECTION

Names of Team Members and Disciplines

_____
_____
_____
_____

PLEASE IDENTIFY THE DATES AND TIMES OF DATA COLLEC-
TION AS WELL AS THE SOURCES OF INFORMATION USED IN ALL
SECTIONS. *The questions in each assessment area are only samples;
teams may have additional questions.*

Description of the Community In this description, include pictures,
newspaper articles, and direct quotes from residents. Omit names for the
purpose of confidentiality.

_____
_____
_____
_____
_____
_____
_____
_____
_____
_____
_____
_____
_____
_____
_____
_____
_____
_____
_____
_____
_____
_____
_____

Diagnostic Statement(s) about the Community Write diagnostic statements after the complete assessment is finished.

_____
_____
_____
_____
_____
_____
_____

_____

_____

_____

_____

Focus on Community-based Needs

(1) Patterns of Morbidity and Mortality What are the leading causes of death and disability? Why do people seek health care? Are there unusual patterns of illness and death in the community?

_____

_____

_____

_____

_____

_____

_____

_____

(2) Demographics What are the characteristics on the community related to age, gender, education level, income, and the types of housing that are available? Have the demographics changed over the last 5–10 years?

_____

_____

_____

_____

_____

_____

_____

_____

(3) Environmental Concerns What does the community look like? What types of environmental problems could cause accidents or disease? Are there any areas in the community where the movement of people is restricted due to pollution?

_____

_____

_____

_____

_____

_____

_____

_____

(4) Public Services What type of public services exist related to fire, police, education, sanitation, recreation, and sports in the community? What services need improvement? How do people judge the quality of these services?

_____
_____
_____
_____
_____
_____
_____
_____

(5) Aesthetics What type of art, music, culture, and religion is reflected in the community? Are there variations in the aesthetics related to different generations?

_____
_____
_____
_____
_____
_____
_____
_____
_____

(6) Health-Related Facilities Describe the various health-related facilities: hospitals, CBOs, subacute and custodial care facilities, public health facilities, and home care organizations. What is the response rate for Emergency Medical Services? How do the health-related facilities relate to the characteristics: available, accessible, affordable, appropriate, adequate, and acceptable?

_____
_____
_____
_____
_____
_____
_____
_____
_____

Care Management Techniques

(1) Mix of Client Problems What are the patterns of morbidity and mortality of the community as they relate to the use of resources? Is the community a magnet for certain types of care that may influence the level of care others receive? For example, is the local hospital so burdened with trauma that others do not receive timely emergency care?

_____
_____
_____
_____
_____

(2) Expectations of the Public for Care Do people in the community want care that is not being provided? Do people view inequality in who obtains services?

(3) Competence of Professionals How do health care providers (HCPs) define the type of care that is provided to the community? What mechanisms are available to evaluate the care that is provided in the community?

(4) Accepted Standards of Care How are standards of care set in the community? Do HCPs follow the guidelines set by their professional organizations?

(5) Use of Interdisciplinary Care Plans (ICPs) or Action Plans Which ICPs are in use in the community? How do HCPs learn how to use them safely? Which disciplines are involved in the use of ICPs?

_____
_____

Influences on Resource Allocation Decisions

(1) **Patterns of Resource Allocation** What are the influences on resource allocation? How has this community allocated resources in the past? Is there a plan for resource allocation as it relates to health care delivery?

_____
_____
_____
_____
_____
_____
_____
_____

(2) **Values and Beliefs of the Population**
What are the values and beliefs of the community as they relate to health and illness ?

_____
_____
_____
_____
_____
_____
_____
_____

(3) **Reliance on Local, Regional and Federal Government Funding** In what ways does the community rely on government funding for health care services? What are alternate sources of funding for the community?

_____
_____
_____
_____
_____
_____
_____

(4) **Influence of Special Interest Groups on Resource Allocation** What special interest groups exist in the community? How do they influence health care decision-making?

_____
_____
_____
_____

_____
_____
_____
_____
_____

(5) Patterns of Insurance Coverage What is the make-up of the population as it relates to insurance coverage?

_____
_____
_____
_____
_____
_____
_____
_____

Validation of Services by the Client

What is the process for involving the consumer in health care decision-making? Are there sufficient patient/client representatives working in facilities? Are there ombudsman services for clients in agencies providing care?

_____
_____
_____
_____
_____
_____
_____
_____
_____
_____
_____
_____
_____
_____
_____

Expertise of the Nurse/Interdisciplinary Team

How are care providers oriented for their work responsibilities? What types of continuing education services are available for HCPs?

_____
_____
_____
_____

_____
_____
_____
_____
_____
_____
_____
_____
_____
_____
_____
_____

Evaluation of the Community Assessment Project

What were the benefits and limitations of completing the community assessment project with respect to the personal resources of the work group/team?

_____
_____
_____
_____
_____
_____
_____
_____
_____
_____
_____
_____
_____
_____
_____
_____

THE COMMUNITY AS CLIENT

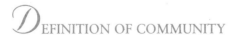

NATURE AND TYPES OF COMMUNITIES

All of the efforts of the community health nurse are directed to improving, protecting, and maintaining the health of the community. The community is the focus of all care provided by the community health nurse whether nursing care involves an individual, a family, an aggregate, or the community as a whole.

The community is the context in which the interactions between individuals and their environment occur. A community is not necessarily restricted by geographical boundaries, yet it has definition and function. The nature of the community is explored in this chapter. The community is defined from a variety of perspectives. Each perspective enables the community health nurse to appreciate the multiple dimensions of the community. As the nurse becomes familiar with the community, it becomes possible to view the community and appreciate the community as a client. Thus, the nurse becomes the provider of skilled and purposeful interactions and interventions with and for the community. First, it is important to define the community and become familiar with the community itself.

DEFINITION OF COMMUNITY

There is no single definition of the community to best reflect its nature and complexity. A community refers to people in the context of their environment as they continuously interact with each other and the environment. Just as there are a myriad of perspectives from which to define a human being so too are there a myriad of perspectives from which to define a community.

Anatomy and Physiology of a Community

Human beings can be examined through a clear understanding of their basic structure (anatomy) and function (physiology). The anatomy of a human being is characterized by body systems or parts, while the physiology of a human being refers to the functioning of these systems or parts. The heart and circulatory system are part of the basic anatomy of the individual while the circulation of blood carrying oxygen and nutrients to human tissue is the function of the circulatory system. The anatomy of the community refers to its structure, which includes the people and the physical characteristics of the community. The people are defined by their demography, including age, sex, gender, race, and other parameters. The physical characteristics of the community include the terrain, the types of commercial, residential, and industrial land use, and the geographical boundaries. The function of a community refers to the utilization of community resources by the people, the linkages between people and the resources, and the unique patterns of people living in their environment.

The structure and function of a community are illustrated by the following example. The structure of a deserted community is defined by the stores that are boarded up, the schools that are vacant, and the houses that are in disrepair. A community cannot sustain itself unless it has the resources needed for food, protection, recreation, and education. Without these vital resources, people may eventually relocate because their needs cannot be met. Others will sustain themselves as best they can, living with deprivation. Still others will seek solutions for their needs outside of the community. The vitality and health of the community in this example are, therefore, limited by the lack of available resources for people to function.

Observing the interactions of people with their environment, analyzing the essential structure of the community, and determining the utilization of resources are ways in which to understand the nature of a community. Using the framework of anatomy to learn about the people and physical characteristics of the community and using the patterns of utilization of resources to comprehend the functioning or physiology of a community, provide one view about the nature of the community.

Gemeinschaft and Gesellschaft Communities

There are other ways in which to appreciate the complexity and diversity of a community. Over 100 years ago, Tönnies (1887; translated by Loomis, 1957) defined human associations as either Gemeinschaft or Gesellschaft in nature. All intimate, private, and exclusive living together was understood as life in Gemeinschaft. Gesellschaft was thought of as public life, or the world itself. Extrapolating from this sociological framework and applying it to the study of communities, it is possible to contrast a Gemeinschaft community with a Gesellschaft community. Consider visualizing these communities with either a horizontal structure (Gemeinschaft), emphasizing locality, or vertical structure (Gesellschaft), emphasizing specialized interest. "Gemeinschaft community relationships are intimate and face-to-face, not discrete and segmented. . . . [they are] concerned with the whole person. In Gesellschaft, the dominant image of relationship [is] that of contract, not habit or custom. The authority of such a society [is] based on the legal, rational ideas of consent, volition, and contract. Persons related in a sense of specific obligation" (Hall & Weaver, 1977, p.156).

In a Gemeinschaft community, the resources of the community are closely linked and in close proximity with each other. Providers and consumers are aligned through common interest and mutual participation. Health care and other services can be accessed and more effectively reach community members in need. This is accomplished because there is a high degree of cohesiveness and familiarity within the community. The members of a Gemeinschaft community are known to each other. For example, if a family's home is destroyed by fire, the family would be cared for by the Gemeinschaft community. The local church or synagogue would call upon its members to provide emergency housing. The neighbors would organize to develop a system whereby one family per day provides meals for the dislocated family. The school community organization would make a contribution from its emergency fund for the family to replace personal items. A Gemeinschaft community is able to mobilize its resources efficiently, expeditiously, and through a network of familiarity. The level of intimacy among community members is mobilized into a generalized community response.

> **Gemeinschaft** is translated from the German as community, mutual participation and common interest.

The Gesellschaft community is characterized by hierarchy, bureaucracy, and a vertical organization. Status, rank, and authority define power within the community. In a Gesellschaft community, actions are accomplished through a hierarchical structure and inevitably involve bureaucratic "red tape" and waiting periods. Individuals are not well known to each other. For the family made homeless by a destructive fire, a social service agency may assist the family to relocate to a transient hotel with others in similar situations. The hotel may be located in an unfamiliar area, leading to a feeling of isolation. Public assistance for financial needs or food stamps for emergency food may be allocated but only after the appropriate applications are completed and identifications verified. During the waiting periods for service, the family may not have access to needed supports.

> **Gesellschaft** is translated from the German as society or company.

In both types of community, the family's needs are addressed, but the experience is qualitatively and quantitatively different. A Gemeinschaft community has a horizontal organizational structure in which the available services are proximal and related to each other. The presence and interrelatedness of services to each other are the defining characteristics of the community. The associations among members and resources create a kind of living organism characterized by openness and equality. The Gesellschaft community has a vertical organizational structure in which services may be distant and superficial. The relatedness in this community is to resources outside the community. Associations among members and resources are public and perhaps more mechanical and hierarchical.

The designations rural, suburban, urban, international, or global should not be confused when determining if a community functions as a Gemeinschaft community or a Gesellschaft community. It is possible, for example, for a large urban community to function as a Gemeinschaft community. A community health nurse making home visits in a high-risk, crime-ridden, urban community may feel safe and protected when the members watch from their windows in an effort to protect the nurse on visits to care for homebound people on the block. A "community watch" creates a safe and nurturing environment in which the nurse is valued as someone necessary to help those in need. The world can become a global Gemeinschaft community through the media and mass communication, enabling individuals to assist children in developing countries to fight disease and impoverishment. A Gesellschaft community may be illustrated by a suburban community in which members feel isolated in their homes, rarely interacting with their neighbors in adjacent houses. Members may shop in large, impersonal stores at malls outside their community where they are not known to the shopkeepers. The idea of applying Gemeinschaft and Gesellschaft associations to communities can help in appreciating the diversity of community types and functions.

Typology of Community Structures

Warren's Classification of Communities

Integral community
Parochial community
Diffuse community
Stepping stone community
Transitory community
Anomic community

Typology is a classification system. Neighborhoods are classified into different types portraying the wide spectrum of community patterns of social function and interaction.

Warren (1977), recognizing the nature of interactive patterns within the community, provides another framework in which to view the community. Warren considers the pattern of communication, the type of leadership, and the decision-making capabilities exhibited by the community as identifying a specific type of community. Warren developed a classification system (i.e., a typology) of communities that defines leadership, cohesiveness, self-sufficiency, and its ties with the larger community or society. Variance among communities is explained through this classification system, which identifies inherent differences among communities or neighborhoods.

Six community types are illustrated by Warren, ranging from cohesive and organized to apathetic and disorganized. The nature and type of community influence the interactions of the community health nurse; therefore, these factors play a significant role in the health services provided. The delivery of effective health services to individuals, families, and groups by the community health nurse contributes to the health of the community. The nurse who is knowledgeable about the particular type of community is able to develop a partnership with its leadership, communicate effectively with members, and plan for the implementation of programs needed to address needs.

Integral Community   The individuals in an integral community have frequent face-to-face contact. The norms, values, and attitudes of the neighborhoods support those of the larger community. Neighborhoods are cohesive, but people also belong to groups outside their area of residence. When problems arise that cannot be handled internally, the leadership of an integral neighborhood helps its members to reach out for assistance. One example of an integral community could be a small rural community in which the members participate for the good of the town. This is an active community, and the members are known to each other. They belong to many organizations, including block clubs and Parent Teacher Associations (PTAs). Members also belong to some groups that are not in the neighborhood. The integral community is a very open and interacting neighborhood (Warren, 1977).

In an integral community, the community health nurse may make a presentation to the community board about a potentially harmful environmental substance about which the community should be alerted. The nurse then works with the community to develop strategies to protect its members. The integral community would actively problem-solve with the community health nurse about health issues and concerns.

Parochial Community   People in a parochial community also have face-to-face contacts, but there is an absence of values or behavioral ties to the larger community. These neighborhoods tend to be protective of their status, often screening out values that do not conform to their own and enforcing their own beliefs within the neighborhood. Isolation from the larger community is encouraged. A parochial community can be united by culture, ethnicity, or religion, for example. In parochial neighborhoods, the populations are both physically and organizationally separated from the rest of the community. Despite the positive identification that may take place among the residents, there is a weak orientation to the larger community. Sometimes, the conflicts between the values and goals of the isolated neighborhood and the larger community may produce further estrangement from the larger community and discourage participation in functions important to the larger community (Warren, 1977).

In a parochial community, the community health nurse is sensitive to the protective stance of the members after carefully determining the value system of the community. Developing a health program that reflects the values of the community is a key to its success. Determining "gatekeepers" within the community who could expedite health programs and identify at-risk populations is an important strategy. Respect for the power structure of the community can give the community health nurse the support needed to implement community-based health services.

Gatekeeper is a powerful member of the community who permits access to people, information, and resources and who monitors input, output, and movement within the community.

Diffuse Community   Individuals within a diffuse community interact infrequently with each other and have few ties with the larger community. There is often a lack of shared norms, values, and attitudes. A primary tie among neighbors is geographical proximity to one another. There may be little or no leadership in these areas, and when leadership exists, it is often not representative of the entire community. An active elite and an organizational network, which tend to ignore or subvert the values of most residents, may be encountered. Such a situation may produce intra-neighborhood conflict. A program of neighborhood improvement may fail because of a lack of internal neighborhood cohesion and inaccurate communication of the existing norms since the leadership is not representative of the members, even though the leadership is part of the neighborhood (Warren, 1977).

In a diffuse community, the community health nurse would attempt to find a common need that can be addressed communally and can pull members together over a shared agenda. The nurse functions as a magnet or in some way identifies an issue that serves as the glue with which to bring community members together.

Stepping Stone Community A stepping stone community is characterized by the rapid turnover of its residents, creating a weak sense of identity within the neighborhood. Members are willing to give up ties established in the neighborhood if other commitments and opportunities arise; they strive to attain a higher social status. Residents of these areas do, however, have close ties to the larger community and do interact regularly with neighbors. Leadership is usually not effective because of the high rate of mobility; conflicts arise between the needs of the local neighborhood and the values of social mobility (Warren, 1977).

Examples of stepping stone communities are political and educational communities. The political center or the educational institution serves as a hub in the community. The members of a political community may be politicians, advocates, lobbyists, and their families and associates. The members of an educational community may be the faculty, students, staff, administrators, and their families and associates. Members move out of a stepping stone community after a specified time or when a particular purpose has been accomplished (e.g., a politician's term of office expires or a graduate student achieves an academic degree).

In a stepping stone community, the interventions of a community health nurse may need to be short-term, given the turnover in this kind of community. Health goals that are immediately achievable should be constructed to enable the members to experience feedback, thereby reinforcing success.

Transitory Community The people in a transitory community fail to participate in or identify with the local community. People keep to themselves because links with others may interfere with the goals of the individual and the family. There may be a widespread feeling of mistrust in this type of neighborhood. Any neighborhood structure is absent except when trying to avoid participation or local entanglements. There are many examples of transitory communities, including prisons and homeless shelters. The transitory community also provides a model of urban anonymity. Families experiencing the stress and strain of achieving their tasks may have limited energy and minimal opportunity for participation in neighborhood issues (Warren, 1977).

A transitory community presents special challenges to the community health nurse because trust must be established before access into this community is allowed. The community health nurse must work diligently to build rapport through understanding and acceptance. Valued actions speak louder than words, thereby establishing the nurse's professional credibility. Demonstration of useful, meaningful, and relevant efforts prove to the community that the nurse is able to make a valuable contribution.

Anomic Community Anomic communities are completely disorganized; residents lack participation in and a common identification with the neighborhood or the larger community. There is a high level of apathy in this neighborhood. Socialization is unlikely to influence or alter the values of its residents. There is little interaction among residents within the neighborhood or between the neighborhood and the larger community. Leadership is largely lacking. A community in which there is social unrest, violence, and economic impoverishment may exemplify an anomic community as residents engage in passive behavior and display alienation (Warren, 1977).

The anomic community is perhaps the most difficult community with which to work since pervasive apathy provides few if any pathways to its core. The rewards of working with this type of community are often limited because of its dynamics. The community health nurse must learn to accept even small changes as significant and meaningful. The community health nurse offers organizational skills, provides contacts, and establishes links between members and with helping organizations within and outside the community. As needs are addressed and the inner resources rekindled, the community health nurse may find a willingness to generate small efforts for health concerns among the members.

Functions of a Community

The health of the community can also be measured by the way it functions. Communities are rich and varied in their nature and complex in their operations. The various frameworks for understanding a given community help the community health nurse develop with members needed health programs responsive to the identified needs.

The boundaries of a community identify it and provide for its integrity. Boundaries that are permeable enable input from the larger community or society and also enable members in partnership with other members to contribute to the larger community or society. Boundaries that filter input and allow for output help to maintain the integrity of the community. The community health nurse must learn to negotiate these boundaries to gain access to the community and to engage with the members in the partnership of health planning, referral, use of available health and social services, and health resource development. Great care must be taken to reinforce the professional credibility of the nurse and the shared goals for developing a community alliance.

Communities perform a variety of functions, some of which are common to all communities. Table 6-1, using the reference points of Higgs and Gustafson (1985), defines the various functions of the community: utilization of space; means of livelihood; production, distribution, and consumption of goods and services; protection of its members; education; participation; and linkages with other systems providing for the needs of its members when the community is unable or elects not to carry out its function.

A community performs functions for its members. These functions are diverse and include providing industry and commerce, fostering socialization, maintaining safety and social control, adapting to changes in the

Major Functions of a Community

Utilization of space
Means of livelihood
Production, distribution, and consumption of goods and services
Protection of its members
Education
Participation
Linkages

⬛

TABLE 6-1

MAJOR FUNCTIONS OF A COMMUNITY

Utilization of Space

Utilization of space refers to provisions for housing and places for socialization and recreation.

Means of Livelihood

Means of livelihood refer to opportunities within the community for employment and the community's ability to provide for its members.

Production, Distribution, and Consumption of Goods and Services

Production, distribution, and consumption of goods and services concerns business and commerce within the community. It also refers to the ability of the community to enable basic transactions for the materials and services on which members of the community rely to perform their activities of daily living.

Protection of Members

The protection of members means the community is capable of creating and enforcing norms and controls that allow the community to function. It also refers to the prevention of physical disasters that can threaten the community and its members.

Education

Education concerns schools and other resources for the socialization of adults, children, newcomers, as well as providing an environment of ongoing enrichment of the community.

Participation

Participation refers to the community's communications, social interactions, and supports.

Linkages

Linkages refers to connections made to other systems to meet the needs of its members when the community is unable or elects not to carry out its functions.

NOTE: From *Community as a Client: Assessment and Diagnosis* (pp. 112–113), by Z. R. Higgs & D. D. Gustafson, 1985, Philadelphia: F. A. Davis. Adapted with permission.

surrounding environment, and providing mutual aid and support. The health of a community can ultimately be determined by examining the functions of a community and their effectiveness.

A healthy community fosters a commitment to the community. Groups are able to identify their interests, thereby facilitating social organizations. Communication flows effectively among groups. The community contains conflict yet allows for group and individual differences and deviance.

Members are free to participate in community activities. Mechanisms for facilitating interaction and decision-making among community members are possible. A healthy community also negotiates and manages the community's relationships to the larger society. Meaning is derived as members interact, define their values and social structure, and create networks of support to enable the members to grow and develop.

Affiliations within a Community

Affiliations within communities are diverse and may define communities within the community. While people may be affiliated by sharing a common geographical area (e.g., neighborhood, village, town, city), they may also be affiliated because they share a common life style, value system, culture, or interest (e.g., Amish, Hasidic Jews). A cultural community may extend across countries and join members internationally in a common set of beliefs and practices that bond the members to each other and create a community that is grounded in its beliefs and life style. Communities are also defined by social affiliations or memberships (e.g., American Nurses Association, National Student Nurses Association). A common health issue or common experience can create a profound bond that is stronger than any cultural or geographical boundaries (e.g., People With AIDS Coalition, Survivors of Suicide, Parents of Murdered Children). The attachments among affected people provide support that is inaccessible through traditional organizations. Individuals may also identify with each other through a common problem or through a solution (e.g., environmental groups concerned with global warming or the scarcity of wildlife).

Community as Partner

Nursing models are significant to community health nursing in appreciating the nature of the community. The community-as-partner model refers to the community as "a group, population, or cluster of people with at least one common characteristic (such as geographical location, occupation, ethnicity, or housing condition)" (Anderson & McFarlane, 1996, p. 261). The target of this model is the community as a whole. The total community is viewed as a partner in care. Congruent with the principles of primary health care, this model supports the community's competence to deal with its own problems, strengthen its own level of health, and act to defend against stressors. The community is viewed as a system, comprised of a central core that defines the people, their values, beliefs, and history and eight subsystems that define the functional aspects of the community. The eight subsystems are: the physical environment; education; safety and transportation; politics and government; health and social services; communication; economics; and recreation. The nursing process is used to guide nursing care of the community.

Community as Caregiver

The community can be viewed as a caregiving agent. Not unlike an individual engaging in self-care or a family providing a caring context for its members, the community is also a living system with the potential to render a caring environment for its members. The members of a community contribute through their individual and united efforts to the community's ability to care for its members. A caring community is the fostering of an environment that supports its members. Consider the following journal entry about a caring community written by a baccalaureate student during her senior practicum in community health nursing.

CASE HISTORY: A CARING COMMUNITY

On a typical weekday morning, the streets of Branton are congested with people, cars, buses, and double-parked trucks. Thick clouds of smoke and the tops of some of the tallest building in the world outline the skyline of a major city, which is approximately 20 min away. Branton, a small community within the outskirts of the city, is a place where a student nurse would never expect to find an absolutely perfect example of a community supporting one of its members—that is, a true "textbook" case, a case that a student may read about as part of an assignment but never expect to see in real life! Well, my expectations proved to be incorrect. It was in the community of Branton that I witnessed the finest example of community support. Branton was the support and lifeline of a developmentally disabled 62-year-old man who had multiple medical and psychosocial problems and no family member in close proximity. The community was his family, in every sense, and he, in turn, was an asset to the community.

It was a cold winter morning, and I was doing my first week of my senior practicum in community health nursing. My preceptor, Ms. Maureen Oliver, R.N., N.P., double-parked in front of a bakery. She asked me to wait in the car while she beeped our next patient, Mr. Timothy Woods. I was not sure why she had to beep Mr. Woods, but I was reluctant to question Ms. Oliver.

While sitting in the car, I recalled the words of my community health nursing professor: "When dealing with the community as a client, a "windshield survey" of the community will aid in the assessment process of the community and facilitate the gathering of valuable data." Thus, I took the time to observe my surroundings. Branton is a small community, only 10–15 blocks. The bakery was on the main street of the neighborhood, a street that consisted of various stores, including a hardware store, beauty salon, dry cleaner, pizza parlor, fruit stand, and gift shop. There were apartments above many of the storefront buildings, typical of many communities that surrounded the city. The streets were clean, and the buildings were

Windshield Survey. This survey is conducted by driving or walking around a community and recording direct observations. Included among the observations are data about the physical environment (e.g., dwellings, open spaces, commercial space, industry, physical boundaries) and the values, beliefs, and religions of the community.

occupied and in good repair, atypical of many of the surrounding neighborhoods of this city. The population included persons of various nationalities, and many different languages could be heard in the streets. The socioeconomic status of most of the people I observed appeared to be lower to middle income.

Ms. Oliver returned to the car with three cups of coffee. I offered to pay for my cup, but she informed me that the bakery always gave her two free cups of coffee for her and Mr. Woods—and one for me today. She told me we needed to wait in the car and look out for Mr. Woods who normally responded to the page within 5 to 10 min. I asked Ms. Oliver to explain. Mr. Woods carries a beeper, and he knows that when he gets a beep with a #1 it is the community health nurse or the social worker, and he comes to meet the health care provider at his apartment, which Ms. Oliver pointed out to me. Mr. Woods lives on the second floor above a row of stores. Ms. Oliver further explained that Mr. Woods did various jobs for many of the stores in the neighborhood and received services in return. He ran errands for the woman who owned the beauty parlor (i.e., bringing her customers coffee or lunch), and in return, he received regular haircuts. He cleaned the area in front of the dry cleaner who, in turn, would clean and press Mr. Wood's clothes. The landlord of Mr. Wood's building allowed Mr. Woods to do odd jobs, which were needed to maintain the property. When anyone in the neighborhood wanted to contact Mr. Woods, they would "beep" him. Although Mr. Woods was unable to read or write, he knew how to respond to his beeper. The beauty parlor paged him with a #2, the dry cleaner with a #3, and his landlord with a #4.

As Ms. Oliver spoke, I continued to observe the busy streets of Branton. Ms. Oliver then pointed straight ahead and said, "Here he comes!" I looked in the direction of her pointed finger and saw a sight I will always remember—a man in his early 60s, meticulously dressed in an overcoat, hat, scarf, and gloves, pulling a small cart that contained a broom, shovel, some plastic garbage bags, rags, and bottles of window cleaner. He was strutting down the street while greeting people with a big smile and a friendly wave. The man exhibited great pride and looked liked a politician campaigning for office. Everyone on the street seemed to know him as though he was the town mayor!

We got out of the car to meet Mr. Woods who was busy locking up his cart to the street sign located directly in front of the door to his apartment. Mr. Woods greeted Ms. Oliver with a warm and friendly hello and led us into his building. Ms. Oliver had explained to Mr. Woods at the end of her last home visit that she would be working with a student nurse for the next 10 weeks and asked his permission to allow me to observe and participate in his nursing care. He was responsive to this arrangement and gave me a warm and friendly welcome as I was introduced to him. He repeated several times that it is important to teach others what you can do so that they can do it too.

Mr. Woods was unable to read and had the developmental level of a school-age child. A care plan for Mr. Woods was developed that was appropriate to his developmental level. Mr. Woods had an intense desire to be independent and was able to learn self-care procedures readily.

Mr. Woods started receiving home care after coronary bypass surgery. After his recovery from this condition, his needs were assessed, and it was determined that he was eligible to receive services of the long-term home health care program. He had insulin-dependent diabetes mellitus, and he had a cystostomy tube in place. Medication bottles were color coded, and Mr. Woods was taught to take a pill from the blue bottle in the morning and a pill from the red bottle before he went to sleep. Mr. Woods was also taught how to care for his cystostomy tube. He demonstrated this care to the community health nurse on her biweekly visits. Mr. Woods tested his blood glucose level two times a day. He used a glucose monitor with a memory feature. It stored his glucose levels for 1 week. Ms. Oliver would record and monitor these levels weekly.

The community health nursing care Mr. Woods received, coupled with the support of his community, enabled Mr. Woods to function at an optimal level in his environment. The community health nursing service provided high-quality care with consistent interventions and evaluation. The members of the community provided acceptance, love, support, and a sense of belonging, all of which are necessary to maintain a high level of wellness. The community health nurse, the client, and the community formed an alliance in caring (Roni Schloss, B.S., R.N.).

Community as an Alliance for Health

Through the unique collaboration taking place among the members of the community, community health nurse, and the interdisciplinary team, a collective is formed enabling a focus on the health of the community. The Alliance for Health Model (see Chap. 5) portrays the community as comprised of interacting forces that are shaped by the community members who in conjunction with the community health nurse and interdisciplinary team are able to exert an influence on these forces. The three interacting forces are the community-based needs, the systems that provide and manage health care responding to these needs, and the influences on decisions for allocating the resources to support the systems of care. The effect of the alliance is a reshaping of the allocation decisions in support of the systems of care that change to address the community's health needs. The Alliance enables consumer and providers of the community to work together to discover the nature of community health needs, the strengths and deficiencies of the systems of care management, and the effectiveness of the allocation decisions to support the health resource of the community.

Focus on Community-Based Needs	Care Management Techniques
Patterns of morbidity and mortality	Mix of client problems
Demographics	Expectations of the public for care
Environmental concerns	Competence of professionals
Public services	Accepted standards of care
Aesthetics	Use of interdisciplinary care plans
Health-related facilities	or action plans

Influences on Resource Allocation Decisions
Patterns of resource allocation
Values and beliefs of the population
Reliance on local, regional,
    and federal government funding
Influences of special interest groups
Patterns of insurance coverage

FIGURE 6-1.

☒

Alliance for Health Model

Self-Definition of the Community

The community health nurse joins with the community in participation and exchange. Through this experience of working with the community, the nurse becomes part of the community. Since each community is unique as well as complex, the community health nurse develops a particular expertise in understanding the nature and type of community that is the focus of care. The community health nurse synthesizes knowledge about communities in general with specific experiential knowledge to develop a self-definition of the community of concern. Appreciating the unique components of the community, including the population of the community and the resources, culture, economics, and geography of the community, assist the nurse in forming an image of the community that is useful in understanding the community as a whole.

$\mathcal{S}$UMMARY

A community is comprised of people in interaction with their environment. A community is a system that performs functions in much the same way a family performs functions for its members. The community can be a caregiving agent, a nurturer, and a sustainer. A healthy community can foster growth of its members through the effective management of its functions.

A community has quantitative and qualitative characteristics that can be assessed and described. How and what to assess in a community is covered in Chap. 8 on community assessment and diagnosis.

As consumers use community resources that goodness of fit between providers or agencies and consumers can be monitored as patterns of health services and patterns of use are analyzed. Finally, a community can attain achievable criteria that measure its degree of health. A healthy community can be defined, and the community health nurse working with the community can identify its health strengths, health risks, and health

Goodness of Fit. This term refers to unions created through understanding and appropriate responsiveness (e.g., providers and consumers join to form an effective alliance; agencies and clients work together so that clients' needs are addressed effectively by agency services).

problems. The community health nurse can develop skills in community assessment, diagnosis, planning, implementation, and evaluation. The actualization of the nursing process in the care of the community as client is delineated in Chaps. 8 to 10.

The focus of all community care is to foster the health of the community. The community health nurse can benefit from an understanding of the nature and types of community from various perspectives, but the key to caring for the community is the ability to create a personal definition of community to guide and inspire community-based nursing practice. Nursing interactions and interventions with the community as client and utilization of the nursing process to intercede with communities is the essence of community health nursing.

KEY WORDS

Demography
Gatekeeper
Gemeinschaft
Gesellschaft

Goodness of fit
Typology
Windshield survey

QUESTIONS

Directions: Choose the one *best* response to each of the following questions.

1. In understanding the community, the nurse considers which one of the following parameters to be most important?
   A. Place and location
   B. People in interaction with environment
   C. Socioeconomic resources
   D. Power structures

2. The anatomy and physiology of a community can be likened to its
   A. structure and function.
   B. history and leadership.
   C. health risks and problems.
   D. health services and providers.

3. The characteristics of a Gemeinschaft community are
   A. bureaucracy and "red tape."
   B. status and rank.
   C. common interest and mutual participation.
   D. authority and vertical structure.

4. Affiliations that help members of a community to form a common bond include

   A. racial tension.
   B. ethnocentricism.
   C. geographical distance.
   D. culture.

5. The function of forming linkages within a community refers to

   A. providing housing and places for socialization.
   B. making connections to other systems to meet the needs of membership.
   C. enforcing norms and controls.
   D. enabling socialization and enrichment of the members.

Questions 6 to 11

DIRECTIONS: The group of questions below consists of lettered choices followed by several numbered items. For each numbered item, select the appropriate lettered option with which it is most closely associated. Each lettered option may be used once, more than once, or not at all.

Match each type of community with a defining characteristic.

A. Rapid turnover	6. Integral community
B. Mistrust	7. Parochial community
C. Protective	8. Diffuse community
D. Disorganized	9. Stepping stone community
E. Cohesive	10. Transitory community
F. Lacking shared norms	11. Anomic community

ANSWERS

1. *The answer is B.* The most important parameter for understanding the community is people in interaction with the environment.

2. *The answer is A.* The anatomy and physiology of a community can be likened to its structure and function.

3. *The answer is C.* A Gemeinschaft community is characterized by common interest and mutual participation.

4. *The answer is D.* Culture is an affiliation that joins members of a community to form a common bond.

5. *The answer is B.* Forming linkages within a community refers to making connections to other systems to meet the needs of members.

6–11. *The answers are: 6-E, 7-C, 8-F, 9-A, 10-B, 11-D.* An integral community is characterized as cohesive. A parochial community is characterized as protective. A diffuse community is characterized as lacking shared norms. A stepping stone community is characterized by rapid turnover. A transitory community is characterized by mistrust. An anomic community is characterized as disorganized.

ANNOTATED REFERENCES

Anderson, E. T., & McFarlane, J. M. (1996). *Community as partner: Theory and practice in nursing* (2nd ed.). Philadelphia: J. B. Lippincott.

This detailed text provides multiple frameworks for viewing the community as a system, including primary health care, epidemiology, demography, research, ecology, advocacy, and culture as well as the community-as-partner model. A complete community assessment is illustrated as well as exemplars of community as partner.

Hall, J. E., & Weaver, B. R. (1977). *Distributive nursing practice: A systems approach to community health.* Philadelphia: J. B. Lippincott.

This is a classic community health nursing text that provides a strong systems theory framework for viewing the community and guiding community health nursing practice.

Higgs, Z. R., & Gustafson, D. D. (1985). *Community as a client: Assessment and diagnosis.* Philadelphia: F. A. Davis.

This is an important reference text covering conceptual approaches (e.g., epidemiological, descriptive, systems, adaption) to community assessment and clinical judgment for community diagnoses. Case studies in community assessment and the application of various nursing theories are useful.

Loomis, C. P. (Ed.). (1957). *Tönnies: Community & society (Gemeinschaft und Gesellschaft).* East Lansing, MI: Michigan State University Press.

This is a translation from the German of Ferdinand Tönnies' 1887 classic treatise in sociology, entitled Gemeinschaft und Gesellschaft, *detailing the work of this eminent sociologist. The editor proclaims the purpose of* Gemeinschaft und Gesellschaft *was to develop scientific concepts that could be used as tools to grasp the historical process.*

Warren, D. I. (1977). Neighborhoods in urban areas. In R. L. Warren (Ed.), *New perspectives on the American community: A book of readings.* Chicago: Rand McNally.

This is another collection of Roland Warren's work on American communities. In his chapter on neighborhoods, Donald I. Warren defines a neighborhood and outlines a typology of neighborhoods, including their roles in social change.

COMMUNITY AS CLIENT

The idea of caring for a community as a client is complex. Many of the same clinical skills used in caring for an individual or a family can be used in caring for a community. At the outset, it may seem impossible to extrapolate clinical skills used in caring for individuals to the level of the community, but it is possible. The use of the nursing process in the care of communities is covered in Chaps. 8 to 10, and the specific skills are detailed. This chapter provides a framework for viewing the community as a **unit of care**. The focus of this chapter is on community-based health care when the community is the client system.

COMMUNITY AS A SYSTEM

The community operates as a system. To understand the nature of the community, the component parts typically are analyzed. However, breaking the community into its component parts may help the community health nurse to understand the components but does not necessarily give the whole picture of the community. Trying to identify the whole takes a degree of expertise in working with the community.

To appreciate this property of wholeness, the community health nurse must analyze the component parts of a community, their qualitative and quantitative attributes, and the interrelatedness of these components. It is the dynamic interconnectedness among the components, their attributes, and their interrelationships that begins to explain wholeness. The nature of wholeness is, therefore, defined as being more than and different from the

Unit of Care. This is the target for the delivery of nursing services that can be either an individual, family, aggregate, or community.

sum of its parts—that is, the sum of the parts is less than the whole. The relationships of the parts to the whole are instructive in trying to comprehend the individual as a human system, as well as the community as a whole living system.

An individual cannot be explained by understanding the body systems of the human being apart from the culture of the individual, the religion of the individual, and the family of the individual. Although each component (body systems, culture, religion, family) describes a component part of the individual, it is not until these components (as well as a multitude of other components) interact with each other that the unique pattern of a particular individual is formed. The whole individual is unique, complex, and multifaceted. A community cannot be fully understood by examining its separate component parts either. The people, the resources, the topography, the history, and other components of the community interact to comprise the community as a whole living system. The individual, the family, and the community are interconnected and part of each other's systems. The interactions and interrelationships among these systems are characteristic of their wholeness (Fig. 7-1).

Thinking about human systems and the notion of wholeness is challenging. The community health nurse is challenged to identify indicators of wholeness and to plan and organize care that is supportive and sensitive to the whole community. Characterizing the wholeness of the community enables the community health nurse to identify accurately its health

FIGURE 7-1.

🔳

Interacting Human Systems

Rings of concentric circles explain the interacting relationships among individuals, families, and communities. The inner circle represents the individual. The individual is part of and contributes to the proximate circle that defines the family and significant others. The family is part of and contributes to the ever expanding outer ring of the community. The community includes friends, neighbors, and aggregates large and small that identify and support the family and its individual members.

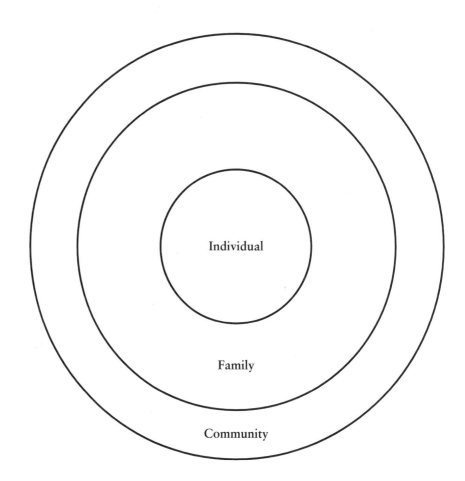

Individual

Family

Community

strengths, risks, and problems. Available community resources and community population characteristics are also identified. The community is considered the target of service when the nurse addresses community health concerns. The community health nurse focuses on facilitating healthful changes that benefit the community. The intent is to try to benefit as many members of the community as possible and improve the overall health status of the community. Pursuing the goal of improved community health is done with the client, which is the community.

As wholeness is understood, it is possible to imagine that the wholeness of a human system could never be reduced. If every human system is inherently holistic then attributes of the system may, in fact, reflect its wholeness. Even though culture alone could never fully explain the holistic nature of an individual, family, or community, culture may be an indicator of wholeness. Until the exact nature of holistic indicants are determined and the characteristics of wholeness critically defined, the component parts of systems and their attributes are examined in order to speculate about their interactions. To comprehend the whole community as a living system, the component parts of the community are investigated, the qualitative and quantitative attributes of the components are analyzed, and the components and their attributes are related to each other.

The capacity of caring may be a holistic indicator—that is, the wholeness of a community may be reflected in its capacity to care about its members. When engaging the community as the client, the community health nurse becomes part of this caring capacity of the community, influencing the health potential of the whole community as positively as possible, given the constraints and obstacles that impede community health.

$\mathcal{V}$IEWING THE COMMUNITY

One way of looking at the community is to focus on the individuals, families, and aggregates within the community. There is a reciprocal relationship among these component parts and the community as a whole. Interventions that support the health of individuals, families, groups, and populations within the community also support the community's health. A change in the health of an individual, a family, or a group affects the health of the community. Community health is reflected in the health of its subsystems or component parts. For example, reducing the risks of a target population within the community, improving the health status of families, and restoring the health of an individual improve the health of the community. Individuals, families, and communities are linked and influence each other. Further, if a community's health is depleted, the individuals, families, and populations within that community are affected and their health is compromised. This interrelatedness is an illustration of community wholeness.

The community health nurse can circumscribe a community of interest when addressing specific health concerns. Boundaries can be contracted or expanded to focus on a particular unit of care. For example, a nurse may identify an aggregate of preschool children as a community to assess and

Aggregate. "An aggregate is a group of people who share some common aspect, such as age, economic status, cultural background, gender, race, area of residence, chronic illness, and so on" (Swanson & Albrecht, 1993, p. 568).

analyze their health care needs and the resources available to address their needs. This group of children can be considered a community within a community. An analysis of all preschool children in the United States may be designated as the unit of care. The boundaries of a community can be flexible and can expand or contract to enable the community health nurse to work collaboratively with a community of interest in addressing specific health concerns.

Multifaceted Communities

Appreciation of the many faces of a community guides the nurse in determining the focus of health care as well as the location of health care services. Communities can be hamlets, villages, counties, urban areas, states, nations, as well as schools, houses of worship, occupational sites, apartment buildings, prisons, and cultural groups. The component parts of these communities are individuals in relationships and family or group networks.

Some communities are defined by geographical configurations such as rivers, streams, and mountain ranges; physical forces and the power of nature circumscribe the boundaries of a community. Geopolitical boundaries may also define a community. School districts often create their own lines of service, resulting in children living on the same block but attending different schools. Cultural, religious, or racial bonds can shape a community and provide an image as well as define a jurisdiction. Not only is space used differently, but dress, food, values, and behaviors can vary considerably from one community to another even though the communities may be in close proximity.

The many faces of community are important for the community health nurse to appreciate and accept. Capturing the essence of a community's wholeness is connected to appreciating the persona of the community. Diversity within communities is the essence of the multifaceted nature of community.

Diversity within Communities

A healthy community is one that accepts the diversity of its membership, not allowing differences to separate or alienate members from each other. In some communities, people of different racial, ethnic, and religious groups live together in harmony; in others, a group's desire for privacy and homogeneity is accepted and respected by the larger community. However, when racism, discrimination, and forced isolation alienate members from each other, misunderstanding and hostility result. A community riddled with racism and discrimination can then be viewed as fragmented and unhealthy. In such a community, members are isolated and limited from full participation in the community by virtue of their heritage or culture. This form of alienation damages the ability of the community to be whole and healthy. The capacity for the appreciation and acceptance of diversity is a way to view the community and its responsiveness to its members.

Vulnerable Communities

The community health nurse directs special attention to the health care needs of community groups that are underserved and vulnerable. This valuing is a key to the nature of community health nursing. These groups are often ignored or treated as superfluous by the larger society. One of the greatest challenges of caring for the community as a client is linking all members in need of health services to available resources and advocating for those unable to represent themselves or unable to access health services. Although community health nurses serve the health needs of the entire population, they are especially sensitized to the special needs of people with few, if any, resources. The community health nurse attempts to reconnect members who are disconnected from the health care system. The integrity of the community rests on its ability to care about all of its members.

Linkages within Communities

Community health nurses know how communities operate, how to access health care, and which are the best resources for specific health problems; they also serve to link people to needed resources. The goal of the community health nurse is to achieve a "goodness of fit" between people and resources so that health needs are addressed. A multiplicity of needs is assessed through a partnership between the nurse and the client. No one in the community is superfluous to the community health nurse, who should be prepared to address the needs of all clients.

With knowledge of community resources, the community health nurse can help even those who are cut off or alienated to make connections that will benefit their health. Because there is an identified need does not mean that the client is ready to utilize care or wants the community health nurse to facilitate that linkage. The client may view the situation very differently from the community health nurse and may not perceive a need for help, or the client may perceive a need for help but seek a different solution than the community health nurse's recommendation. Validation of perceptions and mutual agreement on an identified plan are key to expediting effective linkages. The community health nurse must be knowledgeable about community resources to facilitate an effective linkage once the client and nurse reach a mutual agreement.

Preventive Intervention within Communities

The community health nurse views the community as a client with health care concerns requiring all levels of preventive intervention. Given an epidemiological framework, the community health nurse is aware that health care concerns are complex and multidimensional. Interventions are focused at all three levels of intervention: primary, secondary, and tertiary (Leavell & Clark, 1965). Every health care concern potentially includes all levels of prevention that guide intervention. The community health nurse with this expansive view of health is able to help the community realize a multitude of actions to address health concerns and problems.

Viewing the community from a primary prevention perspective, the community health nurse works with the community to promote and protect the health of the community and its members. This may entail educational outreach to community groups or arranging for influenza vaccinations for a particular population within the community. From a secondary prevention perspective, the community health nurse helps the community by providing screening opportunities for the early detection of illnesses, expedites the treatment of illnesses, and limits disabilities that may result from illnesses and health problems. Blood pressure screenings at community libraries and mammography screenings offered via mobile vans reaching out into the community are characteristic of this type of intervention. For interventions geared at tertiary prevention, the community health nurse assists the community to identify health care resources that focus on rehabilitation and resocialization and provide care for members and their families who experience chronic and terminal illnesses. The community health nurse may advocate for public service reform, which may result in structural changes to sidewalk curbs enabling access for people using wheelchairs and may provide community education about hospice care and services for families coping with terminal illness.

These levels of prevention provide a trajectory from which to view the community. The community health nurse is always concerned with primary prevention intervention, ever mindful of the importance of health promotion and protection as an ideal to be realized.

If a community is at risk for spontaneous forest fires, the efforts of the community health nurse would be concerned principally with fire prevention strategies (primary prevention). If uncontrolled fires break out, the community health nurse would be involved in triage and the treatment of those injured as well as assisting with the design of a surveillance method to detect new fires early to limit possible damage (secondary prevention) The rehabilitation of injured community members, the revitalization of community resources, and the rehabilitation of destroyed lands would comprise the recovery phase (tertiary prevention). Thus, the community health nurse is concerned with the promotion and protection of the health and well-being of both the unaffected and affected community members as well as the environment.

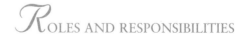

ROLES AND RESPONSIBILITIES

Whenever possible, the community health nurse views the community from the vantage point of the community itself. Whether a community health nurse is making a home visit to an individual, providing family-based care in a managed care setting, or organizing a community safety program, the community health nurse must remain aware of the fact that the practice is based on the client's turf. The community health nurse often intervenes in family history, beliefs, culture, and dynamics. At the same time, the nurse attempts to effect a family-based plan of care, interceding with an array of community agencies, protocols, and hierarchies. The nurse can support, facilitate, teach, advocate, screen, and offer management skills, but the ultimate goal is decisions for action that come from the community, if they possess the ability to be self-directed.

Community-based services are best delivered directly to the community, eliminating as many obstacles and barriers to care as possible. Community outreach is key. To illustrate, if screening for window guards is an agreed-upon strategy to prevent the death of young children from accidental falls from windows, then community health nurses, in conjunction with other health care providers, would best accomplish this task by going door-to-door. In this way, the service is brought directly to the homes of families with young children. First, widespread community education targets families with young children. Families are not expected to travel to a health center to ask for information about how to install window guards, but rather, the community health nurse and other members of the health care team bring that service directly to the families' homes to increase the likelihood that these families will install window guards. The community health nurse would also use the window guard screening as a method of case finding to learn about other health problems or concerns of the family. Screenings are also a way to link community members to health care resources and services.

*I*NTERDISCIPLINARY APPROACH

Community health care needs are often complex and require the skill and expertise of a wide range of health care providers, including community health nurses. The blending of disciplines is referred to as a multidisciplinary or interdisciplinary approach. An interdisciplinary approach permits the synthesis of a full range of skills, talents, and experiences of a variety of health care providers. The community as client through its representative members also brings its expertise to the team and participates fully in the process of planning the changes for improved health.

The community health nurse plays a pivotal role in the team approach. The community health nurse coordinates the assessment, planning, implementation, and evaluation processes and creates alliances for the improved health of the community. The community health nurse is best prepared to represent the client in this process through the nurse's holistic appraisal of the clients's experience and need. Roles commonly performed by the community health nurse enhance this process. The community health nurse is skilled in individual and group therapeutic communication, serves as a communication link to coordinate services, and is proficient in health education and guidance strategies. The community health nurse provides liaison skills between formal and informal systems of care. The community health nurse facilitates transitions between systems of care by use of the discharge planning process that enables the delivery of coordinated and seamless care. The discharge planning process assures the continuity of care as clients transfer from various settings and levels of care. Continuity of care assures the coordinated delivery of ongoing services as needed.

The role of communication facilitator for interdisciplinary team members and community members is referred to as being a communication broker. The community health nurse functions in this role to represent and negotiate exchanges between community members and multidisciplinary team members to effect a health care plan. This role is most often fulfilled by advanced practice nurses—that is, nurses with a master's degree in nursing (ANA, 1993). These community health nurses are prepared to direct their expertise at community health planning and resource development.

$\mathcal{E}$XTENDING KNOWLEDGE OF THE COMMUNITY

Part of the expertise of the community health nurse is a foundation in nursing research. This perspective provides a rich opportunity for verifying and extending knowledge of the community and its members. Epidemiological data are used to monitor and predict patterns of morbidity and mortality and to generate population-based data, which are used to evaluate the need for community-based health services and the responsiveness of the community to address these needs. Nursing research includes the development of strategies to meet the needs of community members, particularly underserved populations. Data are used to understand the health status and health problems of populations and to measure the cost-effectiveness of interventions. Research assists the community health nurse to analyze the needs of the community and use community resources that serve the community. Research provides the community health nurse with information to make healthful changes that benefit the whole community.

The community health nurse views the community as client and gears all interactions and interventions to support the community in achieving its health goals. Being goal-directed is an indicator of health. Goals for health can be identified through a collaborative partnership between the community and the community health nurse. The active involvement of clients and communities in the whole spectrum of care is key to the assessment of the need for care, the design of health care programs, specific interventions, and the evaluation of outcomes. This partnership between providers and consumers of care is the foundation for community-based care. The community health nurse transfers knowledge and skills to the community. Community participation assures the likelihood of care choices that are culturally sensitive and pertinent to the community and its members.

$\mathcal{C}$OMMUNITY-BASED HEALTH CARE

The National Nursing Research Agenda (National Institute of Nursing Research, 1995) identified six challenges to the development of community-based health care strategies based on the work of Krout (1986, 1994). The six challenges are: availability, accessibility, affordability, appropriateness, adequacy, and acceptability. These six challenges concern the provision of care as well as the reception of care. The perspectives of both the providers and the recipients of care may vary considerably. Therefore, both perspectives consider and respond to these challenges. Implicit in these challenges, and equally essential, is the importance of cultural sensitivity and relevance. Culturally sensitive and relevant care is imperative to realize fully and measure accurately service utilization and health care outcomes.

Descriptions of the six challenges to delivering community-based care are summarized below (National Institute of Nursing Research, 1995, p. 19). The challenges must be addressed as community-based health care strategies build on the concepts embedded in primary health care and should be taken into account when planning successful community-based care:

- Availability refers to the number, types, range, and frequency of health and social services offered.
- Accessibility refers to the ability of persons to make use of services, encompassing distance, effort, cost, and awareness of the services. Accessibility includes attention to qualities such as the comfort level of persons entering the health care system.
- Affordability refers to the ability of consumers to pay for services and the mechanisms to secure payment for programs (e.g., voluntary contributions or fees).
- Appropriateness refers to the ability of the health care program to provide the services that are needed, desired, and performed.
- Adequacy refers to the ability of a program to allow persons to enter at the levels they need.
- Acceptability refers to the congruence between the service and the expectations, attitudes, values, culture, and beliefs of the target population. Acceptability is paramount, for if health care is not acceptable to the target population, the services provided will not be effective.

Six Challenges to the Development of Community-Based Health Care (National Institute of Nursing Research, 1995)

Availability
Accessibility
Affordability
Appropriateness
Adequacy
Acceptability

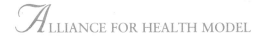

ALLIANCE FOR HEALTH MODEL

Partnerships or linkages among providers, consumers, and insurers of health care are necessary for the development of community-based health care strategies. The Alliance Model for Community Health Assessment (see Chap. 5) blends community-based needs, systems of care management, and resource allocation decisions together for the most coordinated and responsive fit. The expertise of the interdisciplinary team in partnership with the community shapes the response and creates a "goodness of fit." The idea of linkages or alliances is the core concept in understanding the community and in serving the health care needs of communities. Through effective linkages among providers and consumers and those making decisions about funding health services and resources, there is a sharing of knowledge, skills, and power. Therapeutic linkages must be forged between consumers and health care resources so health care needs can be met.

Constructive linkages created among community members strengthen the fabric of the community and reflect the health condition of the community.

Community-based health care is an integrated system of care. Community-based health care includes the three levels of prevention: primary prevention (involving health promotion and health protection); secondary prevention (encompassing screening, early detection, treatment of acute illness, and limiting disability); and tertiary prevention (including restorative care, a focus on chronicity, and care in terminal illness). Community-based health care traverses a continuum of care that is a client-focused alliance supportive of a seamless system of care that uses a comprehensive array of services to improve the health of the community.

POPULATIONS AT RISK AND AGGREGATE-BASED CARE

Community health nurses direct a major portion of their attention to populations at risk within the community. A population at risk is defined as people with high vulnerability to certain health problems. The identification of populations at risk is key to improving the health of the community as a whole. At-risk populations are targeted for direct services to reduce their health risks and to improve their level of health. Populations at risk are aggregates with characteristics or behaviors that increase the likelihood for developing diseases or health disorders. As the health risks of these aggregates increase, increased demands are made on the health care system for services and programs to address these needs, which result in increased health care costs. When segments of the population experience health depletion, they generally become less effective contributors to the community, resulting in reduced community productivity. Individuals and aggregates at high risk also suffer a diminished quality of life.

The community consequences for untreated populations at risk can be devastating. The community becomes depleted when its members are unable to achieve their individual and collective health potential. Changes in the health status of individuals and families affect the health of the entire community. Beneficial community health changes usually require simultaneous changes at the social level. To maintain or improve the community's health, all of its resources are mobilized and often services must be added to address undertreated conditions and underserved populations.

The community health nurse is concerned about the total population of the community and directs services both to people who use available health care resources as well as to those who do not use these services. Some members of the community are skilled at resource utilization while other members of the community are unable to locate a way into the health care system and as a result are disenfranchised and superfluous to the system of care. The community health nurse attends to the needs of all members of the community but is especially focused on people at risk and people unconnected to the available health care resources. The community health nurse respects the decisions of people who by choice do not wish to participate in health care decisions or to use the resources of the health care system.

The community health nurse should be knowledgeable about health risks associated with aggregates, particularly those risk factors that can be modified to reduce the risk for given health conditions. The community health nurse uses demographic data and patterns of morbidity and mortality to identify risk patterns. The leading causes of illness and death are monitored for trends that reveal opportunities for health teaching, health guidance, screening, case finding, and community-based risk-reduction strategies. The community health nurse is aware of interventions for reducing, modifying, or eliminating significant risk factors. Central to intervention strategies is recognition of the fact that morbidity and mortality patterns can be altered through personal life-style changes. Life-style change is important to risk reduction for the top-ranking causes of death. Consider the controllable risk factors for the leading causes of death in the United States: smoking, hypertension, obesity, elevated serum cholesterol levels, and alcohol and drug abuse. These are all modifiable through personal risk-reduction strategies, like smoking cessation, blood pressure control, weight reduction, proper nutrition selections, and alcohol and substance abuse treatment. When the community health nurse promotes the health of individuals, their families, and significant others in high-risk populations, the health of the entire community improves. The community health nurse is caring for the community as client.

To monitor population-based health data, the community health nurse can refer to epidemiologic and demographic sources. Documents such as *Healthy People 2000: National Health Promotion and Disease Prevention Objectives* (1991), *Healthy People 2000 Review 1994* (1995), and *Healthy People 2000 Midcourse Review and 1995 Revisions* (1995) provide detailed goals and priorities for the nation's prevention agenda. These reports indicate that concerted action is required to strengthen the public health system at state and local levels to assure the delivery of services that keep the population healthy. The stated goals call for payment systems that reward providers and health plans that keep people healthy. Systems for data management are also required to provide information on patterns of disease, emerging diseases, immunization rates, and utilization practices and cost-effectiveness of preventive health services. These data are used to direct public policy to promote health and assist individuals to select healthy life styles. The *Healthy People 2000 Midcourse Review and 1995 Revisions* highlights three goals of *Healthy People 2000*. The first goal is to increase the span of healthy life for all Americans, placing emphasis on healthy years not just longevity. The second goal is to close the gaps in health status and outcomes between ethnic and racial minorities and the total population—that is, reducing health disparities among Americans. The third goal is a commitment to assure universal access to preventive health services as part of primary care. Although consensus can be achieved about what essential services should be made available, one of the major barriers to the delivery of these services has been the decline in the percentage of Americans with health insurance coverage. *Healthy People 2000* details 22 priority areas

TABLE 7-1

PRIORITY AREAS FOR HEALTH PROMOTION ACTION

Physical activity and fitness	Food and drug safety
Nutrition	Oral health
Tobacco	Maternal and infant health
Alcohol and other drugs	Heart disease and stroke
Family planning	Cancer
Mental health and mental disorders	Diabetes and chronic disabling conditions
Violent and abusive behavior	Human immunodeficiency virus (HIV) infection
Educational and community-based programs	Sexually transmitted diseases
Unintentional injuries	Immunization and infectious diseases
Occupational safety and health	Clinical preventive services
Environmental health	Surveillance and data systems

NOTE: From *Healthy People 2000: National Health Promotion and Disease Prevention Objectives* (p. 7), by U.S. Department of Health and Human Services, 1991, Washington, DC: Author. Reprinted with permission.

for health promotion action (Table 7-1). The community health nurse works with documents like *Healthy People 2000* to align local community efforts with national and state targets and to improve the health of communities as well as the collective community, the United States.

GAINING KNOWLEDGE OF THE COMMUNITY

There are multiple sources of data available to learn about the community. Chapter 8 details the process for uncovering information about the community, including the community health nurse's own personal assessment, using the senses and observation skills. A helpful community resource for gathering community data is the key informant in the community. A key informant is someone who is knowledgeable about the population and services of the community. A key informant is willing to talk with someone from outside the community and share this knowledge. The community health nurse keeps in mind that key informants present information about the community from their own unique perspectives. Data are validated as additional sources confirm the findings.

The community health nurse asks for the key informant's perception of actual and potential health problems, characteristics of the population, values and beliefs of the community, the usefulness and appropriateness of community resources to the members, and community strengths. The description of evidence that accompanies the personal views of the key

Key Informant. This is a member of the community who is willing to share knowledge about the community, including information about the population and services of the community, with an outsider.

informant is especially valuable. The community health nurse asks how the key informant came to such conclusions. Also instructive is the key informant's perspective on how community health problems could be remediated and solved.

Key informants may also serve as gatekeepers to the community. Gatekeepers enable outsiders to access a client system just as opening a gate permits access to a home or building. In a community, the gatekeeper monitors input and output of the community and enables the community health nurse to gain entree to the community. Gatekeepers are not necessarily also key informants. The difference is the key informant is wiling to communicate about the community with someone outside the community. The gatekeeper may not necessarily communicate information about the community and its resources but does exert power in community structures that permit access and the ability to move about in the community. Key informants and gatekeepers serve vital roles in the community and are instrumental in assisting the community health nurse to gather information about the community.

SUMMARY

The richness of a community can be realized on completion of a careful community assessment and a meticulous application of the nursing process in caring for communities. This chapter is designed to reinforce the importance of viewing the community as a client system. The community health nurse cares for human systems and works to improve the level of health of all individuals. To achieve this mission, the community health nurse directs all nursing actions toward the community as a whole. Data on the health strengths, risks, and problems of the community are analyzed. The strengths of the community provide the energy to mobilize and deal with health risks and problems. Community strengths are identified to foster a sense of pride and accomplishment and create the linkages from which alliances can be formed. Multiple data sources are used to gather information about the community's ability to function and provide for its members. The community health nurse searches for key informants and gatekeepers that allow access to the community and that help to forge alliances for community health. Information about the community provides an action agenda that the community health nurse puts to use in partnership with other members of the health care team and with members of the community to address health care needs.

KEY WORDS

Aggregate	Key informant
Communication broker	Unit of care

QUESTIONS

DIRECTIONS: Choose the one *best* response to each of the following questions.

1. The property of system wholeness is best exemplified by which of the following statements?

    A. The sum of the parts equals the whole.
    B. The whole is constructed of equal and complementary parts.
    C. The whole is more than and different from the sum of the parts.
    D. Wholeness is not definable.

2. One of the challenges of delivering community-based care is the acceptability of the rendered services. Acceptability refers to

    A. congruence between the service and the expectations of the target population.
    B. number, types, range, and frequency of health and social services offered.
    C. ability of consumers to pay for the health care services.
    D. provision of services that are needed and desired by the target population.

3. The best definition of a population at risk is

    A. people who rely on social services for financial support.
    B. people who live far away from health care providers and hospitals.
    C. people who face many obstacles obtaining the necessities of life.
    D. people with an unusually high vulnerability to certain health problems.

4. The three stated goals of *Healthy People 2000* include all of the following except

    A. increasing the span of healthy life for all Americans.
    B. decreasing the prevalence of all communicable diseases.
    C. closing the gaps in health status and outcomes between ethnic minorities and the total population.
    D. assuring universal access to preventive health services as part of primary care.

5. A key informant in the community is someone who is knowledgeable about the community and

    A. keeps outsiders from entering the community and gaining access to community information.
    B. presents a biased view about the community, which is problematic for understanding the community.
    C. is willing to talk with someone from outside the community and share knowledge.
    D. uses knowledge to plan and develop health care resources for the community.

ANSWERS

1. *The answer is C.* The sum of the parts is less than the whole because the whole is more than and different from the sum of the parts.

2. *The answer is A.* Acceptability refers to the congruence between the service and the expectations, attitudes, values, culture, and beliefs of the target population. If the health care is not acceptable to the target population, the services provided will not be effective.

3. *The answer is D.* The best definition of a population at risk is people with an unusually high vulnerability to certain health problems.

4. *The answer is B.* Decreasing the prevalence of all communicable diseases is an important goal of public health programs, but it is not stated as one of the three goals of *Healthy People 2000*.

5. *The answer is C.* A key informant is someone who is knowledgeable about the population and services of the community and is willing to talk with someone from outside the community and share this knowledge.

ANNOTATED REFERENCES

American Nurses Association. (1993). Advanced practice nursing: A new age in health care. *Nursing Facts*. Washington, DC: Author.

This fact sheet provides data that substantiates how advance practice nurses (APNs) can be a critical link in the solution to America's health care crisis. Almost 140,000 APNs are carving out new roles in delivering timely, cost-effective, quality health care, especially to chronically underserved populations such as the elderly, people living in poverty, and those in rural areas. The efficacy of the emphasis on health promotion and disease prevention has already been proven. Cost-effectiveness relates to such factors as the employment setting, liability insurance, and the cost of education, especially as compared to physicians.

Krout, J. A. (1986). *The aged in rural America*. New York: Greenwood Press.

This book documents and analyzes the status and experiences of the elderly living in rural environments and investigates how they compare to the elderly living in more urban settings. Patterns analyzed include demographics, economics, work, retirement, leisure, physical and mental health, housing, transportation, and formal and informal support systems and services.

Krout, J. A. (Ed.). (1994). *Providing community-based services to the rural elderly*. Thousand Oaks, CA: Sage.

This book brings together information from both researchers and practitioners on community-based services for the rural elderly. It presents detailed and specific information on a wide range of community-based services that are needed by and available to elders living in rural areas. The book focuses on exploring how these services can be developed and provided given the realities of the rural setting, resources, and populations.

Leavell, H. R., & Clark, E. G. (1958). *Preventive medicine for the doctor in his community: An epidemiologic approach.* New York: McGraw-Hill.

This landmark text on preventive medicine includes review of the basic principles and the application of these principles to varying health conditions and to organized community action. It is recognized as the finest resource for explaining the natural history of disease and the levels of prevention. The information on the epidemiological approach and its contributions to preventive medicine are often quoted in community health publications.

National Institute of Nursing Research. (1995). *Community-based health care: Nursing strategies.* Bethesda, MD: Author.

This is a report of a National Institute of Nursing Research (NINR) Priority Expert Panel on nursing strategies for community-based health care. It is one of a series of expert panels instituted by the National Center for Nursing Research (NCNR) in conjunction with the development of the National Nursing Research Agenda (NNRA). It describes the concepts and definitions of community-based care, and it explores health in rural and urban America.

Swanson, J. M., & Albrecht, M. (1993). *Community health nursing: Promoting the health of aggregates.* Philadelphia: W. B. Saunders.

This is a community health nursing text that provides an aggregate approach to family and community health practice. It documents how existing social injustices prevent the realization of health as a right for all people. The authors focus on specific aggregates in the community and address the special health needs of selected aggregates.

U.S. Department of Health and Human Services. (1991). *Healthy people 2000: National health promotion and disease prevention objectives.* Washington, DC: Author.

This document serves as a guide to the nation's health goals targeting the year 2000 for achievement. It profiles the American people and the national progress in promoting health and preventing disease. It includes a discussion of the economics of prevention and the challenges and health goals for the year 2000, identifying health promotion, health protection, preventive services, and surveillance and data systems as priority areas. It analyzes the nation's health in relation to age groups and special populations.

U.S. Department of Health and Human Services. (1995). *Healthy people 2000 review, 1994.* Hyattsville, MD: Author.

This text presents a review of tracking data for all 300 original objectives and 223 special population subobjectives, utilizing tables, graphs, and narratives to describe progress toward the year 2000 targets.

U.S. Department of Health and Human Services. (1995). *Healthy people 2000: Midcourse review and 1995 revisions.* Washington, DC: Author.

This text is a report on the accomplishments following the release of Healthy People 2000: National Health Promotion and Disease Prevention Objectives *and the challenges remaining in preventing premature death and in improving health as the year 2000 approaches. It is a detailed progress report on the 22 identified priority areas and the consortium action being taken at the state level and through private and voluntary activities.*

COMMUNITY ASSESSMENT AND DIAGNOSIS

The nursing process defines interactions and interventions with client systems, whether that system is an individual, a family, an aggregate, or a community, and supplies a logical framework for the provision of nursing care. The nursing process involves four phases: assessing, planning, implementing, and evaluating. Nursing diagnosis, the culmination of assessment data, clarifies the health condition or problem needing nursing intervention. Essentially, the nursing process is a systematic way of determining a client's health status, isolating health concerns and problems, developing plans to remediate them, initiating actions to implement the plan, and finally, evaluating the adequacy of the plan in promoting wellness and problem resolution. Application of the nursing process to the community as client is the focus of this chapter.

This chapter explores the multiple dimensions of the assessment phase of the nursing process and concludes with examples of how to write nursing diagnoses that reflect the unique health needs and problems of the community. Further, the community is viewed from the perspective of its strengths as well as its health risks and problems. The nursing process should not be restricted to the identification of problems but also should reflect the rich and varied capabilities and strengths of a given client system. It is a process that involves critical analysis of significant data that are shaped by the perspective of the discipline of nursing. The nurse, client, and members of the interdisciplinary team work collaboratively in health problem recognition, planning and implementing care strategies, and evaluating their effectiveness. Lastly, the Alliance for Health Model provides the organizational structure for understanding the contributing and interacting forces that comprise the community. The components of this structure are: community-based needs, systems of care management, and the influences that determine

Community Assessment. This is the process of searching for and validating relevant community-based data, according to a specified method, to learn about the interactions among the people, resources, and environment. The term community assessment is used to denote one phase of the nursing process, the assessment phase, applied to the community as a client. The term may also be used more generically to encompass the entire nursing process as applied to the community.

Community Diagnosis. This is a statement of need, problem, risk, or strength of the community derived from a thoughtful analysis and synthesis of assessment data. A community diagnosis forms the basis for community-based interventions.

CHAPTER OUTLINE

resource allocation decisions. Each component of the Alliance for Health Model is detailed as the phases of assessing and diagnosing a community's health are revealed. Members of the interdisciplinary team add each of their own unique perspectives to the assessment process. Team members identify variables that strengthen the assessment process.

Assessing a Community

A community can be defined in many ways, but the idea of people interacting with each other and with their environment is key to understanding the community. The community health nurse and members of the interdisciplinary team are members of the community as health care providers. Interactions among clients and health care providers allow the identification of needs and the formation of an alliance to promote, protect, and treat the health of the total community.

Assessing a community as a client is not very different from assessing an individual client, family, or group. The nurse uses a wide range of knowledge and skills to uncover meaningful data that describe and reflect the identity of the community and its current health status. This critical appraisal takes into consideration the varying components of the community, their interactions, and the attributes, both qualitative and quantitative, of each component.

Community Observation

Clinical Impressions

The community health nurse must become immersed in the community in order to gather important information about it. After considering the critical issue of personal safety and determining the most efficient means of transportation, the community health nurse must venture into the community for the best perspective. Traveling by foot wherever possible is the most informative; however, in some areas, a community health nurse may travel by bus, train, car, bike, boat, horse, or rickshaw. The community health nurse may want to consider locating an individual within the community willing to serve as a guide for this information-gathering phase; this decision will be based on the nurse's level of comfort and security in the community, the terrain and obstacles to consider in negotiating it, language and cultural issues, and the availability and willingness of community members to offer this service.

It is important to move through the community in a way that is natural to its members as a way of joining with the community. Sometimes gathering data through observation from a car, train, or bus is referred to as a "windshield survey." Data collected in this way are impressionistic; that is, the community health nurse is recording images of the community, using critical observational skills, just as she or he does when observing an individual client who comes for health care. The nurse considers the over-all impression that client makes. The client may be appropriately dressed for the weather and appear clean and well-kept or may be underdressed for the weather and appear disheveled and confused. The client's skin color may be pale or cyanotic. There may be bruising or open wounds. Lips may be dry, swollen, or crusted, and eyes may appear clear or inflamed. The client may appear breathless, diaphoretic, or limp. Eye contact may be direct or avoided. These clues provide avenues for further exploration, alerting the nurse to potential concerns requiring further validation. After all, the nursing process is a method of investigation that, with the valida-tion of the client, leads to the clarification of health status and, ultimately, the identification of health concerns and problems.

As the community health nurse travels through the community, obser-vations are made about what is seen. Are there people on the streets? Do they engage in conversation with each other? What do the people look like? How do they dress and behave? Are the shops and stores open for business? Are there vacant buildings? Are buildings boarded-up or have locked metal doors? How does the air smell? Are there aromas of indige-nous foods from local restaurants or foul odors from garbage dumps? Are the foods new and delicious when the community health nurse stops for lunch at a busy restaurant, street corner vendor, or farm stand? Does graf-fiti decorate buildings, or have community members painted murals? Are there loud noises from an industrial plant or does quiet characterize the community? Are fumes or smoke being emitted from commercial estab-lishments? Do signs advertise school/community meetings or say "keep out?" What kinds of active businesses are frequented by community mem-bers? Are there apartment buildings, single-family homes, attached houses, farms, high-rise apartments, or a combination? Are the streets filled with potholes, or are ditches overflowing with sewage? A skilled community health nurse can decipher a great deal of information about the commu-nity from this simple form of inspection. Later, data can be gathered to validate these impressions.

Using the Senses

The community health nurse uses every sense (i.e., sight, smell, sound, taste, touch) to observe the community. The senses are employed to appre-ciate the experience of being in the community. Assessment is a process of becoming familiar or getting acquainted with the community. The nurse sees aspects of culture and communication; smells the quality and distinc-tiveness of the air; listens to the sounds that characterize the natural ebb and flow of community interchange and movement; tastes the foods that characterize the ethnic composition of a community; and touches and is touched by the people through eye contact, handshakes, and by providing physical care. The nurse attempts interchanges with local shopkeepers or restaurant proprietors in an effort to gain a complete understanding of the community. Local newspapers or fliers give the nurse a sense of the issues and activities that reflect the community. The community health nurse takes in the community and tries to be part of it.

Safety

It is most important that the community health nurse feels safe and secure in the community setting. If the community health nurse feels at risk or in physical danger, it is important that the nurse take precautions to leave the area safely and to reenter the community with an escort or at a time of day deemed more appropriate for safe passage. Morning hours are generally safer than mid-to-late afternoon hours. It is wise to consult with the local health department or Visiting Nurse Association (VNA) to learn if there are designated areas where an escort is advisable or "no visit" buildings or zones in the community. It is always best to be well informed rather than unknowingly enter an unsafe area.

The nurse must be concerned about personal safety as well as community safety. However, when building a relationship with a community, it is essential that the community health nurse communicates a desire and willingness to be in the community. If the nurse is anxious or fearful that feeling is transmitted to the community members and alienates the nurse from the community members, preventing a successful completion of the assessment. The community health nurse must convey an acceptance and willingness to join the community and appreciate its unique personality. However, safety and security must be considered for the nurse to navigate effectively and constructively in the community setting.

$\mathcal{E}$XAMINATION

Sources of Information in the Community

Telephone book
Health and social service agencies
Library
Government agencies
Chamber of Commerce
Key informants
Staff members at community agencies

Locating Resources

Further investigation of the community verifies the community health nurse's impressions and provides a knowledge base about the community, how it functions, its strengths, risks, health issues, and problems. There are multiple **sources of information about the community** from printed matter, such as statistical data, media, key informants, historians, agencies, and community service organizations, just to name a few. The most helpful initial resource is the telephone book. Community telephone books often provide a brief but instructive history of the community. Usually providing important dates, founders, and the early development of the community, the telephone book provides a beginning sketch of the community. Also listed is the array of health and social services available in the community.

Some communities may have a wide range of health and social services, including the VNA and other nurse-managed health centers. Other communities may host few if any health resources. Hospitals and emergency services are important to note. The community health nurse must gather a personal directory of available health and social service resources; these are important agencies to visit for they provide the infrastructure for whatever health care delivery system is available or lacking in the community.

The library, if available, is a rich source of vital information about the history and development of the community. Crucial reference material includes census tract data, which provide the most recent vital statistics available about the community. These data will reveal information about population size, age and sex distributions, race and ethnicity patterns, socioeconomic status, and housing characteristics, among other demographic variables tabulated in the census. The librarian is a key informant who can guide and assist the community health nurse in uncovering a wealth of resources about the attributes of the community.

Other important sources of data include the local Chamber of Commerce and governmental agencies. These agencies provide the official perspective on the community. The Chamber of Commerce is interested in marketing the best features of the community and is particularly useful to the community health nurse in uncovering some of the many strengths of the community. The Chamber of Commerce is a key networking agency generally aware of the other agencies and offerings within the community. The local governmental agencies may be the mayor's office, the village clerk, or the sheriff's office. These agencies can familiarize the community health nurse with the official government structure of the community. Knowledge about the official chain of command and the way local government functions is critical to understanding funding allocations and tax-supported agencies, which serve the members of the community. Forming a rapport with government officials and becoming known as a health resource within the community are part of the reputation that the community health nurse wants to foster.

Identifying key informants in a community is a special challenge. Key informants can be located in many unexpected places such as beauty parlors, barber shops, hardware stores, or bars. Elders of the community can be especially helpful as they often willingly spend many hours familiarizing the community health nurse with the changes that have taken place in the community. Elders are a rich resource about the ebb and flow of community life and have a sage perspective on the evolution of the community and its influential members. Elders can be found in a variety of places, including senior citizen centers, nursing homes, playing chess in the park, or volunteering at the community center. It is important for the community health nurse to seek representation from members of all age groups and cultural/ethnic groups in the community. Likewise, it is important to seek staff members at community agencies who are familiar with the community to be as inclusive as possible in representing the health needs of the community as accurately and fully as possible.

If language is a barrier to effective communication, the community health nurse must locate members of the cultural group who can serve as translators. Language should never be an obstacle to learning about the community and its members. The community health nurse must be creative and clever in overcoming barriers and obstacles that would otherwise impede communication. Demonstrating an authentic interest in learning about the people and their environment and accurately comprehending the issues and concerns that affect their health potential and day-to-day lives are the missions of the community health nurse.

$\mathcal{F}$OCUS ON COMMUNITY-BASED NEEDS

Patterns of Morbidity and Mortality

Biostatistics is "the science which deals with the plans and methods of collecting, tabulating, and analyzing numerical facts and figures in the life sciences" (Leavell & Clark, 1965, p. 95).

Vital statistics is "the study of data from birth and death registrations" (Leavell & Clark, 1965, p. 95).

Community assessment becomes more focused and definitive as the data sources specify health threats and dangers. The community health nurse must become conversant with biostatistical data. **Biostatistics** and **vital statistics** are the tools that the community health nurse and members of the interdisciplinary team use to assess and diagnose community health problems. These same measures are used again as part of the evaluation phase of the caregiving process to judge the correctness of diagnoses and the effectiveness of treatments initiated in response to identified needs. Thus, biostatistics are used as part of the assessment and evaluation phases of the nursing process. Birth and death rates; age and disease-specific mortality rates; and morbidity, prevalence and incidence, rates are analyzed. Each rate is instructive in understanding more about the population of the community and the health threats and problems it faces. An elderly population may have high mortality rates and high disease-specific mortality rates (e.g., for cancer and cardiovascular disease). Longevity may signify a lifetime of good health, resulting in death in old age, or it may signify the opportunity to live longer only to develop and die from chronic illness. Prevalence rates are important to appreciate the nature and types of diseases that affect this population. If a community has a preponderance of young members, age-specific death rates, targeting infants and young children, are most impressive. Incidence rates for infectious disease may prove helpful in understanding patterns of acute illness and specific attack rates for idiosyncratic conditions. Birth rates help the community health nurse and members of the interdisciplinary team to anticipate the demands that will be placed on child care agencies and schools in the community; they also provide an opportunity to develop plans to promote and protect the health of these new members of the community. Day care health policies may need to be created particularly with regard to the prevention of diarrhea and the importance of universal precautions. Child care workers need to be educated about infant and toddler growth and development and the importance of stimulation to foster the development of language skills, fine and gross motor skills, and socialization skills. This kind of community health planning comes from a careful assessment of population and health statistics, which allows the community health nurse and the health care team to act proactively on behalf of the health of the community.

Demographics

Vital statistics help the community health nurse identify specific health challenges faced by the members of the community; these data instruct the nurse about the degree of vitality present in the community and the degree to which the members are depleted by illness and health threats. Demographic data also help the community health nurse to learn as much as possible about the characteristics of the population.

Locating demographic data is an investigatory process. The key to success is the community health nurse's ability to seek out reliable sources of information from a variety of agencies. The community health nurse wisely uses data already produced for surveys and institutional reports from official as well as voluntary and private agencies. The community health nurse tracks down information and extracts useful findings, which become part of the overall assessment of the community, identifying a wide array of information without initiating a new study. While the community library is generally a good place to start this investigatory process, agencies such as family service associations, counseling centers, disease-related agencies (e.g., heart or lung association, or AIDS education programs), schools, or major employers are among the agencies the community health nurse can tap for official reports. The local health department is also a key source of information as well as the mayor's or governor's office, which may have conducted reviews on the health status of the area or special reports on health-related topics.

Local politicians also conduct extensive research on communities within their jurisdiction and are usually willing to communicate with their constituencies about areas of mutual concern; health care issues may be among their top priorities. Local surveys may have been done on breast cancer rates or the extent to which homelessness is a problem, thereby citing population figures and housing patterns. The police departments or fire departments may also produce surveys about the effectiveness of their departments, which may include population statistics as they view members of the community for crime, accidents, or disasters. Although the objectives and purposes of the various reports and inventories collected by the community health nurse may differ from the objectives of the nurse's self-generated surveys of the community and its members, these sources do contain useful statistical data.

Housing patterns also help define a community. The nurse may care for a community population that resides in a senior citizen planned community or a high-rise building for low-income individuals and families. Homelessness is often a hidden problem in a community, often ignored or minimized because homeless residents rarely ask for assistance. Yet, people who are homeless must be counted, and their problems are a high-priority issue for the community health nurse. Thus, the community health nurse must seek information about people who are homeless from other sources, including the community members.

Basically, demographic data are countable data, that is, information that can be counted and converted into rates, ratios, and other forms of statistical data. The figures that result add to the community health nurse's repertoire but do not constitute the totality of the data. Because the nurse attempts to learn about the whole community, she or he breaks the community down into reasonable components in order to describe and explore it. The components of a community have qualitative and quantitative attributes. Demographic data help the community health nurse learn about the quantitative attributes of the various components.

Public Services

Safety and security are essential components of living and growing in a healthy way. In fact, safety may be the most elemental concern of human systems. The importance of safety and security cannot be underestimated in terms of their importance to life, growth, development, and health. Just as an individual needs to feel safe, so too does a community need to feel safe to act for the protection of its members. In many urban communities that are riddled with crime, the members of the community are frequently the most likely victims. For example, drive-by shootings or gang wars may result in the random deaths of community members who unknowingly enter danger zones. In communities coping with high rates of drug addiction, members may be robbed or their homes ransacked during a drug addict's effort to locate cash or valuables for drug purchases.

The community health nurse must become a known entity with public safety officials not only to foster actions on behalf of personal safety (for the nurse) but also to form an alliance with others about promoting public safety and health. It is especially wise to visit the local police and fire departments. In some communities, these public services may not be official agencies but rather volunteer operations. Neighborhood watch, private security companies, auxiliary police, and Guardian Angels are among the community servants who volunteer to patrol and protect the community. In many communities, firefighters are trained volunteers who respond to fire and emergencies, providing emergency medical services and, in conjunction with area hospital emergency personnel, providing emergency outreach services.

The community health nurse must keep in constant contact with agencies and individuals committed to protect the community. Sometimes the nurse needs an escort into the community and relies on public safety for assistance. At other times, the nurse may identify a community member with a handicapping condition that requires special accommodations in case of an emergency or fire. The nurse can alert police and fire departments about the special needs of this individual so that these departments are prepared to act if evacuation is indicated. Assuring the safety of its most vulnerable members as well as maintaining a continuous level of safety for all members is a responsibility of the whole community.

The community health nurse keeps lines of communication open with public service agencies concerned with community safety. Thus, the nurse becomes known as an agent for health, one who is able to contribute to the broad understanding and specific actions of community safety. The official agencies are also key informants able to contribute data about measures of community safety. Crime rates are illuminating in attempts to understand the specific kinds of threats to a community's well-being. Analysis of specific crimes and identification of vulnerable victims enlighten the nurse about those members who are at high risk and the protective strategies that must be implemented to protect these members. In some communities, elderly members may be victims of abuse by families members experiencing financial strain and stress. In other communities, children may be murdered in random and uncontrolled street violence. Robberies and petty theft may be on the rise in communities with unchecked drug problems and few drug rehabilitation facilities. In still other communities, adolescent gang members may be at war over profits from illegal drug deals, and deaths may occur from bullet or knife wounds. In an otherwise peaceful residential community with a low crime rate, the number of reported homicides may be unexpectedly high because of bodies being dumped off the highway that links a crime-ridden urban center with the suburban residential area.

Learning about the occurrence of fires in a community is instructive to the community health nurse. The fire department may experience a high number of false alarms, which requires investigation because of the personal threat to firefighters and the cost to the agency when the firefighters respond to a prank. Fires may be frequent during cold weather months when families use ovens or unsafe electric heaters to warm their homes if fuel costs are too high. Mobilizing an official response may involve an alliance of agencies, given the complexity of the problems. The fire department may join with the local visiting nurse agency, the housing authority, the social service office, and community leadership to respond to this threat to community members and the community at large.

Public service involves more than community services to provide safety and security in the community. Public service is a broad term that represents all services in the community supported by tax dollars. Some of the other important services provided through public support include sanitation, recreational facilities (e.g., parks, community centers), educational programs, and much more. Knowledge of these services can be obtained through local governmental offices, including village halls, local politicians, and government centers.

Without question, community sanitation is as basic to community health as personal hygiene is to an individual. Just as the nurse would be concerned with a client's ability to provide for her or his own personal hygiene so does the community health nurse exhibit concern about the state of community hygiene or sanitation. If an individual client could not provide for personal hygiene and a support system was lacking to expedite a plan to address this need, the nurse and client may agree to the placement of a home health aide for assistance with these tasks. So, too, in a community, if the official systems are lacking or constrained in allocating resources for community hygiene, a community response may be mobilized to address this issue. It is not unusual in many communities to see signs along a highway identifying the names of local community groups responsible for maintaining the cleanliness of sections of the highway. The local scout troops may volunteer to clean up a beach or park so that members can enjoy the seasonal pleasures of these public resources.

Community sanitation is directly linked to community health. Garbage, stagnant water pools, sewage leaks, and industrial dumping are among the community health problems that can result in disease and a depleted sense of community well-being. The community health nurse must diligently look out for community sanitation problems. These insults to the health of the community often can be rectified through official and volunteer efforts. Often, it is the community health nurse who can make a case for remediating these sanitation problems. The community health nurse, with an understanding of the natural history of disease and the pathogens that cause disease, can make a striking case for the urgency of treating and removing community sanitation problems. For example, lay members of the community may not realize that an uncontrolled pigeon problem is not just a community nuisance but also a potential source for psittacosis. The community health nurse is well versed in the nature of community outbreaks and those diseases that have environmental agents.

Community public services may also include concrete services that provide for socialization and pleasure for the community. Parks, recreational facilities, and community centers are among the services that communities may admire most and that attract others to the community. Knowledge of free and sliding-scale services for recreation and socialization provides the community health nurse with a vital list of resources for referral. The nurse knows best how to identify with the client and the extent to which the health needs involve the need to socialize. The community health nurse fosters the connection between community members and community resources capable of addressing their needs. If the nurse maintains contacts with these agencies, the referral can be expedited even more efficiently.

Aesthetics

Aesthetics is a broad area of interest, involving the valuing and definition of art and encompassing the significance of culture and religion in the community. The assessment of aesthetic and cultural meaning for a community is always instructive. Communities can be homogeneous in their affiliations or represent great diversity. Regardless of the degree of likeness and shared beliefs and values, learning about these associations is essential to appreciate the aesthetic dimensions of community life.

Generally in a community or in subgroups within the community, there is a dominant belief system that can be identified and described; however, there is also diversity. For example, people who believe in a particular religion will share a core of tenets, yet individuals interpret the world and identify their personal beliefs and values quite individually. This diversity is usually accepted by other members of the group. The community health nurse is challenged to learn about the mainstream values and beliefs of a community as well as appreciate the individual differences among community members.

The idea of beauty, for example, is not only "in the eye of the beholder" but also a reflection of a community's persona. One community may exclaim with great pride over the colors, design, and hidden meanings of the graffiti that decorate public places while another community may hire civil servants to paint over graffiti to restore the community's sense of aesthetics. Places of beauty or objects of beauty are intended to inspire and help members transcend their day-to-day existence through the artistic experience. Art helps us access what might be thought of as incomprehensible. Tolstoy in *What is Art?* wrote: "The business of art lies just in this: to make that understood and felt which in the form of an argument might be incomprehensible and inaccessible. Usually it seems to the recipient of a truly artistic impression that he knew the thing before but had been unable to express it" (1898, p. 178). Therefore, in accessing the community's sense of aesthetics, the community health nurse learns about the inner meanings of community life, which are otherwise inaccessible.

Walking or driving through the community is an aesthetic experience. The nurse uses every sense by visualizing, hearing, smelling, tasting, and touching the character of the community. Some communities are spectacular in their sense of an aesthetic presence. Parks, beaches, magnificent gardens, statues, or architectural wonders may be among the aesthetic symbols that engender community pride and appreciation of the surroundings. In other communities, the aesthetic sense may be vacant or bleak. Community apathy may prevail in an environment starved for this kind of nurturance. In still other communities, the sense of aesthetic may be strange or foreign to the community health nurse, in which case, the nurse must appreciate the divergence of his or her personal experience and valuing from that of the community. Stepping back with the intention of appreciating these differences is the best strategy, and being nonjudgmental is the best starting point. For example, a noxious smell may simply be an unknown aroma coming from a popular restaurant in the community. The nurse must work to develop an appreciation for that smell and work on an attitudinal shift from categorizing it as noxious to perhaps pungent or simply characteristic of a particular style of cooking valued by community members. The community health nurse must learn to recognize the smell and refrain from judging the odor or the food consumed by community members.

Almost every aspect of life is influenced by culture. The vastness of cultural influence is found in art, music, dance, theater, religion, dress, eye contact, speaking distance, nutrition, exercise methods, birth control choices, sexual orientation, sexual practices, and much more. What is allowed in terms of practices and beliefs in a community is the kind of information the community health nurse must gather to appreciate the aesthetic domain.

In homogeneous communities, conformity and continuity may be valued and even required for membership. The constancy of values and beliefs in a homogeneous community may be its signature and serve as a guide to its members and bind them to each other through a shared sense of expectations. In a heterogeneous community, an important signature of its health is the extent to which differences and deviance are allowed. The degree to which the beliefs and values of others can be incorporated into community life reflects the health of the community.

As part of the community assessment then, the nurse is concerned with taking in a sensory impression of the community, carefully separating personal expectations from the objective collection of data about the aesthetic characteristics of the community. Then, the community health nurse begins an inventory of agencies and places that provide for the aesthetic components of community life. Key among these are houses of worship. The community health nurse must get to know about all of the religious institutions in the community—from storefronts and buildings used for weekly services to the most sophisticated and well-endowed institutions. The community health nurse must know about the belief systems that each religion espouses as well as make contact with the leadership of each denomination. Forming a relationship with religious leaders enables the community health nurse to access the membership. The confidence of the leadership in the nurse is a necessary endorsement to enable the nurse to deliver a health message to the congregation effectively. Also, religious leaders are often most aware of members with special needs or problems with which the nurse may be able to assist either directly or by referral. This is a kind of case finding made possible by the cooperative relationship the community health nurse develops with clergy.

Cultural events or clubs are other ways of learning about the aesthetic component of a community. Parades, community fairs, art exhibits, theater, concerts, and parks are important aspects of the cultural life of the community and represent times and places for socialization for the members of the community. Social gatherings enable community members to meet their affiliation needs, to be entertained, and to reach outside of themselves and their immediate families to join in the larger life of the community.

Cultural events enable participation in the larger social system. The community health nurse often encounters individuals and families isolated from the larger community. If the community health nurse is aware of welcoming events or places in the community for socialization and entertainment, these can become sources of referral as the nurse attempts to link community members to the social context of their lives. The nurse must be mindful of the cost involved and assure that cost does not become an obstacle to prevent more isolated community members from joining in some aspect of community social life. To some extent, joining this larger social context provides meaning in the lives of community members and the potential for forming social alliances with other members of the community. Opportunities for socialization enable the formation of a social network. Being part of a social network affords social support, which is important for personal health and development.

Each community is marked in some way with aesthetic meanings. The community health nurse becomes an observer of special symbols of meaning in a community. For example, a small park may be constructed in memory of a child victimized by a crime. The park may symbolize the responsibility of the community to protect its most vulnerable members. It may also render a political statement about the urgency of enacting laws to protect the children of the community from the malicious intent of others. Driving along the streets of the community, the community health nurse may come across bouquets of flowers or religious symbols tied to a tree marking the place where a community member died as a result of a driving while intoxicated (DWI) accident. Cemeteries are important community landmarks. Walking through a cemetery is a kind of community history lesson. The community health nurse can learn about religion via the stones used to mark the graves and community epidemiology as death reveals much about a community and its members.

Assessing the aesthetic component of a community is an adventure. It enables the community health nurse to gather data that reveal what the members of the community value and believe, how they practice these beliefs in their lives, and the doctrine and tenets that guide them as characterized by their culture and religion. The aesthetic domain is crucial to the health of individuals, families, and communities. Aesthetic assessment rests on the ability of the community health nurse to gather data objectively without imposing value judgments but rather critically acquiring knowledge that provides access to the ways of life and beliefs of the community.

Health-Related Facilities

Health and social service facilities form the health care infrastructure of a community. Every resource has the potential to provide the community health nurse with a network of referral sources and with personal connections. The nurse must be able to establish collegial relationships with a variety of health care and social service providers. The community health nurse works collaboratively with members of the interdisciplinary health care team and members of the community to create an alliance for health within the community.

Every time the nurse encounters a community health and social services agency, an assessment of the agency should be carried out. Through agency assessment, the community health nurse develops an expert level of knowledge about the health care infrastructure of the community. The community health nurse can follow-up on these assessments with a letter informing the contact about the nurse's involvement in the community and the mission and goals of nursing interventions. A professional card should be included so that communication can continue. The community health nurse should request brochures and helpful information about the agency as well as the professional card of the contact.

The efforts of the community health nurse involve linking members to their communities. The "goodness of fit" between people and available resources is facilitated by the community health nurse. The community health nurse knows not only where the agency is located, what it looks like, what their intake procedure is, the cost, the hours of operation, and whether they provide transportation, but also the name and telephone number of the contact to initiate these services. Preferably, the community health nurse has a personal relationship with the contact person based on mutual commitment, goal sharing, and a track record of effective referrals. For example, it is very effective to pick up the telephone and speak with the director of the day care center directly to explain that a developmentally delayed child of an teenage mother could benefit from the nurturing environment of the community-supported day care center.

The best way for the community health nurse to learn about health-related services is to visit them and forge personal relationships with the personnel in these agencies. The key to comprehending the workings of a health-related agency is a thorough agency assessment. The guide that follows can serve as a format for agency assessment (Fig. 8-1). An agency assessment enables the community health nurse to collect essential information about community agencies. These data can be entered into a community resource directory created by the community health nurse as each community agency is identified. This personal directory is an invalu-

FIGURE 8-1

Guide to Agency Assessment

Name of Agency _____
Address _____
Directions _____
_____
Telephone number _____
Contact person _____
Hours of service _____
Catchment area _____
Services provided by agency _____
_____
_____
_____
Population served by agency _____
_____
_____

Self-referral and/or referral source required _____
_____
Fee for service _____
Insurance coverage accepted _____
Transportation provided _____
Information client must bring for application of service _____
_____
_____
After initial contact, when will client be eligible for services _____
_____
Outreach available _____
Does agency make referrals _____
How is agency funded _____
Additional information _____
_____

able tool for the nurse in identifying helpful and frequently used referral sources. Additional anecdotal data can be added to the directory as ongoing relationships are forged with certain referral sources. As the directory grows in size, the community health nurse becomes more knowledgeable about the community and able to expedite meaningful and effective referrals in addressing the health needs of the community. The directory also can assist the community health nurse in evaluating community services and in identifying gaps in service in the community. The community health nurse generalist in conjunction with community health nurse specialists (prepared at the master's level and higher) can become involved in health planning and community resource development to create agencies to address unmet needs of the community members.

Suppose the community health nurse wanted to formulate a community-based diagnosis related to the focus of community-based needs, a sphere of the Alliance for Health Model. The nurse would like this particular diagnosis to reflect the strengths of the community. The following diagnosis has been accepted by the North American Nursing Diagnosis Association (NANDA) [199–1996].

Potential for Enhanced Community Coping

- **Definition:** A pattern of community activities for adaptation and problem-solving that is satisfactory for meeting the demands or needs of the community but can be improved for management of current and future problems/stressors.
- **Defining Characteristics**
  Major: Deficits in one or more characteristics that indicate effective coping.
  Minor: Active planning by community for predicted stressors; active problem-solving by community when faced with issues; agreement that community is responsible for stress management; positive communication among community members; positive communication between community/aggregates and larger community; programs available for recreation and relaxation; resources sufficient for managing stressors.
- **Related Factors:** Social supports available; resources available for problem-solving; community has a sense of power to manage stressors (NANDA, 1995–1996, p. 55).

It is clear from this diagnosis that the community is viewed as a resource of many strengths. The community is able to cope, that is, to meet the demands it encounters and use the active planning and problem-solving processes of which it is capable when confronted with issues. Members of the community communicate effectively with each other and larger systems. There are resources for recreation and leisure and ways to deal with stressors. The community possesses available support systems. Finally, the community is empowered to manage itself.

CARE MANAGEMENT TECHNIQUES

Mix of Client Problems

To ascertain the mix of client problems found in the community, the community health nurse moves from data collection to data analysis. Community health nurses move beyond the individual appraisals they conduct on identified clients in the community to ask: To what extent are the needs identified in this client characteristic of others in the community? In asking this question, the community health nurse is shaping aggregate client data. Looking for commonalities in clients' needs is the basis for population-based health care. The shared or common needs of a population of the community or of the community itself require a wider scope for intervention and strategies that invariably involve agency level interventions.

The community health nurse tries to uncover health care needs of aggregates in the community as well as represent the total population of the community. However, many members of the community do not access health care services, the reasons for which are variable. For community members who have no health insurance or have minimal or restricted coverage, the cost of health care is prohibitive. Also, a lack of available neighborhood health resources, lack of transportation, the cost of transportation, dissatisfaction with the quality of health care, fear of diagnosis and disability, or nonrecognition of symptoms are other common reasons for not accessing health care services. Thus, the community health nurse should attempt to identify members who use the health care system and those who do not. Clearly, case finding is a hallmark of community health intervention.

The mix of clients in the community, therefore, must be represented by knowledge generated about the population from available census tract data, demographic data, studies on use of services, surveys, and investigations involving the population. The community health nurse must learn as much as possible about the people of the community. As data are analyzed, expectations about the demands on service and the trends for future services can be extrapolated. Uncovering population-based health problems is the key to understanding the case mix of the community.

Public's Expectations for Care

Consumerism to a great extent defines the nature of the relationship between public expectations for care and the actual care rendered. Consumers and providers engage in a relationship through which health care is transacted. Each side of that relationship brings expectations to the nature of this transaction. Consumer expectations should be uppermost in providers' minds as the dialogue moves through its various phases. The consumer and provider are partners in a dynamic relationship about health, whether personal health, family health, or community health.

Providers of care, like community health nurses and other members of the interdisciplinary team, have a responsibility to serve as advocates for consumers. Advocacy involves informing and supporting consumers in the decisions they make about their health care. Sound health care decisions take into consideration the expectations and the adjustments that must be made as health care is negotiated. The provider serves this opportunity for consumer **empowerment** by clarifying consumer expectations in relation to the concrete services providers can offer. The following example is illustrative.

CASE STUDY: A CLASH IN CULTURE

Parents of high school students in a given community protest the school's plan for human immunodeficiency virus (HIV)/acquired immunodeficiency syndrome (AIDS) education because they feel that children should be taught about sexuality and birth control at home. The parents refer to their cultural orientation, family values, and beliefs, which define the importance of separating sexual instruction from the dissemination of health information to their children. The school nurse is aware of sexual activity taking place among the students and believes the implementation of a sexual education program employing the state's AIDS curriculum is an imperative public health measure. This transaction is defined as a clash of cultural expectations. The consumers expect the school to respect their culture and beliefs, and the provider expects the cooperation of the community regarding a public health threat. Cooperation and collaboration are imperative in this situation.

Empowerment. "If power is the ability to predict, control, and participate in one's environment, then empowerment is the process by which individuals and communities are enabled to take such power and act effectively in transforming their lives and their environment" (Robertson & Minkler, 1994, p. 300). Empowerment embodies the idea of partnerships or alliances between professionals and individuals or communities, as opposed to traditional hierarchical provider and consumer relationships.

A forum that enables the expression of the varying points of view may facilitate communication. Perhaps a task force of selected parents, students, public health officials, and the school nurse can be established to investigate the underlying concerns and to develop a consensus for a cooperative outcome. If the nurse proceeded with the educational program over the protestations of the parents, the community would be alienated, and students perhaps pulled from school. If the nurse eliminated any references to sexual behavior and condoms in the educational sessions, the students' health might be jeopardized. Clearly, a cooperative effort must take place in that gray zone defined by the expectations of consumers and the expertise providers bring to the health care transaction.

At the community level, consumer expectations for care can be identified and clarified through mechanisms like community advisory boards, public forums, consumer membership on trustee boards, public announcements offering "800" numbers for call-in participation, surveys, and discussion groups. Mechanisms that foster open communication and opportunities to voice expectations as part of the problem-identification and problem-solving process create the foundation for cooperative community-based planning. The role of the provider involves education and advocacy.

Competence of Professionals

To say the health care arena is dynamic is an understatement. Change in health care technologies and environments is occurring so rapidly it often seems that technology is outpacing the professional's ability to reshape practice and employ the various technologies effectively. The community health nurse cannot rely on yesterday's theories and clinical expectations. Competence is an evolving ability to meet clinical challenges, apply clinical research, and use technologies to enhance health and humanity. Consumers need to know that providers have the appropriate credentials and are employed by agencies that stand behind them. Assurance of professional competence must always be an issue.

As part of an assessment, the community health nurse should inventory the professional resources found in the community by becoming familiar with the providers that could comprise the interdisciplinary health care team. The community health nurse must learn about the credentials and missions of other professionals in the community. Interdisciplinary relationships are constructed out of knowledge and respect for each other. The ability to collaborate for the sake of the health of the community requires that the nurse believes in the importance of the interdisciplinary team.

Insecurity in one's professional capabilities and limitations can result in turf protection. Boundaries can be drawn between health professionals in an effort to self-protect, but effective collaboration is based on the absence of boundaries between the professions. Recognition that similar goals and values can join professionals in a common mission—that is, promoting, protecting, restoring, and maintaining the community's health—is the foundation upon which interdisciplinary collaboration rests.

The community health nurse recognizes that pooling professional resources is a productive strategy for solving community-based problems. For example, the community health nurse may identify a group of elderly people who meet at a senior citizen site. In conducting an assessment of the members, nutritional concerns may arise as a common deficit. The community health nurse must be knowledgeable about the nutritional demands of aging but may not be specifically prepared to remediate some of the more complicated deficits. The community health nurse should seek consultation with a geriatric clinical nurse specialist, a geriatric nutritionist, and a geriatrician. This kind of collaboration fosters mutual respect and taps the specialized knowledge required to care for clients with challenging health problems.

Consultation could lead to other forms of collaboration. For example, this potential team of professional providers may coordinate their efforts to design a nutritional service for geriatric clients in the community, including finding additional funding to expand a limited Meals on Wheels program that serves a restricted number of the homebound elderly population. Sharing one's competence with other members of the interdisciplinary team and asking for consultation as well as providing consultation enhance the community health nurses's network of support, identify mentors, and assure the community of the highest level of professional competence.

Standards of Care

Standards of care provide minimal as well as optimal parameters from which to measure quality health care. Each professional group can refer to its own standards as the benchmark for professional performance in the discipline. Community health agencies are also evaluated periodically to assure the public that high standards of care are rendered to the public. The community health nurse is able to equate his or her practice to professional standards for the discipline. The American Nurses Association (ANA), American Public Health Association (APHA), National League for Nursing (NLN), American Association of Colleges of Nursing (AACN), and Association of Community Health Nurse Educators (ACHNE) are among the official agencies that have standards, statements, and criteria available to the community health nurse to serve as guidelines of clinical scope and to measure performance.

The community health nurse uses these standards to reflect on and improve personal practice and also as points of discussion concerning supervision. Supervision is part of every professional's practice. No one is exempt from the supervisory scrutiny and feedback about practice skill, efficiency, and appropriateness. The community health nurse also contributes to the agency's efforts to achieve and maintain standards set by accrediting commissions. In this way, the community health nurse advocates for quality care for consumers by assuring that agency accreditation and personal evaluations are upheld.

Consumers can be taught objective measures of evaluation and become knowledgeable about the evaluation processes for agencies and individual providers. Consumer participation in these evaluation procedures is essential. Consumer input can be facilitated if the community health nurse advocates for this level of community involvement in community-based health services. The community health nurse is vigilant to assure that consumer surveys are conducted and included in evaluation reports. Consumer participation signals the professional and agency interest in assuring a partnership approach to the delivery of health care and quality in the management systems responsible for the care.

Interdisciplinary Care

Quality health care cannot be discipline-specific because clients are complicated human systems with a variety of complex needs that cannot be fully addressed by any one discipline alone. While each discipline has a unique vantage point, specialized skills, and a commitment to quality care, the recipients of health care (i.e., individuals, families, groups, communities) benefit when health care is seamless, comprehensive, and well coordinated with the client's needs providing the motivation.

Consumer-focused care is not defined by turfs or disciplines but is dedicated to assuring that health needs are clarified and addressed as appropriately as possible. The plan of care emerges from a coordinated effort between the interdisciplinary members of the team and is validated by the client. The onus of responsibility for coordination and collaboration with and for the client rests with health care professionals. Quality health care is client-focused and provided from an interdisciplinary or transdisciplinary perspective. The key to the success of interdisciplinary care planning is identifying members of other disciplines with a "like" philosophy and a willingness to work collaboratively. The community health nurse contributes to the holistic plan of care. The nurse shares the nursing perspective, derived from professional nursing standards for quality care, serving the best interest of the client and addressing measurable outcomes of care.

Community health nurses discuss anticipated and expected outcomes with clients in an effort to close any gaps in the health care plan. The community health nurse contributes to the plan by representing the community's needs, through careful assessment and thoughtful analysis of assessment findings. These data are then validated and form diagnostic statements that capture the community's health concerns and validate the community members' experience.

A nursing diagnosis that refers to the ability of the community to manage a therapeutic regime at the community level has been approved by NANDA (1995–1996) and is written as follows:

INEFFECTIVE MANAGEMENT OF THERAPEUTIC REGIME: COMMUNITY

- **Definition:** A pattern of regulating and integrating into community processes programs for treatment of illness and the sequelae of illness that are unsatisfactory for meeting health-related goals.
- **Defining Characteristics:** Deficits in persons and programs to be accountable for illness care of aggregates; deficits in advocates for aggregates; deficits in community activities for secondary and tertiary prevention; illness symptoms above the norm expected for the number and type of population; number of health care resources are insufficient for the incidence or prevalence of illness(es); unavailable health care resources for illness care; unexpected acceleration of illness(es) (NANDA, 1995–1996, p. 58).

This diagnosis refers to the deficits in available community-based programs for the treatment of illness. In other words, the infrastructure for illness care, including hospital and community agencies dedicated to the treatment of illness, providing both secondary and tertiary prevention care, is insufficient to address the population of people in the community affected by illness. Health care resources may be insufficient or unavailable to address the ills of community aggregates.

$\mathcal{I}$NFLUENCES ON RESOURCE ALLOCATION DECISIONS

Patterns of Resource Allocation

The community health nurse has a keen understanding of the types of resources in the community. Conducting agency assessments has provided the framework for learning about the nature and variety of health care resources in the community and how they are funded. The community health nurse must also find out how decisions are made to fund or support these resources. For example, some agencies are publicly supported. Some agencies are supported by grants or awards and have circumscribed periods of time in which to accomplish their given goals and objectives. Agencies may be voluntary and rely on their charges to support their efforts. Other agencies may be proprietary and be motivated to create a profit. Managed care agencies may be motivated to contain costs and deliver a predetermined amount of service. At the community level, the nurse is interested in learning about how decisions are made to fund or support available agencies as well as plan for new agencies.

Understanding the funding mechanisms and determining what steps are necessary in the approval process for implementation can help the community health nurse to determine how health care resources are allocated. Some communities have health care planning boards that serve as clearinghouses for decision-making about the allocation of community resources. The planning board may not directly fund the health care agency's request for expansion or redistribution of services, but it will approve or disapprove the request based on the need for such services in the community. If a planning board exists, it could be expected to monitor health care resources. The intent of monitoring is to attempt to prevent the duplication of health care services in a community and to assure that health care services are distributed to the target population. Needless to say, the community health nurse would be a valuable member of such a planning board, bringing nursing expertise and knowledge of the community and its health care resources. Nursing involvement at this level of community health planning is essential. The nurse represents the community's needs and serves in an advocacy role.

Values and Beliefs of the Population

The community health nurse has already developed clinical impressions about the values and beliefs of a community through careful observation as part of the windshield survey. Clinical impressions must be validated. One way to validate aggregate values and beliefs is to mobilize community leaders for dialogue about the the health values and beliefs in the community. Appreciating the various voices and the varied points of view they represent is crucial to validating an accurate community impression. Community values and beliefs signify what is important to a community. The education and protection of the youngest members may be a priority, therefore, giving the community health nurse a sense of direction in specifically analyzing pediatric data and the availability of child care and educational resources. The community may evidence deep concern for protecting the environment from contaminants and harmful carcinogens. The community health nurse would work with local environmental agencies to gather data about potential and actual threats to the local environment and learn about sources of contamination. The community may value a strong commercial hub in the community but fear its demise as large shopping complexes seek community approval for their building plans. The community health nurse may be sensitized to the local shopkeepers and join with them to gain community support for their survival.

In addition to mobilizing community leaders for a clearer understanding of community values and beliefs, the community health nurse becomes knowledgeable about the religious and cultural affiliations represented in the community. The nurse becomes familiar with prescribed doctrine and dogma that provide the basis for member affiliation and unite members in shared values and beliefs. Life-style choices are directly linked to health status and choices about health care utilization. Religion and culture are powerful informants of life ways. The community health nurse wisely listens for clues that validate the values and beliefs of members of the community.

Government Funding

The community health nurse should be familiar with the health-related facilities in the community that are funded by governmental sources, whether at a local, regional, or federal level. These institutions are meant to be responsive to all members of the community, regardless of the ability to pay for services. The community health nurse must always look for sources of free care in the community to address the needs of people without health insurance or with minimal forms of insurance. Free care is a precious commodity, often rare and sometimes nonexistent. However, government-sponsored agencies are generally unable to turn clients away. The community may have a city or county hospital facility, or the health department may sponsor an information and referral network, communicable disease clinic, well-child care including immunizations, and other health services.

Consumers are recipients of health care and, therefore, are one party in the delivery of health care. Providers are the second party in this constellation; they render care, representing a wide range of health care professionals. The insurers or the health care insurance industry are the third party in this constellation. For the community health nurse to join with the interdisciplinary health care team and ultimately carry out a plan of care with the community, the nurse must be mindful of this three-party constellation and possess a clear understanding of the role of public health through publicly supported institutions and tax-supported health insurance. Until (or if) the United States adopts a single-payer system of health care, which provides basic health services to all people, the community health nurse must scrutinize the community carefully for sources of health care that are free or calculated on a sliding scale to link members of the community without health care coverage to systems of care. So part of the community assessment must account for government-supported community-based health care services.

Special Interest Groups

Special interest groups are part of the community and have a united voice to represent their needs. These groups may be strong allies of the community health nurse. The nurse can lend his or her support to their goals by contributing nursing expertise and offering health information and consultation. Members of special interest groups may offer the nurse access to their members and be supportive of the nurse by releasing helpful community data or by participating in health surveys that will generate useful information about this segment of the population. Special interest groups, however, by their very specialized focus, are not representative of the community at large. The community health nurse can appreciate the perspective of the special interest group and realize that this is an important but focused perspective.

Health Insurance

As discussed earlier, insurance is the third party in any health care transaction among consumers and providers. The community health nurse needs to know the percentage of people in the community with and without health insurance. Among the people with health insurance, the community health nurse should be aware of the type of coverage. One of the biggest obstacles to securing health care is cost. If members of the community do not have coverage for costly health care, they delay seeking care, do not seek care at all, or secure some alternative, less costly treatment.

People who do not use the health care system are a particular challenge to the community health nurse. Outreach is the answer to this challenge. Community health nurses bring services to clients in their own environment. Community health nurses expect to bring care to the client's home, to neighborhood centers, to community-based programs, to community health fairs, and to the streets frequented by clients. Case finding becomes the best strategy for identifying clients in need of care and for generating data on hard-to-reach populations. The community health nurse is interested in learning about the total population, not just about the people seeking care.

When the members of a community are unable to access health care because of inadequate or absent health insurance they become a vulnerable community with limited capacity to cope with the threat of illness. This reduced coping capacity leaves the members at risk.

NANDA has approved a community diagnosis that refers to the coping capability of the community when dealing with high levels of stress and perceived vulnerability. This type of community diagnosis reveals the compromised capacity of the community to deal with stressors. Stress experienced at the community level is often the result of poor or faulty decisions made about the allocation of health care resources, leaving the community in a deficit condition with inadequate resources to address its health problems. The NANDA community diagnosis is as follows (1995–1996).

INEFFECTIVE COMMUNITY COPING

- **Definition:** A pattern of community activities for adaptation and problem-solving that is unsatisfactory for meeting the demands or needs of the community
- **Defining Characteristics**
  Major: None.
  Minor: Community does not meet its own expectations; deficits in community participation; deficits in communication methods; excessive conflicts; expressed difficulty in meeting demands for change; expressed vulnerability; high illness rates; stressors perceived as excessive.
  Related Factors: Deficits in social support; inadequate resources for problem-solving; powerlessness (NANDA, 1995–1996, pp. 55–56).

In this situation the coping capacity of the community is compromised, and the community is unable to mobilize itself to meet the demands placed upon it. The community may be depleted by the number of cuts in health services and, therefore, unable to cope with the health problems of the community. In some communities, as public facilities are cut and facilities are re-engineered, the community is decimated by the inadequacy of its own resources. When people are left without resources, they cannot survive and neither can the community.

COMMUNITY ANALYSIS

Data collection forms the groundwork for community assessment. The thrust of data collection is informative and descriptive. The community health nurse is able to define and describe components of the community. This view enables the nurse to see the community from a holistic perspective and appreciate the complexity of the given community and its members. Moving beyond descriptions, the community health nurse relates varying findings from detailed observations and probing examinations and begins the process of data analysis. The goal of analysis is a clear picture of the health strengths, risks, and problems of the community. Further, the community health nurse seeks to bring together a "goodness of fit" between community health needs and community resources through an understanding of how health care is managed and how health care resources are allocated. The three spheres of the Alliance for Health Model overlap as the fit between community needs, systems of care management, and decisions for resource allocation are in synchrony. The thrust of community analysis is to determine how these three circles relate to each other. Ultimately, the community health nurse tries to synthesize these findings into coherent statements called *community-based diagnoses*, which crystallize the nature of health risks and problems encountered in the community and delineate pathways for appropriate interventions to reduce risks and ameliorate problems. Community-based diagnoses are validated with members of the interdisciplinary health care team and community members so that actions taken are formed out of an alliance for the sake of the health of the community. The intent of interventions are discussed in Chap. 9. The nursing process as applied to the community is used as a guide to community-based caring.

COMMUNITY DIAGNOSIS

As illustrated, the data gathered during the community assessment phase of the nursing process are pooled, and further analysis is conducted. During this phase, the goal is to formulate meaningful diagnostic statements that define the health strengths, health risks, and health problems of the community. Diagnoses are really clinical judgments or conclusions about human responses to actual or potential problems or processes that are drawn out of the assembled data.

NANDA approved the following definition for nursing diagnosis at the Ninth Conference: "A clinical judgment about individual, family, or community responses to actual and potential health problems/life processes. Nursing diagnoses provide the basis for selection of nursing interventions to achieve outcomes for which the nurse is accountable" (NANDA,

Patterns of NANDA-Approved Diagnoses

Exchanging	Moving
Communicating	Perceiving
Relating	Knowing
Valuing	Feeling
Choosing	

1995–1996, p. 7). **NANDA-approved diagnoses** are categorized into nine patterns: exchanging, communicating, relating, valuing, choosing, moving, perceiving, knowing, and feeling. The order set forth by NANDA for developing diagnoses specifies the formulation of a definition; followed by the defining characteristics of the diagnosis, including major and minor defining characteristics; and finally a list of related factors. The definition is a clear statement of the health condition. Defining characteristics are generally objective indicators of the conditions. Related factors are described as factors that "appear to show some type of patterned relationship with the nursing diagnosis" (NANDA, 1995–1996, p. 7). Related factors may precede the condition, be associated with it, contribute to it, or ameliorate the condition. New diagnoses are submitted for consideration, and it is hoped that continuous revision will take place. Very few of the accepted diagnoses are written at the community level. Submission of community-based nursing diagnoses will hopefully be expanded.

NANDA-approved diagnoses related to the community are limited since the thrust of NANDA's taxonomy focuses on individuals. The three NANDA-approved community diagnoses presented in this chapter are: Potential for Enhanced Community Coping, Ineffective Management of Therapeutic Regimen: Community, and Ineffective Community Coping (NANDA, 1995–1996). The community health nurse is challenged to write community-based diagnoses that are derived from assessment data and take into consideration the three spheres of the Alliance for Health Model: community-based needs, care management techniques, and influences on resource allocation decisions.

The community health nurse, in valuing and appreciating the community truly as a client for care, represents the needs of the community and encourages care managements systems to respond to these needs and serves to influence resource allocation decisions to improve and protect the health of the community. Clarity in diagnostic statements sensitizes the interdisciplinary health care team to the importance and urgency of attending to community-based health issues and problems and to appreciating the remarkable strengths of the community as a resource for health.

The community health nurse can sensitize members of the interdisciplinary health care team to think beyond the individual and the family as clients for care and to think about the community as a client. Refining and extrapolating from diagnoses focused on individuals and families to the community can prove to be an interesting and meaningful challenge. Consider, for example, the following NANDA diagnoses and how they can be envisioned as community-based diagnoses.

CASE HISTORY
INDIVIDUAL-FOCUSED DIAGNOSIS:
ALTERED NUTRITION: MORE THAN BODY REQUIREMENTS

"The state in which an individual is experiencing an intake of nutrients which exceeds metabolic needs" and is characterized as weight 10 percent over ideal for height and frame (NANDA, 1995–1996, p. 13).

COMMUNITY-FOCUSED DIAGNOSIS:
HIGH OVERWEIGHT PREVALENCE

Data to support this diagnosis include: "One in three adults (34%) and one in five adolescents (21%) in the United States are overweight . . . the prevalence of overweight has increased over the last decade for adults and adolescents. Overweight is especially prevalent among certain racial and ethnic groups; for example, nearly half of black women and Mexican-American women are estimated to be overweight" [U.S. Department of Health and Human Services (DHHS), 1995, p. 28]. The diagnosis conveys the pervasiveness of the overweight problem, in this case, the community of the United States.

From this diagnosis, it is clear a reversal of this trend must be orchestrated. Community-based actions are needed on many fronts, including nutrition and physical exercise. Community-based efforts to help people reduce fat consumption, including the use the Food Guide Pyramid and regular physical activity, are in order. Community partnerships to pursue these undertakings will comprise the community-based interventions to address this diagnosis.

CASE HISTORY
INDIVIDUAL-FOCUSED DIAGNOSIS:
IMPAIRED GAS EXCHANGE

This is defined as "the state in which the individual experiences a decreased passage of oxygen and/or carbon dioxide between the alveoli of the lungs and the vascular system" (NANDA, 1995–1996, p. 26).

COMMUNITY-FOCUSED DIAGNOSIS:
IMPAIRED RESPIRATORY HEALTH: EXPOSURE TO AIR POLLUTANTS

Healthy People 2000 (1991) objectives call for a reduction in human exposure to criteria air pollutants by increasing protection from air pollutants so that at least 85 percent of people live in counties that meet Environmental Protection Agency (EPA) standards. Progress made in this area has been attributed to the Clean Air Act of 1990, which "has helped increase the proportion of people living in counties that meet EPA standards for air pollution from 49.7% (which was the baseline) in 1988 to 76.5% in 1993" (DHHS, 1995, pp. 81–82). "Impaired Respiratory Health: Exposure to Air Pollutants" may be a particularly pertinent diagnosis for a group of workers exposed to the inhalation of toxins on their jobs. Workers may be at an industrial site where exposure is concentrated or may be exposed to toxins as they spray herbicides at a variety of locations each day.

CASE HISTORY
INDIVIDUAL-FOCUSED DIAGNOSIS:
SPIRITUAL DISTRESS (DISTRESS OF THE HUMAN SPIRIT)

Defined as "disruption in the life principle which pervades a person's entire being and which integrates and transcends one's biological and psychosocial nature" (NANDA, 1995–1996, p. 49).

COMMUNITY-FOCUSED DIAGNOSIS:
SPIRITUAL DISTRESS: COMMUNITY

Consider the sense of distress and disruption created when a disaster strikes a community and the inherent community response. Terrorism and acts of random community violence rip into the lives of all community members who express concern about the meaning of life and death and their belief systems. Threats to community safety can evoke widespread distress in communities. The distress can be pervasive and transcend the differences that separate people. People can be spiritually united in time of disaster as communal security and the precious nature of community life itself are threatened. Joblessness and poverty may be the sources of spiritual distress for the community. In this case, the oppression of economic insecurity and the sense of failure that comes with lack of work productivity and economic dependence pervades the life of the community, resulting in community distress.

These are a few examples of diagnoses that were formulated to reflect conditions of individuals that can be extrapolated to reflect conditions in the community. Hopefully, the reader is challenged to contemplate community-based diagnoses and to think beyond the individual and the family to view the community as a client and to engage in community-based health care.

In relation to the number of approved diagnoses describing human responses to actual and potential health problems or life processes for individual and families, relatively few diagnoses relate to the community. Community health nurses are challenged to submit community diagnoses for inclusion in the NANDA taxonomy. The community health nurse is in the ideal position to make the strengths, risks, and problems of the community knowable to all nurses and members of the interdisciplinary health care team.

Diagnoses can be written to reflect the strengths or capabilities of a community. For example, a community with a low infant mortality rate provides access to quality community-based prenatal care centers and a coordinated referral initiative through the local high school and community youth groups. The prenatal centers provide educational outreach and case finding to encourage early initiation of prenatal care. Further, the local community health nurse provides postnatal home visits twice weekly during the neonatal period and provides comprehensive follow-up on the mother and infant as well as educating the parents about infant growth and development and infant stimulation. The infant mortality rate for this community is the lowest in its state, and the community leaders and agencies take great pride in protecting the health of their most vulnerable citizens. Children are valued, and parenting is supported to promote and protect the health of infants, their families, and ultimately the community. A community diagnosis stating, low infant mortality rate, would reflect these health-seeking behaviors.

The health risks found in a community can also be characterized through community diagnosis. A large geriatric population residing in a housing project may be at risk for a threatened influenza epidemic. The community health nurse may recognize this community health threat and mobilize the community leaders in the geriatric community to use effective means of communication to reach this population and to justify the importance of an immunization program. The community health nurse may encourage health care professionals from surrounding health care facilities to join in a cooperative effort to immunize the senior citizens and curtail what could become a devastating epidemic, resulting in morbidity and mortality for this community aggregate.

The health problems of a community can be portrayed in a community diagnosis. Weapons-related violent death may be an endemic problem in a given community. The high incidence of human violence is a desperate expression of community ill health. Although there is a serious gap in knowledge and understanding of the causes and prevention of violent behavior, the impact of violent behavior on communities can be addressed. A diagnosis of high incidence of weapons-related deaths may result in school and community-based interventions, including updated training for health care professionals both to identify potential perpetrators of violence and address the needs of victims of violence (DHHS, 1995).

Community diagnoses assist the community health nurse to focus assessment data into meaningful statements about the state of the community's health strengths, health risks, and health problems. Interventions are generated from these diagnostic statements. The community health nurse is ever mindful of the importance of considering the three spheres of influence in assessing the community.

Summary

The community is a client system. The community health nurse is challenged to look beyond the individual members of the community and the family members of the community to view the community itself as a client for care. Communities are complex. They have personalities, resources, strengths, risks, and problems. The community health nurse identifies the health strengths of the community and uses these strengths to balance the risks and problems of the community. The community health nurse engages in a process of community assessment to uncover the dynamics of the community. The assessment is a comprehensive scrutiny of the community as a whole. The community health nurse uses all of her or his skills and knowledge to accomplish this assessment. The data are collected through observation, inspection, and examination of the community. The three spheres of the Alliance for Health Model are used to guide the assessment of the community. Each sphere reveals the varying dimensions of the community. The community health nurse and members of the interdisciplinary team with community members analyze the interrelatedness of the three spheres—community-based needs, care management techniques, and resource allocation decisions—to determine the strengths, risks, and health problems of the community. The degree to which the three spheres overlap indicate the areas of strength in the community. The degree to which the three spheres are not connected and interrelated indicate the areas of risk and health problems in the community. The assessment phase of the nursing process, when applied to communities, provides the community health nurse with sufficient data to formulate meaningful community diagnoses and to begin to formulate plans for community intervention to promote and protect the health of the community.

KEY WORDS

Aesthetics
Assessment
Biostatistics
Demographics
Diagnosis
Empowerment

Goodness of fit
NANDA taxonomy
Resource allocation
Single-payer system
Third-party payer

QUESTIONS

DIRECTIONS: Choose the one *best* response to each of the following questions.

1. A windshield survey provides the community health nurse with which of the following types of data?
   A. Demographic
   B. Vital
   C. Impressionistic
   D. Morbidity

2. To develop a community assessment, the *first* step for the community health nurse is to determine
   A. what pertinent studies have already been done.
   B. the percentage of people within each age category.
   C. the morbidity and mortality rates in the community.
   D. the willingness of community leaders to participate in the study.

3. If health care providers and health care consumers are considered two of the three parties in the health care system, what is the third party?
   A. Hospitals
   B. Health maintenance organizations (HMOs)
   C. Department of Health and Human Services (DHHS)
   D. Insurance companies and programs

4. Community-based diagnostic statements define
   A. prevalence rates of disease in the community.
   B. health strengths, risks, and problems in the community.
   C. the leading causes of mortality in the community.
   D. health problems of individuals and families in the community.

5. The act of community assessment is best defined as
   A. determining the ethnic or racial breakdown of the population.
   B. uncovering the health resources of the community.
   C. becoming familiar or getting acquainted with the community.
   D. locating referral sources by learning about community agencies.

ANSWERS

1. *The answer is C.* A windshield survey is a method for gathering data about the community through observation; data collected are impressionistic.

2. *The answer is A.* The community health nurse first consults sources of data available about the community, like the local telephone book, the library, and the Chamber of Commerce, to determine what pertinent studies have already been done.

3. *The answer is D.* Insurers, whether public, private, or voluntary, are the third party of the health care system.

4. *The answer is B.* Community-based diagnoses are clinical judgments about community responses to actual and potential health problems or life processes and include statements about community health strengths, risks, and problems.

5. *The answer is C.* Community assessment is a process of becoming familiar or getting acquainted with a community to uncover meaningful data that describe and reflect the identity of the community and its current health status.

ANNOTATED REFERENCES

Leavell, H. R., & Clark, E. G. (1958). Preventive medicine for the doctor in his community: An epidemiologic approach. New York: McGraw-Hill.

This landmark text on preventive medicine includes a review of the basic principles and the application of these principles to varying health conditions and to organized community action. It is recognized as the finest resource for explaining the natural history of disease and the levels of prevention. The information on the epidemiologic approach and its contributions to preventive medicine are often quoted in community health publications.

North American Nursing Diagnosis Association (NANDA). (1995–1996). *Nursing diagnoses: Definitions and classification.* Philadelphia: Author.

This text is a compilation of the results of the Eleventh Conference on Classification of Nursing Diagnoses held in 1994. Details of NANDA-approved nursing diagnoses, including definitions, defining characteristics, risk factors, and related factors, are presented. The guidelines for submission of nursing diagnoses are also outlined.

Robertson, A., & Minkler, M. (1994). New health promotion movement: A critical examination. *Health Education Quarterly,* 21(3), 295–312.

Exploring the revolution occurring in the field of health promotion, these authors delve into two concepts critical to this movement: empowerment and community participation. This article explores the multiple meanings of these terms and the implications for practice. Health is viewed as a resource for everyday life, not the objective for living as delineated by the World Health Association (WHO) definition.

Tolstoy, L. (1898). *What is art?* London: Oxford University Press.

This world classic is the most important of Tolstoy's essays on aesthetics. Various definitions of art are examined, all of which for one reason or another Tolstoy finds unsatisfactory. The function of art in classical Greece, and medieval and post-Renaissance Europe, is analyzed, including the differing criteria by which each age has judged its own art. Tolstoy's own definition of art is put forth along with criteria for distinguishing good art from bad.

U.S. Department of Health and Human Services. (1995). *Healthy people 2000: Midcourse review and 1995 revisions.* Washington, DC: Author.

This text is a report on the accomplishments following the release of Healthy People 2000: National Health Promotion and Disease Prevention Objectives and the challenges remaining in preventing premature death and in improving health as the year 2000 approaches. It is a detailed progress report on the 22 identified priority areas and the consortium action being taken at the state level and through private and voluntary activities.

ℵURSING INTERVENTIONS IN THE CARE OF COMMUNITIES

Caring for and about a community's health is the essence of community-based nursing care (Public Health Nursing Section, American Public Health Association, 1980). The community health nurse appreciates the diversity and complexity of factors that influence the community's health. A comprehensive assessment of the community's health leads to the development of community diagnoses. Community-based diagnoses are helpful in providing a specific focus for planning appropriate interventions. The community health nurse collaborates with members of the interdisciplinary health care team and community members to create an alliance that validates the community's health needs and leads to the appropriate interventions. This alliance for community health also determines available systems for care management and considers influences on health resource allocation. The goodness of fit between community health needs, systems of care management, and resource allocation decisions will reveal unmet needs in the community, deficiencies in care management, an absence of community resources, or obstacles to the allocation of available resources.

This chapter focuses on the expertise of the team approach and examines the role of the community health nurse in coordinating efforts to implement successful interventions. Community interventions are therapeutic actions designed to promote and protect the community's health, treat and remediate community health problems, and support the community as it changes over time. Community-based interventions provide a continuum of health services that anticipate community health problems and are responsive to community needs.

ℰXPERTISE OF THE TEAM APPROACH

To be successful, community-based interventions require the concerted effort of many individuals. The community health nurse relies on the expertise of community members and members of the interdisciplinary health care team to put a community-based plan into action. A team approach is illustrated by the following example of a community-based intervention.

If, for example, early detection for the treatment of cancer is considered an important community health intervention, then the community health nurse would have a significant role to play to actualize a cancer screening program. To implement a cancer detection screening program, the community health nurse must first identify a facility that is willing to provide the professional expertise and technological support that is required. Nurses such as clinical nurse specialists, nurse practitioners, oncologists, radiologists, and technicians would be among the personnel at these facilities with whom the community health nurse must interact in the role of liaison with the community.

Publicizing the screening events is another aspect of the intervention that the community health nurse must coordinate. The nurse must create press releases for newspapers and public service announcements for radio and television. The nurse may contact clergy and administrators of churches, synagogues, meeting-houses, and other community centers to obtain approval for distributing publicity fliers at services and meetings. Establishing a good relationship with these community leaders in the planning stages can be very beneficial as it often ensures the proper dissemination of material to their membership. The community health nurse must mobilize the communication system in the community to alert the members of the community about the locations of the screenings, how members can take advantage of this service, and what documentation they need in order to make use of this service.

Since cost is always a significant factor in providing health care, the financial office of a facility such as that proposed here would be instrumental in the processing of insurance and in determining if free care could be provided when insurance is not available. Cooperative ventures with other facilities to conduct a cancer screening program may provide a beneficial cost-sharing possibility.

When several health care facilities join together to conduct screenings, decisions about locations of screenings must be made. The community health nurse can consult with the community relations departments of the facilities and draw on their expertise and contacts in the community to decide the best way to conduct the screening. Arranging for planning meetings and assuring that there is community representation at these meetings is a vital part of organizing such a community-based intervention. Community representatives are encouraged to share their perspective on community health needs and offer advice and caution about how to

The team approach to community-based interventions is instrumental in making the intervention a success.

approach the community. Regularly scheduled meetings assure that communication flows effectively and that all who are involved have a voice and experience the planning phase as responsive to their perspective.

One approach to the cancer screening might be a mobile van that travels through the community to bring screenings directly to the community members. If this was the recommended approach, permits from the cities, towns, and villages that participate in the mobile screening need to be secured. The community health nurse must consult with town officials and police departments to ensure that proper documents are secured and safety issues are resolved. A route for the mobile screening unit will need to be charted. Radio and television stations and newspapers should be contacted to alert the community about the screening.

The value of screening is to locate members of the community as early as possible in the disease process to offer prompt treatment and to limit any resulting disability. Screenings, therefore, must not only provide results to individuals who were screened but also have a system for referral so that necessary treatment is received. Community members will experience a sense of empowerment if they can effect a plan for action based on knowledge of their risk and available resources for treatment. The screening program will only be effective if a system of follow-up is planned. Thus, a community screening program involves the dedicated cooperation of community members, members of the interdisciplinary team, health and community agencies, community officials, and the press and the media. The community health nurse lends support to this process by coordinating the expertise of others in the community, using established networks, and forging new relationships within the community. The intent of the screening is to offer community members referral for possible diagnosis, since screening positive is presumptive, and to secure appropriate treatment as early as possible in the period of pathogenesis. Identifying affected members of the community as early as possible in the trajectory of illness so that treatment can be initiated is an example of a community-based intervention requiring the combined and coordinated efforts of the community health nurse, community members, and the interdisciplinary health care team.

ROLE OF THE COMMUNITY HEALTH NURSE

Most Valued Characteristics of a Professional

Expertise
Reliability
Responsibility
Accountability
Trustworthiness

Working with community agencies and valued contacts from these agencies requires that the community health nurse demonstrate the highest degree of professionalism. The **most valued characteristics** in this professional relationship are reliability, responsibility, accountability, and expertise. The community health nurse is trustworthy and dependable, that is, she or he follows up on the plan of care and maintains the highest quality of care. In fostering collaborative, cooperative relationships, the community health nurse must enlist the expertise of other members of the community to accomplish community-based health interventions. The combined efforts of the community health nurse, community members, and team members are much more effective in addressing the needs of the community than any one discipline alone. The community health nurse can facilitate the merging of the various perspectives and disciplines toward a common goal.

Key to the implementation of a team approach is the capability of the community health nurse as an effective collaborator and as a coordinator of care. Collaboration requires that the community health nurse possess a keen sense of the nursing profession's definition, goals, and functions. The community health nurse appreciates, and is able to communicate, the unique perspective that nurses offer in diagnosing and treating human responses to conditions of health, disease, disability, and death among varied populations. Collaboration also requires effective communication skills. Clarity in communication, given the various perspectives of community and health care team members, is essential in effecting a planned community-based intervention. Decision-making by consensus is the goal of collaboration. Consensus requires thoughtful discussion so that shared goals can be established and strategies determined for their implementation. The ability to deal with conflict constructively and to identify common issues and concerns are among the particular skills required of the community health nurse. Forging alliances is a cooperative undertaking. Turf issues must be resolved in ways that do not limit or detract from alliance building. The community health nurse draws on her or his expertise as a caring professional, combining a broad base of knowledge about health and social problems and the skills to intervene for the improved health of the community.

The community health nurse, in the role of coordinator of care, intervenes at the community level. The coordination role depends on the organizational capabilities of the nurse. The community health nurse must be able to analyze and synthesize data in meaningful and useful ways. Analysis and synthesis are high-level cognitive functions that depend on the community health nurse's practical comprehension of the community, its resources, and its members. The community health nurse draws on clinical knowledge of the community and his or her reputation as a respected and welcomed person in the community. The community health nurse pulls together information and resources to assist the community in addressing its health concerns and problems as well as in maintaining its strengths.

The aim of a coordinated plan of care is the notion of seamless care, that is, care without gaps. The community health nurse is concerned with caring for the whole community, not just the members that avail themselves of health services. Members without access to health care, members alienated from health care, and members without a voice to identify their needs are among the members of the community for whom the nurse cares. Regardless of the success of a community-based intervention, the nurse always asks about those community members who were not serviced. The community health nurse and other team members direct their care to the whole community. The ability to coordinate care enables the community health nurse to focus on reducing gaps in services to all community members.

The key to the successful implementation of collaborative care, relying on community members and the interdisciplinary health care team, is the community health nurse's skill as an effective collaborator, facilitator, and coordinator.

The community health nurse is the voice of the community and its members, particularly championing the needs of the underserved and those without a voice. The intent of this representation is to assure that the needs of all members of the community are considered and, hopefully, addressed. The aim of community-based intervention is to encourage community members to become effective partners in health care. As the community health nurse intervenes to raise the level of knowledge and skill among community members, their power and ability to engage in a participatory relationship in health care increases. The community health nurse transfers professional knowledge and skills to the members of the community. The goal of intervention is to assure that members of the community can care for themselves and mobilize the needed community resources to meet their own needs. Health care providers become valuable and responsive resources of the community and partners in the process.

COMMUNITY-BASED SERVICES

To design a plan of care with an individual client, the community health nurse uses assessment data gathered from the history and physical. This plan includes implementation of treatments and procedures and individualized health teaching and guidance. At the community level, the data gathered from the assessment of the community are used to plan community-based interventions. Community health nurses are involved in the development and implementation of health programs designed to address the health needs, risks, and problems of the community identified through the assessment. The nursing process is applied to the community as client.

The assessment process identifies the kinds of services and programs that are needed in the community. If there is a need for health information to be disseminated throughout the community, a health fair may be an effective strategy. At such an event, information can be liberally distributed to members of the community. Fliers, brochures, posters, and consultation can be offered to members as they enjoy the opportunity to attend the health fair. Information about reducing the risk of heart disease, the warning signs of cancer, protection from falls and accidents at home, and the importance of childhood immunizations are examples of the health information that can be disseminated.

If an assessment process determines that a health alert needs to reach the community, a warning can be issued via mass media, including radio, television, and newspapers. Alerts are designed to warn the community about health threats with the potential to affect the whole or a particular segment of the population. For example, a particular food could be associated with possible contamination, or a heat wave could be expected in which case recommendations to avoid dehydration would be important to communicate. A telephone number for questions enables community members to have their concerns addressed and to report on their experiences. Health fairs and health alerts are among the strategies that can be used to generate interest about health issues in members of the community.

If a particular health problem is identified through the assessment process, different strategies from those used to generate community awareness are used to intervene. The community health nurse serves as a facilitator to mobilize health care resources in the community to address the problem. For example, community assessment data may reveal an alarming number of teenagers in the community who use alcohol to meet their recreational and socialization needs. The community health nurse would arrange to meet with the teens through school-based clubs and groups, consult with the school nurse, and attend the school-community association meetings. The nurse may learn that students, parents, and teachers are particularly concerned about life-threatening situations, such as alcohol-related accidents. If there is interest in organizing a multifaceted response, the community health nurse may serve as a resource to the school-community association to help them select strategies that have a successful track record in other communities, such as Mothers Against Drunk Drivers (MADD) and Students Against Drunk Drivers (SADD), which have effectively responded to the problems of alcohol and adolescence. Safe Home is another program that community health nurses may suggest to the community. In this program, parents and other members of the community commit themselves to support early and ongoing education about alcohol and to provide alcohol-free youth activities.

If teen alcoholism is assessed as a community problem, there will be a need for treatment services. The community health nurse could collect information about the treatment and rehabilitation facilities in the community and share this information with the school and teen groups. Information about Alcoholics Anonymous, Al-Anon, and Alateen meetings can be distributed at the schools. A list of helpful resources, including alcohol treatment facilities (both inpatient and outpatient), addiction intake units, and hotlines/helplines, can be validated by the community health nurse before widespread distribution to community. The local police department could be enlisted to monitor the illegal sale of alcohol to minors. The community health nurse, informed about the available resources through the comprehensive assessment of the community, is now able to organize that information into useful resources and guides for community members. One of the key areas of nursing intervention in the community is to link community members with available resources.

The community health nurse in cooperation with community members and members of the health care team may confront the possibility that the community does not have the necessary resources to address an identified problem. The rise in alcohol-related incidents and accidents may be related to the lack of available recreational and socialization resources for the community's youth. If this is the case, an alliance of interested consumers and providers could create enough community interest for an organized response to that unmet need. For example, the community health nurse could be instrumental in creating a community forum about the idea of creating a community youth center.

The nurse could organize meetings to encourage teens to speak publicly about what they would like to see created. They may be interested simply in a place to congregate without many organized events. In response to this interest, a parking lot could be converted into a place for street hockey

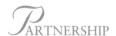

and basketball; a lounge area could be used for gathering and watching videos; or a drop-in center could be established as a place to hang out and meet with others. The youth are often able to define exactly what they want and need from a youth center, while the parents may have other ideas about what the youth center should be. The community health nurse could serve as a facilitator of communication and help the youth and their parents to resolve their differences effectively. Creating a resource that will truly meet a community need takes patience, time, and cooperation.

$\mathcal{T}$ARGET FOR COMMUNITY-BASED SERVICES

Target Population. This is a population that has been identified as at risk because of characteristics or behaviors that increase the chances of developing disease or disorder.

Community-based care is directed at a **target population**, which is often described as a population at risk. Populations at risk are aggregates that possess characteristics or exhibit behaviors that increase the chances of developing disease or a disorder. The community health nurse as part of the community assessment team identifies populations at high risk in the community so that interventions can improve their health status. It is important to identify populations at risk in a community because they place increased demand on the health care system for services and programs. This demand and increased utilization of health care services increase community health care costs. Members with depleted health can experience a diminished quality of life as well as reduced community productivity. The health of the community is reflected in the health of its members. Promoting the health of individuals and families that are part of high-risk populations improves the health of the community as a whole.

The community health nurse needs to know the risk factors associated with each high-risk population in the community, which risk factors can be modified, and the effective strategies for intervention. Interventions are geared toward reducing, modifying, or eliminating specific population risks. The community health nurse analyzes assessment and diagnostic data to identify nursing actions that can be taken across the continuum of care. Prevention interventions can reduce risk in high-risk populations. Primary prevention interventions are concerned with health promotion and protection strategies. Secondary prevention interventions are concerned with early diagnosis, treatment regimens, and limiting disability. Tertiary prevention interventions are concerned with rehabilitation efforts. By analyzing assessment and diagnostic data carefully, the community health nurse can anticipate and respond to community health needs and problems.

$\mathcal{P}$ARTNERSHIP

The idea of community health nurses and other providers of care entering into a partnership with consumers is the foundation of community-based health care (Matteson, 1996). Every community, whether heterogeneous or homogeneous, presents with a complex array of issues, health risks, and health problems. The community health nurse is incapable of addressing and solving all the problems of the community but serves the community best by supporting its strengths and encouraging it to advocate for itself by learning how to use the expertise of health care providers and other members. The responsibilities of the community health nurse and other providers of health care are to serve the community through facilitation, education, organization, consultation, and direct care.

Partnership is built on the ideal of mutual respect and cooperation. The community health nurse seeks to promote mutual respect among all members of the alliance for health. Promoting respect is facilitated when communication flows freely and is channeled constructively for the greater good of the community. Cooperation at the community level is often built on a foundation of successful ventures that make a difference to the life and health of the community. The community health nurse is able to assist progress toward a healthier community by fostering partnerships between providers and consumers and by helping the alliance created through this partnership to identify mutual goals that are achievable through a concerted community effort. Linking community members with resources that address their needs is one of the most important community health nursing intervention strategies. Encouraging partnerships of providers and consumers to address mutual concerns and developing linkages between community resources and community members to address their needs are the key components of community-based care.

Strategies for Community-Based Intervention

Population-based interventions require the community health nurse to extrapolate skills used in the care of individuals and families to the community level. Population-based interventions are focused on aggregates. The goal of population-based nursing practice is to promote the health of the community. In promoting healthy communities, the nurse is responsible for all the people in the community, not only those people who present for services. Population-based interventions are derived from a systematic assessment of the health strengths, needs, problems, and expectations of the people. The community health nurse together with community members determines the course of action and how to best use the limited resources of the community. Evaluation of interventions is also a collaborative effort and feeds back to ongoing assessment of needs and expectations.

Population-based care is defined by the community health nurse's accountability to the people of the community, who as partners in care, forge an alliance with the community health nurse. This alliance results in better utilization of available resources and, when possible, the development of new approaches for improving the health of the community.

Among the types of population-based intervention strategies are health teaching and screening; risk appraisal and risk reduction; advocacy; and health planning and resource development.

Health Teaching and Screening for Aggregates

The community health nurse is inherently a health teacher and counselor. In virtually all clinical situations, the nurse provides health information, education, and counseling (Stanhope & Knollmueller, 1997). To function effectively in providing these services, the nurse must understand the kinds of learning that can be transmitted. Learning is a dynamic interchange between the community health nurse and the community members: the nurse learns from the community members while he or she educates the community members. This dynamic interchange enables the nurse to refine perspective and reshape the focus of the learning experience continually based on a holistic understanding of the people and their health needs and expectations. The nurse learns about the values and beliefs of the community, including the cultural and spiritual influences on health. The nurse learns about the community's capacity to care for its members through members, agencies, and resources, enabling the nurse to build linkages between people with needs and available services. The nurse contributes expertise to the community, that is, knowledge and skills that empower the community to care for itself.

Information is power. Health information empowers communities to promote their own health and protect the health of their members. The transmission of health information through education and counseling is a major component of community-based nursing interventions (Friede, O'Carroll, Nicola, Oberle, & Teutsch, 1997). Identification of learning needs takes place through a systematic assessment, which is validated by the community members. Learning involves more that the simple sharing of information. Imparting information does not necessarily guarantee that understanding has taken place, that the information can be put to use, or that the information will result in a change in health practices. The community health nurse intends to relate information in such a way that the community understands it and behavioral changes result.

The three domains of learning identified by Bloom (1956) and used by nurses as health teachers are: cognitive, affective, and psychomotor learning. *Cognitive learning* is mental processing. The cognitive domain involves the recognition of knowledge and the development of intellectual capabilities and skills. Learning in the cognitive domain begins with the simple recall of information. Comprehension follows, in which recall is combined with understanding. Then, the learning is put to use through application. Self-care is a good illustration of the application of new information for personal health. Moving beyond application involves the ability of people to analyze or break down material into its component parts in order to understand the relationships among the parts. Once broken down, the next level of cognition involves synthesis in which the elements are formed into a new whole. The community puts its own unique twist on learning and finds solutions to its problems. The highest level of cognitive learning, evaluation, takes place when cognitive learning is judged for its usefulness. The nurse and the community members judge the adequacy of solutions and needed improvements.

Affective learning involves emotions, feelings, or affect. This kind of learning deals with changes in values, beliefs, and attitudes. Values are deeply influenced by society, as well as the beliefs and experiences of the families and people who form the community. Values and beliefs can be learned and changed, a process that occurs at several levels. The first level is receptivity when people in the community demonstrate a willingness to be attentive. This is followed by responsiveness when people become active participants by responding or reacting, thereby showing their interest in seeking out more information on their own. As affective learning progresses, the people of the community learn to accept, appreciate, and become committed to the new value. Ultimately, the new value becomes part of community behavior as it is incorporated into the life style of the community.

Psychomotor learning is learning to perform skills that require some kind of neuromuscular coordination. Community members must demonstrate the capability required of the skill, learn how to perform the skill, and practice the skill realizing that mastery is possible when the skill can be performed in a smooth and coordinated fashion. Community health nurses can teach groups in the community how to perform cardiopulmonary resuscitation (CPR) and other lifesaving skills which require psychomotor learning.

Consider, for example, a community-based health concern like human immunodeficiency virus (HIV) and acquired immunodeficiency syndrome (AIDS). Community members may need to learn about the modes of transmission of HIV, methods of protection from the virus, and the trajectory of the syndrome from the point of infection. This kind of learning is cognitive. It is essential that members of the community receive accurate and useful information that clarifies misinformation and enables them to gain a fuller understanding of the syndrome. Members of the community must also learn that people with HIV/AIDS can engage in community life as fully as possible. Engendering acceptance and a willingness to share in the life of the community involves affective learning. Ideally, the members of the community come to believe that all members of the community are valued and important and entitled to their rights. Learning universal precaution skills involving blood and body fluids includes the use of gloves, bleach/water washing for blood spills, and use of CPR masks in an emergency situation that requires mouth-to-mouth resuscitation. This kind of learning is psychomotor because it entails the development of skills. Teaching in this domain requires a demonstrable performance of skills. Over time, the skill is performed capably.

If the community health nurse is able to clarify the learning needs of the people in partnership with them, then the nurse can determine the domains of learning involved and then construct methods for teaching that respond appropriately to the learning need. Cognitive information may be broadcast over the local television or radio stations to reach the greatest number of community members. For example, education about the need for immunization as a measure of health protection could be transmitted in a culturally relevant manner to assist people to seek information for themselves and their significant others. Forming support groups to share experiences involving loss and trauma fosters affective learning; it teaches people that they can become survivors by integrating these losses into their lives and living beyond the trauma they have experienced. Teaching members of the community how to perform the Heimlich maneuver and CPR facilitates psychomotor learning at the community level. A community can decide that all members should become proficient in executing these life-saving interventions. Teaching these skills to groups eventually blankets the entire community with this learning.

Screening programs (U. S. Preventive Services Task Force, 1996) are an efficient and effective way to identify individuals in the community who may unknowingly have a health condition or disease. Screening is categorized as secondary prevention because the stimulus precipitating the health condition or disease has already influenced the interactions of the host, agent, and environment. As a result, the person has entered the period of pathogenesis in the natural history of disease. Screenings can identify a single condition or be multiphasic, thereby involving a battery of tests to detect several disease conditions. The important aspect of screening a particular population is that screening does not provide a conclusive diagnosis; rather, screening is presumptive, identifying individuals who may unknowingly have a problem; further testing is required for a definitive diagnosis. Therefore, the goal of screening is to lead to an early diagnosis of a health condition or disease, which permits prompt treatment to limit the progression of disease.

The community health nurse plays a critical role in facilitating referral for appropriate testing and diagnosis. Without this follow-up and referral, the significance of the screening is invalidated, and the people of the community are left without needed care. Screenings should not be used as substitutes for regular health care since the findings of screenings are presumptive and the focus of a screening is quite limited. The nurse should also caution community members that false-negative results may occur. The community health nurse is aware of the necessity of reaching all members of vulnerable groups and the importance of meticulous follow-up. Screening enables case finding in the community. Case finding is a continuous process, not a one-time project. Screenings in combination with teaching and counseling provide a huge complement of services to the community.

The community health nurse acts as a therapeutic agent for health education, counseling, and screening. The nurse is able to teach and counsel about and screen for a vast array of concerns that the people of the community will find useful, meaningful, culturally appropriate, and beneficial to the community's health.

Risk Appraisal and Risk Reduction

The appraisal of health risk and strategies to reduce these risks are important interventions to promote the health of communities (Pender, 1996;

Woolf, Jonas, & Lawrence, 1996). Risk appraisal is a method used to describe the chances of becoming ill or dying from selected diseases. A risk appraisal generates a probability statement about the likelihood of disease based on quantifying the effect and interaction of influencing variables. For example, risk factors associated with developing heart disease are smoking, hypertension, hypercholesterolemia, and obesity. A risk appraisal called RISKO: A Heart Health Appraisal quantifies these four factors and develops scores for men and women, which result in estimations of risk. RISKO was developed by the American Heart Association (1994).

High blood pressure, high blood cholesterol, cigarette smoking, and physical inactivity are considered the four major modifiable risk factors for heart disease; obesity is a contributing risk factor. Physical inactivity is not part of the statistical base from which RISKO was derived. The RISKO scores measure the risk of developing heart disease in the next several years for those individuals currently showing no evidence of such disease. Risk categories are: lowest risk of heart disease for age and sex; low-to-moderate risk (needing some improvement) for heart disease for age and sex; moderate-to-high risk for heart disease for age and sex (needing considerable improvement on some factors); high risk for developing heart disease for age and sex (needing a great deal of improvement on all factors); and very high risk for developing heart disease for age and sex (should take immediate action on all risk factors). Since diabetes strongly influences the risk of heart disease, additional points are added to the total score for persons with diabetes. This simple hand-scored tool can be used with large groups of people to determine subgroups at the various risk levels for heart disease, which necessitates varying forms of intervention to help populations reduce their risks. Using aggregate risk appraisal data is an important method for impacting the health of populations in the community.

Risk appraisal and risk reduction provide a way in which the community health nurse can assist aggregates to develop a self-care agenda. The success of risk reduction is based on the finding that mortality decreases as the number of health practices increases (Schoenborn, 1986). Health is an elusive and complex condition. The determinants of health include the environment, human biology, health care, and life style. Risk appraisal and risk reduction focus on life style as a major determinant of health. Life-style choices are made everyday. Some of these choices are known to be health depleting or damaging. Health habits have been studied longitudinally. One of the earliest and most significant studies was conducted in Alameda County, California. This study "found that seven specific health habits, commonly referred to as the 'Alameda 7,' were related to both concurrent and subsequent health status and to long-term survival" (Schoenborn, 1986, p. 571). These habits were: having never smoked, drinking less than five drinks at one sitting, sleeping 7 to 8 h a night, exercising, maintaining desirable weight for height, avoiding snacks, and eating breakfast regularly. Educational, racial, and income differences were found for most of the health practices. The people at greatest risk were in socially and economically disadvantaged groups. Studies like this reveal the great disparities that exist in communities and within specific populations regarding health potential.

Health-hazard appraisals are risk appraisals that use clinical and epidemiological data to assess health risks to avert disease and premature death. Lifetime health monitoring is another appraisal that also uses clinical and epidemiological data but provides preventive measures appropriate to different age groups. This appraisal lists recommendations that are age-group specific. A wellness inventory is an appraisal that suggests healthy life-style changes that support wellness. Regardless of the particular method or tool, the idea of appraising risk and developing intervention strategies to reduce risk are important strategies for communities.

The community health nurse is always alerted to identifying persons in the community who are at risk for whatever reason (race, culture, gender, age, economics, geography) to help connect them to services in the community that may be able to address their need for health promotion services. In addition to conducting risk appraisals for populations in the community, the community itself can be appraised for risks for the entire community. Risks such as as air, water, and noise pollution as well as racism are powerful threats to the health of the community. Risk appraisal enables the community health nurse to collect data about the community and its populations, to quantify risk, and then to develop risk-reduction strategies to decrease risk factors. Risk appraisal and risk reduction are important strategies for community health promotion and early detection of health threats and disease patterns.

Advocacy

Advocacy (Kohnke, 1982) is part of the philosophical foundation of nursing and clearly a key component of the community health nurse's practice. It comprises the acts of informing and supporting communities in the hope of achieving their health potential. Advocacy can take on many forms. The nurse can be the voice for individuals without power. Advocacy by representation is the act of standing up for community members whose needs are not being addressed. In order to accomplish this, the community health nurse may attend community board meetings and speak on behalf of those community members who are not linked to the health resources of the community.

The community health nurse can also act as an advocate of the community by demystifying the health care delivery system. Often people in the community do not know how to access services or how to get through the maze of services available. Understanding admission requirements, knowing the kinds of documentation that are necessary for service, and being aware of reimbursable services and the services that address particular problems are pieces of information that the skilled community health nurse can offer community members. Sometimes community members simply need a point of entry into the health care system to benefit from the services. The community health nurse then uses personal contacts at agencies to open doors and enable the community members to partake of services. Ultimately, the community health nurse tries to transform a profoundly authoritarian health care system to one that encourages and supports participation.

Advocacy is a form of empowerment. When the community health nurse advocates for the community, power is shared and ultimately transferred to the community since self-care is the goal of healthy communities. In addition to representing the people's needs and enabling existing resources to be used by the community, the community health nurse also monitors and evaluates the quality of care members of the community receive. Engaging in research that measures outcomes and quality of care is the essence of advocacy. High-quality care, affordable care, accessible care, and responsible care are the goals of community-based health services.

Health Planning and Resource Development

Planned change is a powerful strategy in the care of communities (Bennis, Benne, & Chin, 1985). The community health nurse is challenged to participate actively in the political process that supports the development of health care services that are affordable, accessible, culturally appropriate, innovative, and of the highest quality possible. The community health nurse facilitates the possibility for power created through a collaborative alliance with community members and interdisciplinary team members. This collaboration sets the stage for enabling communities to become truly responsive to population-based health problems and concerns (Table 9-1).

The community health nurse looks to policy makers and community leaders to engage in this process of change for the expansion and development of needed community resources. Systems of care management can be created, which maximize limited resources and expand the boundaries of agencies concerned about health (Shortell, Gillies, Anderson, Erickson, & Mitchell, 1996). Creative solutions to difficult human problems are possible. The ingenuity of the community health nurse in collaborative alliances can result in valuable solutions. The voice of the community health nurse is the voice representing the health of the community. The nurse becomes the translator of community health needs. The community health nurse translates the health care system into an approachable, responsive service for the promotion and protection of the health of the community. The community health nurse becomes involved in health policy and planning so that resources needed in the community can be developed.

CHALLENGES OF POPULATION-BASED CARE

The nursing process, the method used by community health nurses to assure the delivery of quality professional nursing care, has long been focused on individual health, giving limited attention to health concerns of families, aggregates, and communities. The community health nurse now uses the nursing process to care for the entire community. Yet, refinement of systematic assessment, diagnostic statements, intervention strategies,

Planned Change. Planned change is a systematic, purposeful, collaborative effort to integrate change for health in a community through the use of agreed-upon actions

Task Force. A task force is an interdisciplinary alliance of community and professional members acting to represent the community of need and promote and protect community health.

◙

TABLE 9-1

STEPS IN COMMUNITY-BASED PLANNED CHANGE

Assessment of Community Need
- Gather together a task force or group of interested community members representative of the diverse viewpoints, needs, and populations of the community.
- Analyze existing data about the community sources, including morbidity and mortality studies, community reports, and previously conducted surveys.
- Determine the community's history of coping with change and willingness to change.
- Design and conduct a survey of the community to verify impressions of existing data and establish current health patterns and problems, using the Alliance for Health model.
- Agree upon an identified area of need for planning interventions.

Analysis and Planning
- Synthesize all sources of data and identify priority areas of concern to community health.
- Employ knowledge of the community's willingness and style of responding to change in the planning process.
- Develop a plan for intervention, working through a collaborative alliance.
- Identify desirable outcomes that can be used to measure efficacy of planned interventions.

Implementation
- Identify and link possible sources for funding the plan.
- Facilitate a plan through efforts and actions of task force members.
- Carry out the plan collaboratively.

Evaluation
- Use qualitative and quantitative measures to judge outcomes or interventions.
- Identify short-term and long-term consequences of interventions.
- Integrate early evaluation findings to effect continuing implementation.
- Use outcomes to reassess community-based needs.

---

and methods of evaluation are needed. Application of the nursing process in caring for communities must become a skill that all nurses use.

Nurse educators are challenged to formulate curricula and provide clinical learning opportunities in community-based nursing. "Nurse educators need to prepare themselves to practice in an increasingly community-oriented industry. The National League for Nursing . . . describes this phenomenon as '. . . realigning our (professional) allegiance and accountability away from institutions and toward populations'" (Zotti, Brown, & Stotts,

1996, p. 211). The identification of at-risk aggregates is central to community-based care.

The creation of community health care centers for the health of communities in which the community health nurse plays a central role challenges our health care system to become more responsible about the health of community members. Identification of populations at risk and case finding are the core elements of community-based care strategies. Efforts to create legislation reducing risk and saving lives can be undertaken with collaborative efforts between community members and health care providers. Care management and the development of affordable services for aggregates challenge our delivery systems to provide responsive direct care.

The community health nurse is challenged to create knowledge through epidemiological research, which supports and promotes the health of communities and generates population-based clinical data. The community health nurse is also challenged to address the needs of populations as they change. Shifting health patterns and problems that require rapid response for community-based interventions dictate the need for vigilant and responsive community health nurses. These nurses must also be proficient in statistics, geographical distributions, housing needs, environmental alterations, and international health issues and concerns. The community health nurse must also "read" the community as it evolves, to anticipate potential health problems and implement health practices and services to remediate these problems as early as possible.

Community-based care is not only a challenge to the community health nurse and members of the multidisciplinary team but also a challenge to communities. Communities are challenged to regain power and reshape themselves embracing the notion that health is their right.

$\mathcal{S}$UMMARY

Responding to community-based problems takes the cooperation of the community health nurse, community members, and the members of the interdisciplinary health care team. Systems of care management need to be mobilized, and innovative solutions need to be organized. When agencies already exist in the community, the community health nurse can serve as an organizer and facilitator to enlist providers to deliver the needed services. When agencies are nonexistent, the community health nurse can develop an alliance with community members and members of a health care team to advocate for the needed services. The community health nurse can also implore existing services to expand their mission to address unmet needs in the community.

The community health nurse working at the community level is concerned with linking people to resources. The nurse uses skills in health planning and resource development to assist the community in its ability to respond to community needs.

Community-based interventions enhance the community's health through a partnership of providers and consumers. Programs that support the community's health are identified and designed. The community health nurse is ultimately concerned with creating effective linkages between community members and the resources that can address their health care needs. The health of the community improves as the health of populations within the community improves.

KEY WORDS

Advocacy	Resource development
Collaboration	Risk appraisal
Coordination	Risk reduction
Health planning	Screening
Health teaching	Team approach
Partnership	

QUESTIONS

Directions: Choose the one *best* response to each of the following questions.

1. Comprehensive assessment of the community's health leads to
    A. community intervention.
    B. community planning.
    C. community diagnosis.
    D. community evaluation.

2. The goal of community-based interventions is
    A. sharing professional expertise with community members.
    B. resolution of turf issues among disciplines.
    C. service delivery only to those most in need.
    D. self-care through resource utilization.

3. In community-based care, a population at risk is defined as
    A. an aggregate with an increased chance of developing a disease or disorder.
    B. a population of people living far away from a hospital.
    C. people with many obstacles to obtaining the necessities of life.
    D. individuals who rely on social services for financial support.

4. Although all of the following activities can be carried out by the community health nurse, which one is *not* typical of a community-based practice?
    A. Conducting a scoliosis screening for school-age children
    B. Giving first aid to a child injured on a playground
    C. Advocating for a Safe Home program for parents of adolescents
    D. Instituting a first-aid class for teachers in the school system

5. Each role that a community health nurse assumes has its special characteristics. Which of the following are the most important characteristics required of the community health nurse–collaborator role?
    A. Communicates effectively, conflict-resolver, able to form alliances

B. Spirit of inquiry, analytic, scientific orientation
C. Formulates objectives, organized, teaches effectively
D. Risk-taker, public speaker, tenacious

ANSWERS

1. *The answer is C.* Community diagnoses are derived from community assessment data.

2. *The answer if D.* The goal of community-based interventions is to assure that members of the community can care for themselves and mobilize the needed community resources to meet their own needs.

3. *The answer is A.* Populations at risk are aggregates that possess characteristics or exhibit behaviors that increase the chances of developing a disease or disorder. Options B, C, and D are examples of at-risk populations.

4. *The answer is B.* Caring for an individual child is not an example of community-based care. Options A, C, and D refer to interventions with aggregates and are, therefore, examples of community-based care.

5. *The answer is A.* The role of the community health nurse–collaborator requires effective communication skills, the ability to deal with conflict constructively, and a willingness to forge alliances with community members and members of the interdisciplinary health care team.

ANNOTATED REFERENCES

American Health Association. (1994). *RISKO: A heart health appraisal.* Dallas: National Center.

This brochure provides a way to evaluate the risk of coronary heart disease based upon risk factors. Descriptive information is also provided on the prevalence of health, disease, guidelines for reducing risk, and securing additional information from the Heart Association.

Bennis, W. G., Benne, K. D., & Chin, R. (1985). The planning of change (4th ed.). New York: Holt.

This text provides a comprehensive overview of the process of implementing change.

Bloom, B. S. (Ed.). (1956). Taxonomy of educational objectives: The classification of educational goals. New York: David McKay.

The classic work of Benjamin Bloom is frequently referenced when learning is discussed. The domains of learning are detailed.

Friede, A., O'Carroll, P. W., Nicola, R. M., Oberle, M. W., & Teutsch, S. M. (Eds.). (1997). *CDC prevention guidelines: A guide to action.* Baltimore: Williams & Wilkins.

This text is a selection of Centers for Disease Control and Prevention (CDC) guidelines on a variety of public health topics, many of which are not typically covered in medical or public health texts. The guidelines include sections on infectious diseases, maternal and child health/nutrition, cancer, chronic disease, environmental health, injuries, occupational health, and miscellaneous topics.

Kohnke, M. F. (1982). Advocacy: Risk and reality. St. Louis: C. V. Mosby.

This book remains the most comprehensive treatise on advocacy written for a nursing audience.

Matteson, P. S. (Ed.). (1995). *Teaching nursing in the neighborhoods: The Northeastern University model.* New York: Springer.

This book describes the community-based clinical nursing education model developed by Northeastern University College of Nursing, in partnership with Boston's Center for Community Health Education, Research, and Service. It offers practical guidance for nurse educators who wish to respond to emerging trends by innovating community-based learning for students. The Boston center is one of seven consortia around the country supported by the W. K. Kellogg Foundation in its initiative for Community Partnerships for Health Professions Education.

Pender, N. J. (1996). *Health promotion in nursing practice* (3rd ed.). Stamford, CT: Appleton & Lange.

This book provides an overview of major health behavior models and theories that guide health promotion interventions. Strategies for health promotive care are discussed, which spark interest in patient-focused health care systems that meet the health promotion and disease prevention needs of the population. Future directions for health promotion research and theory development are proposed.

Public Health Nursing Section, American Public Health Association. (1980). *The definition and role of public health nursing in the delivery of health care: A statement of the Public Health Nursing Section.* Washington, DC: Author.

This pamphlet presents the position statement of the Public Health Nursing Section on the definition and role of public health nursing in the delivery of health care and explores the dimensions and theoretical framework of public health nursing practice. This work was supported by a grant from the American Public Health Association.

Schoenborn, C. A. (1986). Health habits of U. S. adults, 1985: The "Alameda 7" revisited. *Public Health Reports, 101* (6), 571–580.

This article presents selected findings on the prevalence of seven health habits, commonly referred to as the "Alameda 7," which were shown to be associated with physical health status and mortality in a pioneer longitudinal study initiated in 1965 in Alameda County, California. The Alameda study focused attention on the importance of everyday practices for the maintenance of good health, and ultimately, for longer life.

Shortell, S. M., Gillies, R. R., Anderson, D. A., Erickson, K. M., & Mitchell, J. B. *Remaking health care in America: Building organized delivery systems*. San Francisco: Jossey-Bass.

This book presents the results of a comprehensive 4-year study of the response to growing management care and cost-containment pressures among several health care systems. It examines the success and failures of the current system and provides case study examples and recommendations for developing and implementing a more integrated, cost-effective delivery system.

Stanhope, M., & Knollmueller, R. N. (1997). *Public and community health nurse's consultant: A health promotion guide*. St. Louis: C. V. Mosby.

This book is a compilation of instruments, guides, charts, graphs, and forms that provide public health and community health nurses with cues to aid in caring for individuals, families, and communities. Assessment guides are complemented with detailed indicators of risk, teaching techniques and anticipatory guidance, and screening tools and diagnostic criteria.

U. S. Preventive Services Task Force. (1996). *Guide to clinical preventive services* (2nd ed.). Baltimore: Williams & Wilkins.

This new edition carefully reviews the evidence for and against hundreds of preventive services, recommending a test, immunization, or counseling intervention only when there is evidence that it is effective. The section on screening covers: cardiovascular diseases; neoplastic diseases; metabolic, nutritional, and environmental disorders; infectious diseases; vision and hearing disorders; prenatal disorders; congenital disorders; musculoskeletal disorders; mental disorders; and substance abuse.

Woolf, S. H., Jonas, S., & Lawrence, R. S. (1996). *Health promotion and disease prevention in clinical practice*. Baltimore: Williams & Wilkins.

This book provides clinicians with practical information about how to perform clinical preventive services. The book is organized in the same sequence as the clinical encounter. How to gather information is followed by designing a health maintenance plan targeted to personal health behaviors and risk factors and concludes with putting prevention recommendations into practice.

Zotti, M. E., Brown, P., & Stotts, R. C. (1996). Community-based nursing versus community health nursing: What does it all mean? *Nursing Outlook, 44* (5), 211–217.

This article compares and contrasts community-based and community health nursing practice, challenging nursing schools in the United States to develop curricula and provide clinical experiences in the community and emphasize community development and participation in community assessment.

COMMUNITY-BASED CARE OUTCOMES

Nursing Process. This is an interrelated dynamic sequence of purposeful nursing actions aimed at analyzing and meeting clients' health needs. The steps include assessment, diagnosis, planning, intervention, and evaluation.

Outcome Evaluation. This is a measurement of the results or consequences of a particular action in relation to some criteria.

CHAPTER OUTLINE

The methodology of nursing is the **nursing process.** It is an ongoing, circular process that involves problem-solving, critical decision-making, clinical skills, application of theory, and use of self. When we first learn about a process, it is often easier to examine its phases in a linear progression so that the individual steps of the process can be closely examined. However, complex human systems cannot be fully defined or appreciated through linear progression. This chapter explores the nursing process as a dynamic, rhythmical series of planned actions in which human needs are recognized, appreciated, responded to, evaluated, and assessed.

Human learning progresses along a continuum that ranges from simple recall of information, through understanding concepts, toward the creative use of new information. Evaluation is a high-level expression of learning, which involves critical quantitative and qualitative decision-making. It involves examination against specific criteria and requires judgments to be made as to whether or not these criteria have been satisfied. Evaluation data become the basis for ongoing assessment and revision of plans.

The nursing process can be applied to all client systems: individuals, families, aggregates, and communities. The evaluation phase of the nursing process involves the measurement of client outcomes that result from specific nursing interventions. The community health nurse, in partnership with the client, utilizes outcome criteria to shape and reshape nursing diagnoses, to serve as a basis for intervention, and to provide measurement of ongoing goal attainment. The nursing process, a circular process, is connected as evaluation and ongoing assessment link the process into a whole.

This chapter explores the process of evaluation as it applies to aggregates and communities. It focuses on the outcomes of the nursing process in the care of communities. There is a relative lack of specific criteria that validate the critical role community-based nursing interventions play in the delivery of cost-effective, quality health care. With the advent of managed care, home care agencies aggressively determine individual client criteria to guide home visits and to validate their role. With a renewed emphasis on health promotion, community health nurses are further challenged to substantiate their vital role in improving the health of communities. Outcome criteria are needed to establish the efficacy of nursing care strategies and to provide research data upon which community health nursing practice is validated and funding decisions are determined. Political support of community health nursing services is essential for continued funding of nursing and other related health services that serve the health of the community.

$\mathcal{P}$ROCESS OF EVALUATING A HEALTH PROGRAM

The last formal phase of the nursing process is the evaluation phase. It is in this phase that the nurse makes a judgment about whether clients' needs were met by particular nursing actions. Evaluation is closely connected to both assessment and identified goals. It helps to determine whether there is a need for further data collection or goal revision. The evaluative process should lead the community health nurse to ask qualitative questions about an intervention. It is impossible to determine whether or not a goal has been achieved without supporting evidence. Was the goal met and if not, why not? Was the data assessment complete? Was the goal realistic? Was the goal supported by the client?

Community health nursing is faced with the challenge of moving beyond individual or family-centered interventions to focus on population and community-based care. The community health nurse's competence in assessment, collaboration, coordination, community empowerment, and health program implementation is an essential resource that will help to improve the health of communities. However, the task of validating these services as well as making them operational is a primary responsibility of the community health nurse (Deal, 1994). Educators and nurse researchers are focusing on the development of outcome criteria to evaluate and establish the benefits and cost-effectiveness of community health nursing interventions. Agencies and nursing organizations are networking to establish evaluation criteria based on client outcomes instead of organization or provider activities (Harris & Dugan, 1996). The recent health care shift towards health promotion and population-based interventions provides the perfect milieu for advancement of the role of the community health nurse.

The goal of community-based health care is the delivery of culturally relevant health care that is available, accessible, affordable, appropriate, adequate, and acceptable. Additional elements include an equal partnership between the provider and the population served and an interdisciplinary team approach to care. Just as the nursing strategies aimed at communities are uniquely aggregate-focused, so too are the outcome measures. Measurable **outcomes** of health care services include utilization, improved health status,

Outcomes are measurable changes in the client's behavior attributable to the dyamic interchange between the client system, nursing actions, and intervening variables.

Rural/Urban Continuum. This is a conceptualization of residence that includes very large cities at one end and small, remote rural areas at the other. The myriad of towns, villages, and suburbs lie in between these extremes.

quality of life, health promotion, disease prevention, and satisfaction with health care (National Institute of Nursing Research, 1995). The community as client is intimately involved with all phases of health care: goal setting, program development, and making decisions about expected outcomes.

Populations are dispersed along a **rural/urban continuum**, which relates to the density of population. Place of residence is known to play a significant role in an individual's perception of health. Research focuses closely on the similarities and differences between rural and urban residents and the social, cultural, and health issues that are evident in each setting (National Institute of Nursing Research, 1995).

Evaluation is usually thought of in two categories: *formative evaluation* and *summative evaluation*. Each serves a very different purpose.

The main goal of formative evaluation is providing feedback. It is used during the early working phase of a program. It aims at securing useful information to improve and administer a program. Formative evaluation is ongoing and provides direction for changes in goals or interventions.

Summative evaluation addresses overall effectiveness and goal-attainment. It is carried out at the conclusion of a program and provides data on whether or not overall objectives were met. The analysis of this summative evaluation determines what future interventions are indicated.

The following scenario illustrates the importance of including evaluation in every phase of the nursing process and the need for the community health nurse to remain continuously open to new data.

CASE STUDY: The Importance of Evaluation in Every Phase of the Nursing Process

In a given community, the community health nurse may determine from conducting a community health needs assessment that the adolescent population's nutritional health needs are not adequately met. Upon further inspection of the data and after consultation with a network of school nurses, the evidence leads the community health nurse to conclude that this population is specifically at risk for eating disorders. An eating disorders screening that targets the community's adolescent population is successfully instituted. The resources of the school nurse network, the parent–teacher associations, and other members of the health care team were all mobilized to gain community support. The number of adolescents screened in relation to the total student population was statistically very high.

The true measure of success, however, does not lie with the large percentage of adolescents screened but rather with the quality of follow-up provided to those adolescents whose screening results were positive for the risk of an eating disorder. These students were referred to community facilities that were able to make the appropriate diagnosis and offered needed treatment. However, since change is a slow process, the best indicator of successful goal attainment would be the number of adolescents and families actively involved in treatment after a period of 6 months.

In this example, conditions are ideal. The health problem was recognized as an important adolescent risk factor, the screening was effective in reaching the identified target, and the facilities to diagnose and treat were available and used. The original screening goals were carried out. Under varying community conditions, the process could be very different. If the

⌖

TABLE 10-1

PHASES OF PLANNED COMMUNITY-BASED NURSING EVALUATION

Planning
- Determine if goals and objectives were written in a clear, measurable manner
- Select criteria that will determine to what degree goals are met
- Identify what specific questions will be addressed in the evaluation
- Establish a time framework
- Build in evaluation into every phase
- Assess and plan for the costs involved
- Assure consumer/provider input
- Establish responsibilities
- Build a process for how the findings will be used
- Determine whether or not the evaluation is feasible

Data Collection
- Determine when, how, and by whom data will be collected
- Refine the process based upon your early findings
- Build and use indicators of progress that show movement toward stated goals

Analysis
- Identify who will analyze the data
- Establish mechanisms for analysis
- List interpretations
- Raise as many questions as possible about the findings and relationships with other known data
- Make recommendations and list a variety of courses of action, including the strengths and weaknesses of each

Synthesis and Communicating
- Determine which of the findings will be included in a report and whose responsibility it will be to compile this
- Establish a format
- Make decisions regarding who will receive the evaluation findings

Implementations of Findings
- Refer back to original planning regarding how results of evaluation were to be used
- Establish a process for integration of findings
- Incorporate those responsible for implementation into the process

screening was planned but the parents and school community were resistant to referring the students, efforts would first have to focus on exploring this resistance and building trust. Time would have to be spent gaining community support for an acceptable program. If during the implementation phase it was discovered that the necessary resources for care management were not available to provide follow-up treatment alternatives, the nurse might conclude that adolescent health care was not a community priority. The nurse might focus energy on building an alliance of concerned adolescents and families to increase community awareness of the need for adolescent- focused health services. Political action might be indicated to secure future funding for adolescent health care needs. Ongoing evaluation is the binding thread between each of the phases of planned nursing action. Success does not necessarily mean that original goals were met. In the context of a partnership with the community, planned nursing actions require constant examination, critical judgments, and an open mind.

CHARACTERISTICS AND COMPONENTS OF EVALUATION

The choice of a specific evaluation approach is directly linked to the evaluator's skill at matching up the focus of the evaluation with an appropriate design. No one particular type of evaluation tool meets all needs. Nor is one approach inherently better than the other. This challenge lies in making a good match.

Much of the evaluation of quality care within the health care field today has its history in a structure-process-outcome framework (Donabedian, 1969). From its origins in medicine, Donabedian's theories have been widely adapted to nursing and other health care areas. The delivery of health care to communities is often carried out through **programs** focused at the aggregate level. The evaluation of these interventions is often more complex and sophisticated than evaluation at the individual client or family level. An expanding collaborative view of community evaluation can be conceptualized within the framework of an open-ended structure-process-outcome approach. Familiarity with questions of evaluation that are best addressed in each part of this approach will aid the nurse in maximizing benefits to the client.

Program is a set of structured activities within the health care system aimed at meeting the identified needs of individuals, families, aggregates, and communities. It has as its goals the elimination or reduction of a problem or risk, fostering of strengths, and health maintenance or promotion.

Structural Questions

The evaluation of structure focuses on organization and instrumentalities. It involves facilities, equipment, materials, human resources, and financing. There is an assumption within this approach that the fulfillment of certain conditions in a setting is directly related to the quality of care. This approach is frequently used for the accreditation and certification of agencies. Structural evaluation is usually carried out through an examination of records or direct observation. When analyzing structure, the community health nurse might ask:

- What are the specific responsibilities of nurses in a particular setting?
- What are the numbers of baccalaureate vs. master's prepared nurses?
- What is the ratio of Spanish-speaking nurses to Spanish-speaking clients in a community?
- What is the consumer/provider ratio on the planning board for a community or agency?
- What is the pattern of resource utilization?
- How is the budget itemized?

Process Questions

Process evaluation focuses on the care itself. It examines and judges the elements and details of the actual care provided. There is an appraisal and testing of the belief that certain characteristics of care are directly related to levels of provider performance. Process evaluation focuses on the means by which programs and services are delivered to a community. One level of process questioning addresses an inspection of the fundamental goals and objectives of a program. It reviews the implementation of a program for the specific purpose of fine-tuning. Process evaluation is formative evaluation. Evaluation may be daily or periodic. Program management concerns are addressed while constantly examining the original goals and objectives in the light of a changing environment. Process evaluations obtain data through observations of nurse/client interactions and review of program and community records.

Another level of process evaluation concerns assessing client satisfaction with the services provided. Goodness-of-fit type questions fall into this category and are carried out through interviewing, survey, observation, and testing. Process questioning often involves subjective data and requires a strong input from both client and staff. However, this collaborative approach can lead to innovative and alternative methods of delivering care to communities (Bingham & Felbinger, 1989). When analyzing process, the community health nurse might ask:

- Is there an actual need for this program, as it is designed?
- Is the original budget on target?
- Are contractual agreements between the provider and the community being met? If not, what barriers have been identified?
- Are the needs of the community adequately reflected in the stated goals and objectives?
- What additional staff needs are there?
- To what degree is there observable community support? How can this be increased?
- Which components of the plan seem to pose a problem for implementation?

- Are we reaching the target population? What type of outreach has been attempted? What may be needed in the future?
- What are community perceptions of the program? Is there an image problem?
- Are there time or resource constraints?
- What staff concerns have been identified during the early phases of the program?
- What concerns have community members brought up? Have program changes incorporated this input?
- Are we duplicating services provided elsewhere?
- What changes in the plan are needed to meet the stated objectives better?
- What else is needed to ensure progress?
- Has the original program evolved? If so, how and why?

Outcome Questions

Outcome evaluation assesses the end results of care. It analyzes specific expected and unexpected changes in a client's health status, behavior, attitudes, or knowledge that are attributable to some specific intervention. When most people think of program evaluation, impact evaluation is what comes to mind. As a result of this intervention, what types and levels of change were effected? Evaluations that assess impact are easier to visualize and appear to be more straightforward and recognizable than process evaluations. Outcome evaluation focuses on overall effectiveness. It determines how well the objectives were met in the final analysis. What good, if any, was done? Outcome data can be obtained from clients' or statistical records, interviews with clients, and questionnaires. There is a need for the development of valid and reliable instruments to measure nursing's contributions.

For community health nurses, there is a growing interest in the development of outcome criteria related to health promotion. Clients' choices and expectations from health promotion are important considerations when deciding which outcomes are acceptable. Health behavior and life changes occur systematically over extended time periods. The timing of data collection is critical when evaluating health promotion outcomes since the client's overall well-being will vary at any given time (Gillis, 1995). This necessitates the development of different nursing outcome evaluation tools that are sensitive to assessing changes in wellness.

It is well documented that health is significantly affected by the amount of personal control an individual or community experiences. This level of empowerment includes the ability to alter one's life and environment effectively (Robertson & Minkler, 1994). An expanded view of outcome evaluation, as it applies to health promotion, needs to incorporate methods for assessing changing levels of empowerment and self-responsibility as measures of improved health status. There is a further need for the development of community-based outcome assessment that is culturally relevant. Research is needed to reflect the unique and changing health status of people living in urban and rural settings. When analyzing outcome, the community health nurse might ask:

- What happened to the target population as a result of the activities of this program?
- To what degree were the program goals and objectives met?
- Was the program cost-effective?
- How well did this program actually meet the identified need?
- Was the program design appropriate to meet the needs of the target population?
- Which populations were adequately served? Which were not?
- Which of the impacts require ongoing assessment?
- What were some of the impacts of the program? Short-term? Intermediate? Long-term?
- Which of the long-term impacts can be assessed?
- What is the community's level of satisfaction with the program?
- What types of changes can be directly related to the goals and objectives of the program?
- What other needs arose during the implementation of this program?
- What unplanned effects arose during this program?
- Where client expectations met?

The choice of an evaluation approach is determined by the nature of the questions being asked and the limitations placed upon the evaluation process. Outcome measurement in nursing is still developing. The interconnectedness between process and outcome is being closely examined. A combination of approaches is strongly recommended in the nursing literature. In this way, if outcomes are different from the expectations, changes can be made and situations remedied. The dynamic nature of evaluation can be best explored through an integration of approaches.

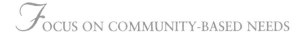

𝒻ocus ON COMMUNITY-BASED NEEDS

The nursing process is employed to respond to and address the health needs of the community when the community is the client. Keeping the Alliance for Health Model in mind, the community health nurse is able to evaluate whether community health care needs are being met (see Chap. 5). Ideally, community-based health care needs are addressed by available systems of care management found in the community. Decisions are made that foster the allocation of resources and that address the community-based need. Effective decision-making allows the appropriate distribution of resources to the community. Key to the appropriate distribution of resources is the importance of equity, the protection of quality services, and the prevention of unnecessary waste and duplication of services. The community health nurse is instrumental in assuring that the community's needs for services are accurately portrayed and validated and in coordinating the interdisciplinary health care team. When there is proper alignment between the systems of care management and allocation decisions, the health care needs of the community can be met.

Figure 10-1*A* shows three circles representing the focus on community-based needs, the systems of care management, and the influences on resource allocation decisions. These three circles are linked, indicating that the community has identified health care needs, systems for care management, and a variety of forces influencing the decisions made for the allocation of health care resources. However, there is little or no overlapping among these circles, indicating that community health care needs are not being addressed by the available systems of care management or by the decision-making process, which influences the allocation of health care resources. If the community health nurse, in conjunction with the other members of the interdisciplinary health care team, joins with community members to validate the community's health care needs and to contribute their mutual expertise, then pressure is put on the circles to increase the area of overlap among them, as illustrated in Figure 10-1*B*. As the overlapping area increases, a greater integration is accomplished. Community health care needs integrate with the systems of care management and resource allocation decisions. When this integration is possible, the forces that influence decision-making are more likely to be responsible to the community, and the health care needs of the community are more likely to be addressed. The gap between needs and services closes.

The evaluation process measures the effectiveness of integration on closing the gap between community health needs, the available service

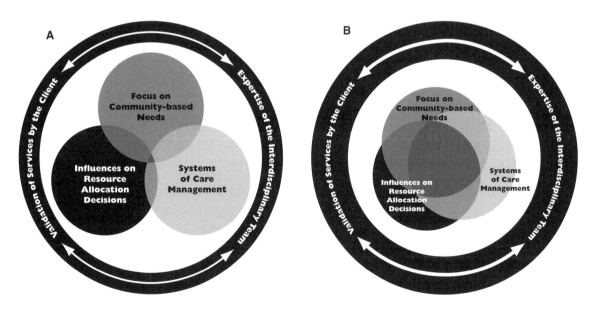

FIGURE 10-1 Movement from a less integrated model of care to a more integrated model of care is illustrated in this figure. The stronger the partnership among the client, the community health nurse, and the interdisciplinary team, the better the oppportunity for integration of the systems of care management and the influence on resource allocation decisions.

delivery system, and the decisions made to allocate resources to address unmet needs. Examination of community-based needs from the perspective of the evaluation phase provides the community health nurse with the outcome measures that promote overlap of the three circles and decrease the gap between community need and community health services. The community health nurse facilitates the evaluation process and ascertains objective measures of community health care outcomes.

Patterns of Morbidity and Mortality

The incidence and prevalence of patterns of illness (morbidity) and death (mortality) in a community are critical measures of a community's health and well-being. The community health nurse should be familiar with the types of illness and the causes of death that affect a community's health. Epidemiologic data are collected to learn about patterns of health, disease, defect, disability, and death in a community. The community health nurse must be vigilant to discover new patterns of illness in a community to assure that members are appropriately treated and restored to the best possible state of health. Case finding can be accomplished through community-based screenings as well as through case-contact follow-ups.

Screening may identify individuals who are asymptomatic, as many health problems can be subclinical at the time of the screening. Screening programs may also identify individuals in the community who unknowingly have a health problem, including infectious or chronic conditions. Screenings are an excellent and relatively inexpensive method for uncovering illness in a community. However, screening does not provide conclusive diagnoses, and therefore, it is imperative for the community health nurse to provide referral and follow-up to all community members testing positive to assure that a diagnosis is made and treatment is initiated.

Case-contact follow-up is a form of surveillance that the community health nurse uses to track illness from one case to another. This detective work involves careful interviewing and tracking leads from case to case. This method is particularly useful in following communicable disease. The community health nurse seeks to identify members of the community who may not be aware that they have entered the period of pathogenesis because they are asymptomatic. The goal is to limit the progression of disease through prompt treatment made possible by early diagnosis. The effectiveness of intervention is measured by the number of screenings conducted against the number of community members considered at risk, the number of subsequently diagnosed cases of illness, and appropriate, prompt follow-up treatment.

Illness that is prevalent in a community requires constant surveillance and case management. Surveillance and management of a disease like tuberculosis (TB), one of the leading causes of death during the early part of the 20th century, are most instructive for the community health nurse. TB, which requires long-term treatment, has always proved a challenge for the community health nurse and other members of the interdisciplinary health care team. Rates of TB are now rising, requiring a redoubling of efforts for people already infected. Multidrug-resistant strains of the bacillus and increased rates of infection, particularly among Asians and Pacific Islanders, Blacks, and Hispanics, pose a great challenge if the *Healthy People 2000* (1995) targets are to be met. Allocating resources that provide community-based systems of care management to reach infected populations requires the steadfast efforts of community health professionals working with community members to achieve this health objective. If TB is spreading and threatening the health of the community, the community need is apparent; however, the systems of care management may not appropriately reach the target population, and decisions for allocation of resources for new and innovative programs to reach the affected population may not be forthcoming rapidly enough to stop the spread of the disease. Figure 10-2 illustrates this potential dilemma. In Fig. 10-2*A*, the need is apparent, but there is little overlap with the systems of care management or the decisions for resource allocation. The community health need is not being adequately addressed by the available systems of care management or by the influences on resource allocation decisions. Outcomes in this scenario are potentially disastrous since community health need is left unchecked. The health of the community is at great risk. The community health nurse would document the lack of available community resources and the deficits in the agenda for funding and resource allocation decision-making. The integration of a care model, which addresses the unmet community-based need, is illustrated in Fig. 10-1*B*.

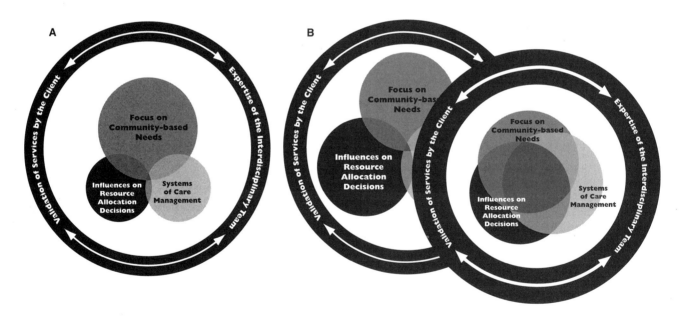

FIGURE 10-2 In this figure, community-based needs are not being met because of problems in the coordination of the systems of care management and the resource allocation decisions. Greater integration is possible through a partnership of the community, the community health nurse, and the interdisciplinary team when they take action together to address community-based needs.

Demographics

Population statistics are instructive to the community health nurse when evaluating the shifting demographics of the community and its available resources. For example, consider a community that has exhibited stability in its population growth over the years. No great influx of newcomers has taken place, but the members have changed from raising children to sending children off to college and other communities to start their own lives. As the population ages, the services it requires change. People who are shut-ins and individuals who are disabled need innovative solutions to problems that interfere with the activities of daily living. Food shopping services could be provided by the food market, a Meals-on-Wheels program could be developed for people shut-in in their homes, or local restaurants could hire drivers to deliver meals to the homes of community residents. Community services are shaped and reshaped to address the needs of the residents. Not all communities transform themselves to respond to the needs of the members. The community health nurse is ever mindful of the match between the shifting demographics and the services available in the community. Innovations, renovations, and alternative styles of delivering services to the members can be developed if demographics and the utilization patterns of services are monitored. This kind of evaluation leads to the development of new and inventive measures to address needs that were previously unknown or unrecognized.

Shifts in the distribution of age in the community are only one kind of parameter to evaluate. A community is reconstituted when cultural groups enter or leave a community. The care administered by health care providers changes as the population changes. The community health nurse seeks culturally sensitive and appropriate care for the varied cultural constituencies of a community. The community health nurse needs to learn about the values and mores of each cultural group, apply the principles of transcultural nursing practice, and measure the effectiveness of the care rendered.

Shifts in the patterns of employment are instructive to the community health nurse when evaluating occupationally related forms of injury. The effectiveness of injury control programs is monitored to establish the appropriateness of resources for the prevention of on-the-job accidents. Identification of new environmental hazards at workplaces signals the importance of ongoing evaluation of occupational health risks. The community health nurse uses demographic data related to patterns of employment to predict the kinds of workplace health programs that promote and protect workers as well as the surrounding community. For example, smoking cessation and workplace wellness programs may be developed in response to identified needs of workers. Outcome measures are devised to evaluate the relative success of wellness initiatives and to strengthen the health of employment settings in the community.

Housing is always a critical community health concern. Safe and affordable housing is one of the most pressing human needs in most communities. The community health nurse evaluates the types and distribution of housing in the community and the degree to which homelessness exists.

The community health nurse expedites referrals for community members in need of housing and addresses the requirements of people with special needs for group homes, residential treatment facilities, or handicap accessible facilities. The community health nurse evaluates the availability of housing in the community to link people with housing needs to housing resources.

Community demographics are a source of data used by the community health nurse to monitor and evaluate the link between the needs of the community and its members and the facilities and services of the community. Shifts in the population and its defining characteristics inform the community health nurse about the needs of the population.

Environmental Concerns

Environmental concerns are multitudinous, ranging from air and water quality, to asbestos and lead in the homes, schools, and workplaces, to the prevalence of violence on the streets. Some environmental health concerns are pressing problems for the community, and as a result, action groups and coalitions form to advocate change and reform. The community health nurse and other members of the interdisciplinary health care team lend support and expertise to the organized efforts of the community. Other environmental concerns may not be known to members of the community and may pose significant risk. The role of the community health nurse is to educate the community and serve as an expert witness to community groups that wish to learn about a community health problem. The community health nurse evaluates progress made toward the amelioration of environmental health concerns. Some environmental health concerns may be specific to a particular aggregate or endemic to the community at large.

The National Institutes of Health and the Centers for Disease Control and Prevention are the leading agencies concerned with environmental health problems identified as part of the *Healthy People 2000* objectives [U. S. Department of Health and Human Services (DHHS), 1995]. Some of the measures used to evaluate the achievement of the environmental health objectives include: the number of asthma hospitalizations, number of outbreaks of waterborne diseases, blood lead levels, standards for air pollution, radon testing, and the release of toxic agents identified on the DHHS list of carcinogens. Other measures involve solid waste disposal and treatment, safe drinking water standards, and household hazardous waste collection.

The community health nurse must be aware of the environmental link to certain diseases. Among the many diseases and dysfunctions that have a known or suspected environmental component are: cancer, reproductive disorders (e.g., infertility) low birth weight, neurological and immune system impairments, and respiratory conditions (e.g., asthma) (DHHS, 1995). Exposure to environmental hazards can be through air, food, and water and may involve pesticides, toxic chemicals, and radiation. Environmental health concerns and their relationship to particular diseases are frequently associated with repeated and cumulative exposures.

Studies concerning breast cancer, for example, can examine a number of environmental risks, including the possibility of exposure to contaminated drinking water, sources of indoor and ambient air pollution, electromagnetic fields, pesticides, and other toxic chemicals. The community health nurse evaluates the extent to which the women and men in the community have knowledge of their possible risks for breast cancer and the effectiveness of community education programs that address these risks.

It is important that the community health nurse identifies particular aggregates in the population at risk for environmental health hazards. Asthma, for example, disproportionately affects children, women, minorities, and people living in urban areas. Evaluation of the impact of prevention programs for these high-risk populations is critical to efforts to reduce the number of hospital days designated for the treatment of asthma and the number of deaths that are attributable to asthma. Community health nurses play a significant role in educating families about the importance of reducing children's exposure to tobacco smoke. Community health nurses, as smoking cessation therapists, are advocates for smoke-free environments. Measuring progress in achieving this goal, at all levels—individual, family, agency, and community—is a critical evaluation procedure.

Public Services

Public service workers and specific services guard the safety of the community. The degree to which the members of the community feel safe is related to the efficient function of these public services. Police, fire, parks, traffic, and transportation departments, public utilities, and auxiliary services are among the most vital public services that, in addition to their varied functions, protect the community and its members. Safety is a basic human need that must be satisfied in order for high-level functioning to occur. A safe community enables individuals and families to focus on functions and responsibilities that support their own growth and the development of the community. An unsafe community abandons its members, leaves them prey to acts of violence and violation, and thwarts their progress toward achieving goals and actualizing their potential. The community health nurse is aware of the importance of assessing indices of safety in the community. When a safe environment is hampered, the community health nurse works with other members of the interdisciplinary health care team and community members to evaluate gaps in public services that require attention and strengthening. In addition, the community health nurse mobilizes public services for individual clients in the community with special needs. The community health nurse will find invaluable personal support from public service providers and their services when confronted with problems of safety while working in the community and when unable to access clients due to unsafe community circumstances.

Evaluating the degree to which a community is safe or unsafe is often difficult. Appearances can be and usually are deceiving. At first glance, an economically deprived community with a high rate of unemployment and members found frequently hanging out on doorsteps can be thought of as a high-risk and unsafe community. Yet, this may be an inaccurate portrayal of this community. In actuality, a community health nurse may be quite safe in this community and find that the members are always cordial and cooperative. The members may go out of their way to make sure the nurse gets safely to the desired destination. Although this is not an organized neighborhood watch community, the neighbors do watch out for each other and for valued visitors in the community. Safety is self-monitored, and members protect each other and the nurse. On the other hand, a middle- to high-income, well-groomed community may appear safe but could pose a safety threat to the nurse. Safety is always a concern for the community health nurse. The nurse is concerned with his or her own personal safety, with the safety of clients, and with the safety of the community at large.

The community health nurse is concerned with the relative presence of the various public services and public service providers in the community. When clients are afraid to leave their homes because they do not feel safe on the street, the community health nurse evaluates the degree to which the police are present in the neighborhood. The nurse uses assessment data that have been gathered about public services to determine what other official or community-based organizations address community safety. An evaluation of their presence in the community is key. Even with police or a neighborhood watch present, the special concerns and worries of a particular population may need to be addressed differently or more vigilantly. Senior citizens may require a safe zone during designated hours to feel safe using an area of the park near their housing complex. Additional services may be necessary to provide protection for some of the most vulnerable members of the community.

The abduction of children is one of the most frightening and devastating losses for a community; it exemplifies the vulnerability of the community and its inability to protect its young members. The community health nurse, with parents and other concerned community members, evaluates the ability of the community to protect its children. The need for safe havens for children to play without fear and without the threat of strangers could result from such an evaluation. The community health nurse could become an advocate for safe playgrounds and the conversion of a public building into space for play groups. Evaluation of the community's safety net could lead the community health nurse in the direction of resource development.

Community health nurses are often involved in public service campaigns to educate and protect the community about potential hazards and safety threats. For example, community health nurses visit families with young children to advise them about the importance of window guards to prevent window fall fatalities. Campaigns like "Children Can't Fly" are aimed at making sure window guards are installed at no cost to families to prevent accidental death.

During the winter months in communities in cold climates, the community health nurse finds the community members who are unable to afford heat or are in buildings with furnace problems. As a result, homes may be heated by an open oven door or gas burners. Some families purchase unsafe portable heaters that are associated with devastating accidents. Community health nurses evaluate household environments for safety threats and contact superintendents and utility offices to advocate for their clients. Senior citizens or individuals with disabilities who live alone can benefit from referral to a public service company that provides a voice-activated call-for-help system. The community health nurse can also register these vulnerable clients with the local fire department so that the department is alerted to their needs and the importance of special equipment should a fire evacuation need to take place in their building. Registering clients with special needs with public service departments like fire and police departments could save lives in case of an emergency.

When organizing services for the community, the community health nurse not only evaluates the need for services but also the quality and appropriateness of the services provided. In the case of infants whose deaths remain unexplained and the resulting autopsy identifies the cause of death as sudden infant death syndrome (SIDS), the public services that responded to the family's call for emergency help require careful evaluation. A person who has discovered a lifeless infant is in a heightened state of vulnerability and confusion and usually responds by calling the emergency number 911. Different communities respond differently. Police officers, fire fighters, and emergency medical technicians are among those who respond. Historically, parents have been held responsible for their infant's death until the autopsy proves otherwise. This unfortunate situation leaves families further devastated. They can even be charged with abuse or murder. In some cases, the infant's bedding, crib, clothing, and toys are taken from the home as part of the crime scene investigation. Many precious items get lost or are never returned to the family. The community health nurse may be able to address the needs of these stricken families through outreach to the families in their homes. Counseling and preventive intervention, which support grieving families as they learn to live with a child's death, are the hallmarks of community health nursing care. Evaluation of the affected families' perception of how they were treated by the first responders could lead to professional education for first responders. Learning about the distinguishing characteristics of SIDS and child abuse as well as expected postmortem signs can help first responders to respond with appropriate compassion and knowledge.

The community health nurse evaluates the responses of public service workers and agencies to the wide range of human needs exhibited by members of the community and by the community itself. The community health nurse is concerned with when, how, and if public service workers and agencies respond to these needs and with the quality of the response. Providing for the safety of the community is the domain of public service workers and agencies. The community health nurse can link community members to public services and translate the needs of the community to public service departments. The community health nurse uses evaluation data to suggest ways to improve the level of safety of the community.

Aesthetics

The aesthetic component of a community contributes to the richness of a community. A community devoid of this aesthetic component deprives its members of opportunities to enhance their appreciation for art and culture. The community health nurse recognizes that the sense of pride in one's community is found in its aesthetic expressions. Community pride is the equivalent of self-esteem for an individual and family. The community health nurse evaluates the presence, absence, and meaning of aesthetic expressions in an effort to appreciate this dimension of community health. Aesthetic expressions are tied to the community's sense of pride in itself, its culture, its religion, and its willingness to support and appreciate art and artistic representations.

Expressions of art and culture in a community may appear foreign and unknown to the community health nurse. The nurse offers a willingness and interest in learning about the meaning of art and aesthetic expression in the community. Beauty can be appreciated through a desire to learn and understand the beliefs and values of others. The community health nurse can learn a great deal about a community's life ways by witnessing a parade or visiting statues, shrines, and museums. The community defines what is beautiful and important to reveal and revere. The evaluation of the aesthetic components of a community is not a judgment of artistic qualities but an effort to determine the presence, absence, and relative meaning of artistic expressions in the community.

If the community health nurse encounters buildings that are vandalized and boarded-up and museums and theaters that are no longer used, he or she may correctly conclude that the aesthetic component of this community is absent. Opportunities for engaging in the community's artistic events are absent, and the community members are missing out on this component of community pride and creativity. The artistic light of the community has been extinguished.

Communities express their aesthetic component differently. In some communities, the array and multitude of artistic offerings require an arts council to provide coordination and to publicize events. In other communities, small galleries feature the work of local artists and artisans. Outdoor exhibits, fairs, parades, and other communal events enable artists to show their work. The aesthetic component of a community has roots in the past and reflects something about the history of the community. Art traverses the past, present, and future and teaches what the community values and believes to be beautiful. Art may be found in the written word, in visual expressions, in shape and forms, in theater and dance, in architecture, and in gardens and landscaping. Beauty can be found in many corners and crevices of a community. A peaceful garden may provide respite from woes; a remarkable building will stand as a work of art just as a sculpture erected in front of it will capture the spirit of its onlookers.

The community health nurse tries to understand something about the community's values and appreciation for art and artistic expressions through an evaluation of the aesthetic component of a community. The community health nurse is nonjudgmental and motivated to learn about the meaning of artistic representations in the community. The sense of community pride is found in its aesthetic component. The richness or lack of aesthetics found in a community is instructive to the community health nurse in caring for the community.

Health-Related Facilities

Health-related facilities are the network of supportive services in a community designed to serve the community's health needs. The community health nurse evaluates the availability, accessibility, affordability, appropriateness, adequacy, and acceptability of these services in the community (National Institute of Nursing Research, 1995). Elementary to this evaluation is knowledge of community health needs. The health-related facilities and services of a community must exist in proportion to these needs. The intent of health-related facilities is to respond to community health needs. Since communities are dynamic so too are their health needs and status. This dynamic state requires that health-related facilities undergo continuous evaluation of their ability to respond to community health needs. The development of goals with target dates enables agencies to measure their relative effectiveness in achieving their goals. Establishing goals is a collaborative process among members of the community, the interdisciplinary health care team, and agency staff. Goals may involve decreasing mortality, reducing the number of cases of certain illnesses, decreasing the number of accidents, improving the environmental quality, and enhancing the ability of health care agencies to reach a particular population or offer a new and valued service.

The community health nurse tries to ascertain if the health needs of the community are addressed by the health-related facilities in the community. If drug addiction is a major community health problem, the community health nurse evaluates the availability of drug rehabilitation facilities and the impact of treatment modalities on the success of the rehabilitation. The nurse must also gauge the community's receptivity to programs like needle exchange, especially in communities with few treatment opportunities. If a community has a large geriatric population and a large caseload of clients with Alzheimer's disease, the community health nurse evaluates the availability of services like adult day care and respite care.

The community health nurse monitors the distribution of health-related facilities in the community. The equitable distribution of services is key to a community's health. Some communities are rich with services but suffer from maldistribution and overlap of services. The health of other communities are threatened by a lack of services. The community health nurse promotes the systematic evaluation of community resources. Objective community data are needed to ascertain if services are, in fact, having the desired impact on community health needs and if desired outcomes are being achieved. Evaluation is an ongoing process. The community health nurse continually validates the appropriateness of health-related facilities that impact the community's health. The results of community health services must be measured in relation to the health needs of the population served.

$\mathcal{S}$UMMARY

The most important element of evaluation is that it informs the community health nurse about the progress or the lack of progress made in achieving community health goals, and it points to the importance of reassessing community health needs. Evaluation leads back to assessment. The community health nurse assesses the needs of the community and considers the systems of care management and the influences on resource allocation decisions. The circles of the Alliance for Health Model provide a framework for the community health nurse to engage in the care of communities. Each component of the model instructs the nurse in the factors and forces that should be considered to appreciate the complexity of the community as the client. The community health nurse cares for the community; the community is the client.

KEY WORDS

Nursing process
Outcome evaluation
Rural/urban continuum

QUESTIONS

DIRECTIONS: Choose the one *best* response to each of the following questions.

1. Formative evaluation is used to

    A. provide feedback information.
    B. validate statistical findings.
    C. eliminate the need for outcome assessment.
    D. assess goal attainment.

2. In a hypothetical community, most residents are older, retired persons, but the community nursing services are focused on mothers and children. What statement concerning the nursing process as applied to this community is relevant?

    A. Basic preventive services must take priority.
    B. Children are a valuable community resource and their health should be protected.
    C. Community needs should be systematically evaluated.
    D. Federal mandates should govern which services are provided in the community.

3. During summative evaluation, the community health nurse would be most likely to ask which of the following questions?

   A. Are there adequate resources to carry this project out?
   B. Is the program working effectively?
   C. Did this program promote a desired change in health behavior?
   D. Am I reaching the target population?

4. The primary reason for community health nurses to become involved in health planning is to

   A. secure legislative power relinquished by other health care professionals.
   B. enhance the health care system's responsiveness to clients' needs.
   C. establish a case for nurses to receive third-party reimbursement.
   D. relieve consumers from the responsibilities of community health planning.

5. Community-based health care evaluation emphasizes all of the following principles *except*

   A. equal partnership with the consumer.
   B. professional territoriality.
   C. research expansion.
   D. integration of service.

6. Empowerment relates most closely to

   A. feelings of control and mastery over one's life.
   B. cultural identification.
   C. legitimizing political power.
   D. conflict resolution.

ANSWERS

1. *The answer is A.* The purpose of formative evaluation is to provide useful information to improve and administer a program.

2. *The answer is C.* The evaluation of community needs is ongoing.

3. *The answer is C.* Summative evaluation focuses on measurement of goal-attainment.

4. *The answer is B.* Community health nurses are invaluable and unique sources of information regarding the health care needs of a community.

5. *The answer is B.* Community-based health care evaluation emphasizes a multidisciplinary philosophy.

6. *The answer is A.* Empowerment is the concept of power defined as the ability to control the factors that determine one's life.

ANNOTATED REFERENCES

Bingham, R. D., & Felbinger, C. L. (1989). Evaluation in practice: A methodological approach. New York: Longman.

This text illustrates the techniques of program and policy evaluation through a series of 20 readings. It provides many examples and design methodologies taken from a wide range of disciplines.

Deal, L. W. (1994). The effectiveness of community health nursing interventions: A literature review. Public Health Nursing, 11(5), 315–325.

This article describes services provided by community health nurses at both the home-based and community levels. It documents the effectiveness of these interventions based on available literature and makes recommendations for future evaluative research.

Donabedian, A. (1969). Some issues in evaluating the quality of nursing care. American Journal of Public Health, 59(10), 1833–1836.

This article expands on the author's original work and focuses on issues surrounding the assessment of the quality of nursing care. Approaches to evaluation are outlined, and technical issues surrounding the nursing audit are discussed.

Gillis, A. (1995). Exploring nursing outcomes for health promotion. Nursing Forum, 30(2), 5–12.

This article takes a critical look at nursing outcomes as they relate to health promotion. There is a focus on the unique challenges faced by nurses as they attempt to identify and measure the factors that influence health behavior changes. The important role of the client's expectations is emphasized.

Harris, M.D., & Dugan, M. (1996). Evaluating the quality of home care services using patient outcome data. Home Healthcare Nurse, 14(6), 463–465.

This article presents the importance of patient outcome evaluation. It defines three types of outcomes and describes how one Visiting Nurse Association used this framework to analyze hospital re-admissions.

National Institute of Nursing Research. (1995). Community-based health care: Nursing strategies. Bethesda, MD: Author.

This extensive report discusses the concept of community-based health care in depth. The needs of health populations along the urban/rural continuum are used as a framework for community health nursing strategies. Emphasis is placed on documenting areas in need of further research.

Robertson, A., & Minkler, M. (1994). New health promotion movement: A critical examination. Health Education Quarterly, 21(3), 295–312.

This article discusses the impact of the health promotion movement of the 1980s. The revised World Health Organization (WHO) definition of health is examined. This article explores the concepts of empowerment and community participation as they relate to health status.

U. S. Department of Health and Human Services. (1995). Healthy People 2000: Midcourse review and 1995 revisions. Washington, DC: Author.

This is a report on the accomplishments following the release of Healthy People 2000: National Health Promotion and Disease Prevention Objectives and the challenges remaining in preventing premature death and in improving health as the year 2000 approaches. It presents a detailed progress report of the 22 identified priority areas and consortium action being taken at the state level and through private and voluntary activities.

CARING FOR PEOPLE IN THEIR HOMES OR WHERE THEY LIVE

OVERVIEW OF HOME CARE CONCEPTS

As discussed in Chap. 2, professional home care nursing began on Henry Street on the Lower East Side of New York City, at the end of the 19th century. The clients of the early community health nurses were generally poor immigrant families who were often at high risk for communicable diseases. The goal of community health nursing was the protection and improvement of the health of all family members. Nurses were concerned with the environment, socioeconomic conditions, and all other conditions affecting individual and community health.

The focus of care has not changed in community health nursing since then, simply its methods of providing care. Today, the community nurse may care for the young mother and her infant with acquired immunodeficiency syndrome (AIDS), the postoperative client, or the elderly person living alone by providing skilled care and supervising the care provided by the home health aide (HHA), attendant, or family and friends. This chapter deals with the community health nurse as provider of home care to the family and individual. How nursing care is delivered may have changed, but the professionalism, commitment, and creativity of the community health nurse are evidenced by the community health nurse working toward keeping the public healthy.

The home visits made by community health nurses are guided today by professional groups like the American Nurses Association (ANA) and accreditation agencies like the Community Health Accreditation Program (CHAP) of the National League for Nursing (NLN) and regulated by state departments of health. Home visits are made to apartments, private homes, nursing homes, homeless shelters, boarding homes, dormitories, elderly housing facilities, and group homes. In most settings, a family member or a friend may assume the role of caretaker. In some situations, family members may not live with the client but may still be involved in caring for the client.

The community health nurse works with the entire family when caring for the client. It is important for the nurse to develop a personal relationship with the family or caretaker as well as with the individual who is the focus of care. It may take a few visits for this relationship to develop, but it is an important component of caring for the client at home. A strong interpersonal relationship allows the nurse and client to communicate openly and honestly about health status concerns.

A home visit is made following a referral from a physician, social worker, discharge planner, or lay person from the community. The goal of the community health nurse is to provide direct care as well as an ongoing assessment of the client. Health promotion, maintenance of both family and individual health, and support services for the dying and for bereaved families may also be goals of the community health nurse. With the advent of hospice care and the increased presence of high-technology care at home, highly skilled community health nurse specialists or hospice care nurses must often visit clients at home. The need for such specialists may be indicated by the initial referral or by a referral made by a community health nurse after visiting the client for sometime.

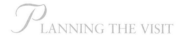

PLANNING THE VISIT

Organizing the Plan

The most common referral of a client to an agency for home visits occurs after an assessment of needs has been made before discharge from a hospital or ambulatory care setting. Today, many discharge plans are developed by case managers, who may be a nurse in a hospital or an ambulatory care setting, a community health nurse, or another health care provider such as a social worker. These plans may generate a referral for home care.

The community health nurse reviews the referral, which includes the physician's directives for care. For Medicare clients, this information is usually communicated to the nurse on a standardized "Home Health Certification and Plan of Care" form (Fig. 11-1). This form (also called a 485) was developed by the Health Care Financing Administration (HCFA) so that Medicare clients were assessed and treated in a uniform way. The 485 form describes a plan of treatment, that is, the care to be provided by the home care team of providers.

After the initial assessment, if changes are needed in the plan of care, the nurse telephones or sends a fax message to the ordering physician for approval. Referrals are made to other providers according to an established internal procedure. New orders and referrals are sent to the physician for his or her signature. Every time the community health nurse provides care to the client, a visit report is completed. Figure 11-2 is an example of a nursing visit report.

Department of Health and Human Services
Health Care Financing Administration

Form Approved
OMB No. 0938-0357

HOME HEALTH CERTIFICATION AND PLAN OF CARE

1. Patient's HI Claim No.	2. Start Of Care Date	3. Certification Period		4. Medical Record No.	5. Provider No.
		From:	To:		

6. Patient's Name and Address	7. Provider's Name, Address and Telephone Number

8. Date of Birth	9. Sex ☐ M ☐ F	10. Medications: Dose/Frequency/Route (N)ew (C)hanged
11. ICD-9-CM	Principal Diagnosis	Date	
12. ICD-9-CM	Surgical Procedure	Date	
13. ICD-9-CM	Other Pertinent Diagnoses	Date	

14. DME and Supplies	15. Safety Measures:
16. Nutritional Req.	17. Allergies:

18.A. Functional Limitations

1 ☐ Amputation	5 ☐ Paralysis	9 ☐ Legally Blind				
2 ☐ Bowel/Bladder (Incontinence)	6 ☐ Endurance	A ☐ Dyspnea With Minimal Exertion				
3 ☐ Contracture	7 ☐ Ambulation	B ☐ Other (Specify)				
4 ☐ Hearing	8 ☐ Speech					

18.B. Activities Permitted

1 ☐ Complete Bedrest	6 ☐ Partial Weight Bearing	A ☐ Wheelchair
2 ☐ Bedrest BRP	7 ☐ Independent At Home	B ☐ Walker
3 ☐ Up As Tolerated	8 ☐ Crutches	C ☐ No Restrictions
4 ☐ Transfer Bed/Chair	9 ☐ Cane	D ☐ Other (Specify)
5 ☐ Exercises Prescribed		

19. Mental Status:

1 ☐ Oriented	3 ☐ Forgetful	5 ☐ Disoriented	7 ☐ Agitated
2 ☐ Comatose	4 ☐ Depressed	6 ☐ Lethargic	8 ☐ Other

20. Prognosis: 1 ☐ Poor 2 ☐ Guarded 3 ☐ Fair 4 ☐ Good 5 ☐ Excellent

21. Orders for Discipline and Treatments (Specify Amount/Frequency/Duration)

22. Goals/Rehabilitation Potential/Discharge Plans

23. Nurse's Signature and Date of Verbal SOC Where Applicable:	25. Date HHA Received Signed POT
24. Physician's Name and Address	26. I certify/recertify that this patient is confined to his/her home and needs intermittent skilled nursing care, physical therapy and/or speech therapy or continues to need occupational therapy. The patient is under my care, and I have authorized the services on this plan of care and will periodically review the plan.
27. Attending Physician's Signature and Date Signed	28. Anyone who misrepresents, falsifies, or conceals essential information required for payment of Federal funds may be subject to fine, imprisonment, or civil penalty under applicable Federal laws.

Form HCFA-485 (C-3) (02-94) (Print Aligned)   PROVIDER

FIGURE 11-1 A sample home health certification and plan of care form from the Health Care Financing Administration.

NURSING VISIT REPORT   ☐ REVISIT ☐ FINAL

A.R. # _____ LIFE NO _____

Date: _____ HCC _____

Name: _____

Instructions Given/Patient or Family Responses: _____
_____
_____
_____
_____
_____
_____
_____

NEW PROBLEMS ON THIS VISIT   NURSING INTERVENTION
(Primary Dx - Other Pertinent Dx including Nursing Dx)   (Indicate time frames for resolution)

☐ New ☐ Ongoing   _____

1. _____   _____
   _____   _____
2. _____   _____
   _____   _____
3. _____   _____
   _____   _____
4. _____   _____
   _____   _____
5. _____   _____
   _____   _____

PLANS FOR NEXT VISIT:_____
_____
_____
_____
_____
_____

Name of H.H.A./PCW/HK _____ Vendor _____ Schedule _____
Supervision _____
_____

Relationship with Patient, Family and Staff _____ Attendance & Punctuality _____
Is there a privately hired caretaker in the home? ☐ Yes ☐ No   Vendor _____ Schedule _____
GOALS - Short Term (and Time Frames): _____
   _____
   _____
   _____
   Long Term (and Time Frames): _____
   _____
   _____
   _____

DISCHARGE PLANS: _____
_____
_____

Visit Frequency: _____ Date of Next Visit _____

Patient's Signature: _____ Nurse's Signature: _____
      WHITE - PATIENT'S COPY   CANARY - BILLING COPY   PINK - DIRECT SERVICE NURSE COPY

FIGURE 11-2 A sample nursing visit report.

Figure 11-3 is a copy of the revisit record that may be used by various therapists in the home. Physical therapists, speech therapists, and occupational therapists, for example, might be involved in the care of various people. An example of a discharge summary or 60-day reauthorization form is provided in Fig. 11-4.

The client's particular environment factors into the actual plan of care. For example, the two clients discussed below appear to have the same needs when discharged from the hospital, but upon returning home, each has different needs. Neither client is mobile, and both need support services related to the activities of daily living (ADLs).

CASE STUDY: THE DIFFERENT NEEDS OF MR. JAY AND MR. SMITH

Mr. Jay has absolutely no home support system, while Mr. Smith has an adequate home support system. In addition to providing skilled care to both clients, the community health nurse needs to recommend an HHA to assist Mr. Jay with ADLs, shopping, and meal preparation.

Mr. Jay relies on phone calls and letters for emotional support and contact with his family and friends who are unable help him physically at home. The community health nurse monitors the relationship between Mr. Jay and the HHA, as well as his relationships with his long-distance friends to see if any adjustments are necessary.

The community health nurse makes every effort to ensure that the support system of Mr. Smith remains intact.

Scheduling the Visit

After assessing the needs of clients within the community health nurse's caseload and conferring with the clients, the community health nurse sets priorities and then schedules visits to each client. For example, if the client is a diabetic and must have insulin first thing in the morning, the nurse must schedule an early morning visit. The community health nurse must cluster visits with clients living in the same location and must learn to project the length of each visit. Some visits may take 30 min, while others may take over an hour, especially when an initial assessment must be made.

After prioritizing visits, the community health nurse prepares a transportation plan. The nurse then calls the client and verifies the approximate time of the visit. Clients may not be available at a particular time because of previous appointments with other health care providers or because the time is not convenient for the client's family. Clients may also simply refuse a visit. If the intention of the visit is, in part, to assess the needs of the entire family, the nurse may need to adjust the visit schedule.

The nurse must also confirm that the equipment and supplies needed for the planned visits are available in the clients' homes. However, the community health nurse must be especially careful to avoid cross-contamination of equipment between clients. It is not the norm for the agency to provide equipment and supplies for clients.

PATIENT NAME		
ADDRESS		
AR NO.	LIFE NO.	COORDINATOR
VISIT DATE	TIME	
	FROM:	TO:
PATIENT SIGNATURE		

REVISIT NOTE - THERAPY

☐ P.T.   ☐ O.T.   ☐ S.T.

PROBLEMS/COMPLAINTS:

TREATMENT/INSTRUCTION GIVEN:

RESPONSE/PROGRESS TO TREATMENT/GOALS:

PLAN: (REVISED GOALS / FREQUENCY / PLAN FOR NEXT VISIT)

COMMUNICATION/COORDINATION: (T/C CALLS / CONFERENCES)

RECORD

D/C PLANS:

REVISIT DATE:

THERAPIST SIGNATURE   COORDINATOR INITIALS

FIGURE 11-3 A sample of a revisit note for therapy services.

NAME		AR NO.
STREET ADDRESS		
CITY, STATE, ZIP CODE		

☐ **60 DAY NOTE** (COMPLETE B, C, D)
☐ **DISCHARGE SUMMARY** (COMPLETE A - F)

ADMISSION DATE	DISCHARGE DATE	COORDINATOR

THIS FORM ORIGINATED BY:
☐ RN ☐ P.T. ☐ O.T. ☐ S.T. ☐ MSW

DIAGNOSIS

CERT. PERIOD
FROM: TO:

A. PATIENT'S CONDITION ON ADMISSION

B. PATIENT'S PRESENT CONDITION, PROGRESS TO DATE

C. SERVICES PROVIDED AND OUTCOMES (INCLUDE FREQUENCY OF VISITS, HHA, SKILLED SERV. ETC.)

D. HOW ARE UNMET GOALS TO BE ADDRESSED

E. REASON FOR TERMINATION (INDEPENDENT, FAMILY TOOK OVER, HOSPITALIZED, EXPIRED ETC.)

F. FOLLOW UP CARE ☐ PRIVATE MD ☐ CLINIC ☐ OTHER (Specify below)

NOTIFIED

☐ COORDINATOR DATE NOTIFIED:___/___/___

☐ PATIENT DATE NOTIFIED:___/___/___

☐ PHYSICIAN DATE NOTIFIED:___/___/___

SIGNATURE

DATE

PATIENT RECORD

CMC 2076 Rev. (9/95)

FIGURE 11-4 A sample of a discharge summary or 60-day recertification note.

Introductory Phone Call

The first responsibility the nurse has to the client is to identify her- or himself as the professional who is planning to make a home visit. This may be done over the phone, although some clients have no telephone, or in person at the client's front door or over the apartment house intercom. The nurse explains the reason for the visit and informs the client if other individuals are also expected, such as another nurse, an escort, a supervisor, or a student. It may be helpful to offer personal descriptions of these individuals so that the client feels more comfortable offering access to his or her home. The nurse should also present official identification to the client at the door.

Review of Previous Visit

Every visit has a set of goals and future plans of care. To prepare for each visit, the nurse always reviews the last progress note and the overall plan, including medications and treatments. At the beginning of the visit, the nurse reviews with the client the agreed-upon goals and treatments. The nurse and client should also review what was helpful about the previous visit and discuss how stated goals were met.

CASE STUDY: TEAMWORK BETWEEN THE NURSE AND CLIENT

Mr. Jacks, a 66-year-old client with a diagnosis of adult-onset diabetes, was recently discharged home following a partial amputation of the left foot. The client was sent home with orders to soak his foot daily in a solution of normal saline, followed with a wet-to-dry dressing. The community health nurse made daily visits for 1 week during which time the nurse taught the client's wife how to perform the care. The nurse reviewed with the wife how to change the dressing, using sterile technique and observing universal precautions. The nurse observed the wife complete the soak and change the dressing. It was agreed that soaking the foot and changing the dressing should occur each day when Mrs. Jacks returned from work. The community health nurse then decreased the visit frequency to three times a week with the consent of the client's physician.

On the next visit, it appeared that the dressing had not been changed. Mrs. Jacks was at work. Mr. Jacks explained that his wife had been unable to change his dressing and soak his foot for the past 2 days at the planned time as she was very busy at work, and when she came home, he was already asleep.

After doing the prescribed care, the nurse reviewed with Mr. Jacks the importance of soaking the foot and changing the dressing. The nurse further explained that the dressing change and foot soak could be done at any time and still be effective.

The nurse and Mr. Jacks agreed that the soaking and dressing changes could be done in the morning before Mrs. Jacks left for work. The nurse phoned Mrs. Jacks to verify that this was possible, and she said that she was relieved, as morning was a better time for her and that she had believed that the foot care procedures could only be performed later in the day. During subsequent visits, the nurse noted that soaks and dressings were done appropriately.

By adjusting the routine, the nurse can often help clients to meet their goals. If a client has been visited previously by another community health nurse or any other health care provider, it is important to determine if a special care routine has been established. This approach not only saves time for the nurse but helps to create a sense of continuity of care for the client.

Establish Visit Time and Location

It is important to negotiate a likely time for the visit and explain that delays may occur. Specifically, the nurse must ask if the client has any other health-related appointments that may make another time more productive. The nurse must also ask about planned visits by friends so that the clients know that they need to be available and not preoccupied with guests when the nurse arrives. The nurse should verify the address and ask about such details as the exact location (including cross streets) and the visibility of the address number or apartment number. One of the most difficult tasks in planning for visits is accommodating the nursing needs and the personal preferences of the client. Some clients need visits that match a plan for medication administration or other treatments. Some prefer morning or afternoon visits. Community health nurses may also need to schedule visits around work schedules of family members and friends of the client, when they are involved in the plan of care.

If the client reports an emergent problem, the nurse should instruct him or her to activate the emergency response team (i.e., call 911) or report to the primary care provider immediately. Clients should not wait for the nurse's visit if they are in distress.

$\mathcal{S}$AFETY

It is imperative that the community health nurse use care and common sense when traveling to and from clients' homes. Safety tips include: (1) carry only the money and supplies that are needed to minimize loss if theft occurs; (2) leave a schedule of your route with coworkers so that they know where you will be; (3) do not change your schedule without notifying the agency; (4) travel with identification; and (5) dress in a uniform or

Questions to Review before the Visit
- What is the purpose of the visit?
- Do you have all the pertinent information you need before making the visit?
- What is the focus of the visit? How does the focus relate to the major diagnoses?
- What are the activities that need to be followed up from the previous visit?
- What literature, research, and teaching materials may be helpful?
- What are the specific things you will teach on this visit? Do you have all the equipment you will need for the visit?

professional clothing. Many home care agencies require community health nurses to wear specific uniforms, while others simply require neat, clean, professional attire, which will blend into the communities served.

Traveling by car, whether personal or company, requires frequent checks to ensure that the car has enough fuel and is in good working order. Using public transportation requires coordination of location with a dependable bus or train route. If possible, the community health nurse should drive around an area to become familiar with the community so that he or she will know where to go for supplies, information, or assistance.

*T*HE VISIT

Setting a Therapeutic Tone and Establishing Goals

The visit provided by the community health nurse gives the client and the client's family the opportunity to receive professional services in their own home. Unlike a hospital visit, the home visit is family-focused and occurs in an environment familiar to the client, that is, the household and the community in which the client is living.

The community health nurse must develop a relationship with the client and the family. This is an important part of the visit. The actual home visit is initiated by a formal introduction of the community health nurse and the agency with which the nurse is affiliated. During the initial visit, the client is provided with The Patient Bill of Rights, and services offered by the nurse, information about the agency providing care, billing procedures, and payment schedules are discussed. The name and telephone number of the home care coordinator are given to the client during the initial visit, thereby assuring that this vital information is documented.

Goals are essential for every visit because they direct the setting of priorities for the visit. Goals and priorities are recorded in the client's record, where they are accessible to any health care provider who visits the client. The most up-to-date information about the client must be written down immediately after the visit.

The intervention phase follows. In this phase, the plan of care and the provision of services, such as wound care and teaching, are implemented. The community health nurse also determines whether referrals are needed and whether there is a need for ongoing nursing visits. Although the frequency of visits is often determined by eligibility for service, agency policy, and insurance coverage, it is the nurse with the physician who must decide if the level of care matches the needs of the client.

At the end of each visit, the nurse reviews what has been done and formulates a plan for the next visit or visits. The visit review helps the client and family (or other caregiver) to identify and assess what has been accomplished and often serves as reinforcement for health teaching. The community health nurse documents the visit by recording it in the progress notes.

Communication

Communication is the most important part of the home visit; it is the key to preventing problems and using resources appropriately. The communication process begins with setting goals and communicating them to the client and ends with recording (i.e., charting) the outcomes. The community health nurse must be skilled in both verbal and written communication.

Sometimes one family member attempts to control communications during the visit. However, every effort should be made to have everyone participate. It is especially important to listen to the client, that is, to hear in the client's words how he or she is feeling.

CASE STUDY:
JANE AND MILLY HARRIS LIVE TOGETHER, AND MILLY DOES ALL THE TALKING

The community health nurse made a home assessment visit after Jane Harris was discharged from the hospital following emergency surgery. The nurse tried to obtain health information to plan the schedule for necessary visits, but whenever the nurse asked Jane a question, Milly answered it. Milly also volunteered health information about her sister that the nurse did not need to include in the assessment.

The community health nurse needs to assist Jane Harris in describing her own home care needs. Milly Harris needs to be thanked for her input but encouraged to allow Jane to speak for herself.

Incorporating family interaction into the details of the visit and plan of care is important. This is often difficult because families do not always maintain geographical closeness, and family members who do not live nearby may feel guilty because of their inability to participate more fully in the client's care. In the following situation, a family member interferes with the visit.

CASE STUDY:
SALLY STITH IS A REGISTERED NURSE AND THINKS SHE KNOWS EVERYTHING

Margaret Stith was recovering at home from a broken hip. Margaret often mentioned how much she missed her only daughter, Sally, who lives 400 miles away "and never visits!" Once, however, Sally was home with her mother when the nurse arrived, although the nurse was not expecting her.

When the nurse discussed Margaret's needs, Sally became very defensive and stated, "You know, I am a nurse! . . . I know what my mother needs, and I do not need you to tell me what is going on!"

Sally Stith needs reassurance from the community health nurse and the opportunity to vent her frustrations about living so far from her mother. The nurse needs to encourage phone contact or letter writing to increase Sally's involvement in her mother's care.

Universal Precautions

The Centers for Disease Control (CDC) require that universal precautions be used in caring for all individuals, as all clients are potential sources of pathogens, bloodborne or otherwise. Universal precautions are practices that nurses and clients must follow for personal safety from infection; they range from hand washing to the wearing of masks and gowns. Universal precautions are intended to prevent contamination of mucous membranes or accidental tissue damage (i.e., needle stick) with an attendant risk of infection. The client's status determines the precautions to be observed. Precautions include face masks, gloves, aprons, glasses, eye shields, or masks, as appropriate. All health care providers must follow universal precautions. Hair and shoe coverings are rarely if ever used in the home.

The community health nurse who fails to follow universal precautions risks professional censure. However, the goal is to achieve adequate protection without overprotecting oneself or unnecessarily isolating the client. Containers for syringes or other sharp objects (i,e., lancets) are usually provided by the agency or a pharmacy. Homemade containers should be constructed of puncture-proof plastic with a screw top lid. A 10:1 water: chlorine bleach solution should be prepared to cover the contaminated items before disposal in the garbage.

Hand-Washing Procedure

1. Ask the client or caretaker where you can wash your hands.
2. Remove soap and paper towels from the bag. (These should be kept in the outer-most or side pocket so as not to contaminate other items in the bag.)
3. Spread out one paper towel to provide a clean field.
4. Place the other clean paper towels on that field.
5. Run the water and then squeeze the liquid soap onto your hands. Do not reuse bar soap from client-to-client.
6. Wash vigorously, rinse, and use the towels on the clean field to dry your hands; use that same paper towel to close the faucets.
7. If there is no running water, use the waterless soap and towels in a similar manner.

Hand Washing

As in other settings, hand washing between clients, that is, at the beginning and end of each visit, is an essential component of infection control in the home. The materials for hand washing are kept in the nursing bag. They include paper towels, liquid germicidal soap, a bag for disposal, and for some situations, a cleaning solution that requires no water.

NECESSARY EQUIPMENT

Contents of the Nursing Bag

The nursing bag is used to carry instruments to be used in a home visit. These include screening instruments (i.e., thermometer, sphygmomanometer, stethoscope), sterile and clean gloves, measuring tape, tongue depressors, sterile disposable syringes, penlight, CPR mask, thermometer shields, large tweezers, sterile cotton swabs, goggles or eye shields, sterile fields, aprons, alcohol swipes, cleaning solutions, materials for record-keeping, and educational materials. The bag generally has several compartments to keep items apart, as much for maintaining cleanliness as for organization. The cleanest areas of the bag are arranged from the inside out; the outermost area is the least clean and includes items such as hand-washing equipment. The bag should never be placed on the floor.

Cleaning Equipment in the Home

It is important to bring as little soiled or used equipment away from the home as possible, thereby lessening the chance of cross-contamination between clients. Although it is best to use disposable equipment or the client's own equipment, if it is necessary to carry away used gear, the nurse should carefully clean it before placing it in the nursing bag. The community health nurse should wear clean disposable gloves and wash used equipment in germicidal soap. Items such as thermometers should be washed in soap and cold water and disinfected with alcohol. Careful planning by the nurse can prevent reuse of supplies in most situations.

Nursing Assessment of the Client

The primary focus of the community health nurse at the initial home visit is the assessment of the client and the family. Traditionally, determining the physical status of a client is considered diagnosing illness, which is within the scope of the physician's practice. However, nurses have also become proficient in using physical assessment techniques, and these skills provide another avenue for data collection by the community health nurse.

Nursing assessment is holistic and, therefore, broader than the medical approach of data collection. It is a systematic process of collecting and analyzing physical, psychological, sociocultural, spiritual, developmental, economic, and life-style information. The nursing assessment provides a basis for nursing diagnosis and for determining a plan of care to achieve the desired outcomes. The processes of assessment, diagnosis, planning, implementation, and evaluation are begun on the first visit and are ongoing throughout the course of the client's care.

The type of assessment model used by the community health nurse is often determined by the employer. It is important for the agency to identify one model that the entire staff can use for data collection. Some home care agencies continue to use the medical model of physical assessment; some use the nursing model of functional health pattern assessment; and many use a combination of both the medical model and the nursing model of functional health patterns.

Bag Technique

1. Never place the nursing bag on the floor.
2. Place the bag on clean newspapers or plastic bags or hang from a door knob.
3. Set up a clean paper towel before hand washing. (See margin note on Hand-Washing Procedure.)
4. Always place nonsterile items closest to the outside of the bag. These include garbage bags, newspapers, and hand-washing equipment, followed by educational equipment, notebooks, and paper materials.
5. The innermost section of the bag contains the equipment used for direct client care.

Community health nursing has traditionally been holistic in scope and practice. However, in today's climate of cost containment, where finances rather than the client's needs may guide aspects of nursing practice, some agencies, which are not concerned with the holistic health care approach, may use an assessment model that addresses only the client's chief complaint. This is often a challenge for the community health nurse. The Alliance for Health Model presented in Chap. 5 provides a structure that aids in the understanding of this challenge and makes suggestions for its possible resolution.

The nurse, as a member of the multidisciplinary health care team, must have a solid grounding in nursing and in physical assessment. This allows the nurse to work as an effective partner of the client and the other health care professionals on the team.

Client History

Each physical examination begins with the health history of the individual client and of the family. The particular items that the nurse chooses to include in the health history depend on the condition of the client and the focus of the visit. The method of data collection also depends upon the needs of the client. For example, a client using a respirator at home may not be able to communicate verbally but may be able to write his or her response. The nurse would supply this client with writing instruments or a letter chart and pointer to accomplish the collection of data.

The health history usually has five parts: (1) identifying data, (2) present illness and chief complaint, (4) current health status, and (5) family history.

Identifying Data   The correct spelling of the client's name; the date and place of the client's birth; and the client's gender, race, marital status, occupation, language spoken and read, most recent health history, and religion are recorded in this part.

Present Illness and Chief Complaint   The community health nurse notes the onset of the present problem, describes its course, symptoms, treatments, and the effectiveness of the treatments. The chief complaint should be stated in the client's words.

Past History   Childhood and adult illnesses, accidents, injuries, operations, and hospitalizations are recorded here.

Current Health Status   The nurse records any medications that the client is taking (whether prescriptions or over-the-counter medications), allergies, tobacco and alcohol use, illicit drug or substance use, diet, Pap smear and mammogram results (for women), last tuberculin test (PPD) or chest x-ray, cholesterol level, stool for occult blood, immunization dates, sleep patterns, exercise, environmental hazards, nutrition, and elimination patterns (i.e., voiding, bowel movements).

Family History A family history includes the cause of death and health status of all members of the immediate family (i.e., the genogram discussed in Chap. 12). Occurrences of diabetes, heart disease, cancer, arthritis, asthma, allergies, mental illness, and substance abuse are all relevant.

Physical Examination

The community health nurse should be proficient in general physical assessment. A general survey and review of systems are performed during the physical examination. Breathing patterns, signs of cyanosis or jaundice, posture, gait, grooming habits, skin turgor, temperature, height, weight, and vital signs are all noted.

The community health nurse notes if the client is over- or underdressed, if there is any indication of poor hygiene, if the client's clothing is disheveled or clean, and if there is any odor of urine or feces on the clothes. The client's speech patterns are also noted; for instance, the nurse notes whether the client's voice is hoarse or if the client slurs his or her words. The community health nurse also assesses alertness, level of consciousness, and presence of lethargy. Many resources exist for the community health nurse to use as a guide in physical assessment (Bates, Bickley, & Hoekelman, 1995; Zang & Bailey, 1997).

The following steps must be taken to prepare the environment, the equipment, and the client for the physical examination. The examination should be completed with minimal stress and without interruption whenever possible, so the environment should ensure privacy and comfort. It is important that the room be warm enough so that exposing a body part for examination does not chill the client.

Lighting should be adequate, and the nurse should have room to work around the bed during the assessment. Lighting and space may be problematic in some home environments, requiring the nurse to spend time in preparing the area in which the client will be examined. Lighting and furniture may need to be moved but only after getting permission from the client. The community health nurse should attempt to keep both equipment and hands warm during the physical examination. The nurse should assist the client with position changes during the examination as necessary.

*P*OSTVISIT RESPONSIBILITIES

A number of questions can help the community health nurse assess the success of the visit. The answers to these questions may motivate the nurse to increase or decrease visit frequency, initiate referrals, move the client to a more appropriate level of care (i.e., hospitalization), or terminate services.

Questions to Review after the Visit
- Did I accomplish the purpose of the visit? If not, why not?
- What information did I gather?
- What were the client's and family's (i.e., significant others) attitudes toward the visit?
- What teaching was accomplished? How do I know what the client and family understood?
- What community resources are available and pertinent?
- What referral or follow-up needs to be planned?

Progress Notes

As in a hospital setting, the progress notes made before, during, and after a home visit are legal documents. All telephone calls to and from the family or client should be noted, even when the client does not answer the phone because these calls indicate the nurse's intent to provide services to the client.

All information concerning the visit itself should also be recorded. This can be done in outline immediately after the visit and then documented more thoroughly in the client's health record when the nurse returns to the agency. Actual hands-on care, assessment, and health teaching to the client or caretaker are all noted. These notes are important for several reasons: they are a source of continuity of care for the client, they provide a legal account of the visit, and they are important for reimbursement.

Each agency has its own method of documentation. As agencies are dependent on third-party reimbursement and these funds are increasingly difficult to secure, documentation of services has become increasingly important. Each agency monitors the progress notes for documentation of service to the client in order to ensure the clinical appropriateness of care and for reimbursement for services rendered. If documentation is written in an unacceptable manner, the agency will not be reimbursed. Therefore, it is extremely important that the progress notes are written clearly and that they indicate the specific reimbursable services rendered and the client's response to care.

In the instance of the nurse giving an insulin injection to the client, clear and precise documentation would include: the amount and type of insulin, where and by whom it was administered (i.e., 15 units of NPH or human insulin, administered subcutaneously by the nurse into the left deltoid region), and a physical description of the injection site (i.e., the skin is intact with no discoloration or change in turgor).

In describing a client with Parkinson's disease with an unsteady gait, the nurse might write: gait unsteady, poor balance, and tremors on the left side, including the leg and arm; client states that he has vertigo when changing from a lying to sitting position. The client requires partial assistance with ADLs from an HHA.

The community health nurse who teaches a client about diet should include in the notes the number of calories required by the client, the client's knowledge about nutrition, and other specific aspects of the diet if they are noteworthy. The client's ability to chew, swallow, and maintain normal bowel function is also part of the nutritional assessment.

Often progress notes are entered into computers for faster access to services as well as faster reimbursement. Computerization of records also makes measurement of clients' outcomes easier to track, and agencies are better able to track clients with special problems as part of risk management. Nurses and other professionals can also be evaluated for the care they give or withhold from their aggregate of clients.

Computerization has greatly influenced the reporting of client-related information. Many community health nurses download client information on a modem or after they return to the agency after making visits to clients. A computerized network of data allows for faster and more complicated sorting of data to evaluate quality of care indicators.

Referrals

The community health nurse may need to refer a client for health care services other than nursing care. Services for which a client may be referred include screening [e.g., hearing or vision testing, x-ray or magnetic resonance imaging (MRI)]; a physician's visit; laboratory tests (e.g., blood, urine); emergency services; physical, speech, or occupational therapy; social work; HHA or homemaker; or nursing home placement. The community health nurse also may refer the client for food support services such as Meals on Wheels. Emergency or crisis referrals may include Adult Protective Services, the American Red Cross (for emergency housing), the Department of Health mental health crisis unit, or the local Domestic Violence Protection agency. Child abuse reporting is mandatory. (There is a national hot line for reporting child abuse at 1-800-635-1522).

The community health nurse shares the rationale for making the referral with the client and often the family. The nurse then notifies the health care professional to whom the client is referred. Many agencies have a standard form for referrals and may have a list of specific agencies to which referrals should be made. All referrals should be cleared with the referring primary care provider. A follow-up phone call or visit is made by the nurse to determine if the client has been seen by the referring agency.

Supervision of Home Health Aides

Overseeing the plan of care for home health aides (HHAs) or personal care workers (PCWs) is an important responsibility of the community health nurse. Workers in the home may have many titles, and the nurse should review the scope of work for each worker so they can provide appropriate assistance. The nurse should determine the level of assistance needed by the client and how this is supplied by the HHA or PCW. This discussion focuses on the work of the HHA.

The delegation of care by the community health nurse to the HHA is governed by the Nurse Practice Act of each state. Most states' Nurse Practice Acts allow nurses to delegate certain nursing care activities to unlicensed individuals; however, there are certain nursing functions that may not be delegated, including the initial nursing assessment and any subsequent assessments that require professional nursing judgment; determination of a nursing diagnosis, goals, or plan of care; and all nursing interventions that require professional knowledge and skill (ANA, 1995).

Delegation does not unburden the community health nurse of responsibility for the care of the client. Therefore, the HHA never performs skilled care. This includes the administration of medication to the client unless otherwise regulated by professional licensing boards or the Department of Health. The HHA can assist clients by bringing their medication to them or by opening a container, but clients must be capable of administering their own medication.

The community health nurse creates the plan of care for the client and sees that it is carried out by the HHA. The plan specifies physical care of the client by the HHA, including meal and dietary needs, positioning of the client, range of motion exercises, ambulation, assisting the client with medications, toileting, dressing, skin and bath care, recording of fluid intake and urinary output, temperature, pulse, and respiration (Fig. 11-5). Figure 11-5 is an example of a worksheet used to guide the work of the HHA or PCW.

( ) HHA ( ) PCW

_____DAYS X _____HOURS VENDOR_____

PATIENTS NAME:_____

ADDRESS:_____

(PLEASE REVIEW PLAN OF CARE WITH PARA PROFESSIONAL AND UPDATE AS NEEDED)

<u>SERVICES TO BE PROVIDED</u>   <u>INSTRUCTIONS</u>

MOUTHCARE:_____

FOOTCARE:_____

SHAMPOO: ( ) BED ( ) SINK ( ) TUB_____

SKIN CARE: ( ) LOTION ( ) MASSAGE_____

NAIL CARE: ( ) FINGERS ( ) TOES_____

BATH: ( ) BED ( )SPONGE ( ) TUB ( ) SHOWER_____

TOILETING: ( ) DIAPER ( ) BEDPAN ( ) URINAL ( ) COMMODE ( ) TOILET_____

DRESSING: ( ) UPPER ( ) LOWER ( ) SHOES_____

OTHER (SPECIFY)_____

MEAL PREPARATION: ( ) BREAKFAST ( ) LUNCH ( ) DINNER ( ) SNACK_____

DIET (FILL IN)_____FLUIDS (AD LIB)_____RESTRICTED_____

FEED PATIENT_____ ASSIST WITH FEEDING _____ ( ) CUT FOOD ( ) PREPARE TRAY_____

WALKING _____ ( ) CRUTCHES ( ) WALKER ( ) CANE ( ) GUARDING   ( ) QUAD CARE

TRANSFERS: ( ) FULL ASSIST ( ) PARTIAL ASSIST_____

TURNING AND POSITIONING: ( ) FULL ASSIST ( ) PARTIAL ASSIST_____

RANGE OF MOTION _____ACTIVE _____PASSIVE_____

CATHETER CARE (SPECIFY)_____

OSTOMY CARE (SPECIFY)_____

MEASURE & RECORD : INTAKE _____OUTPUT_____

MEASURE & RECORD: ____TEMPERATURE _____PULSE _____RESPIRATIONS ____ORAL ___RECTAL __AUXILLARY

MEDICATIONS _____ASSIST _____REMIND_____

VN SIGNATURE:_____DATE:_____

FIGURE 11-5 Plan of care to be carried out by the home health aide or personal care worker.

WORKING WITH OTHER COMMUNITY HEALTH CARE PROVIDERS

Some universities or colleges maintain nursing centers to support ambulatory screening programs or home visiting services for their faculty practice and student learning. They may collaborate with other funding agencies to provide care for needy clients in the community, often at no cost to the client. An alliance between a school of nursing and a community health social service center could provide home care and screening programs to geriatric clients in the community so they do not fall through the cracks of the health care system. These alliances serve clients who, for example, are not sick enough for home care visits but often need the support of a skilled visitor. These alliances are growing in the field of parish nursing. All faith communities are potential settings for lay caregiver support networks.

HOME CARE FOR THE HOMELESS

If the homeless person residing in a shelter is referred to the community health nurse, the visit is carried out just as for any client who lives in his or her own home. However, it is often the staff or possibly other residents in the shelter who provide support for the client rather than family or friends. When an entire family is residing in the shelter together, the family may provide support for the client. However, shelter life may be stressful and may compromise the ability of the family to meet the needs of the client.

The support of clients' needs is often dependent on a great number of variables, for example, the size and type of shelter. Some shelters provide residents and families with long-term stays in order to give them the opportunity to find affordable housing or employment. Others offer limited stays of 30 days. Although some of the homeless persons in shelters are unemployed, many are employed but are simply unable to afford housing. Some have experienced a disaster that destroyed their home (i.e., fire, flood). Still other shelters provide only short-term services. These may include a place to reside during inclement weather or simply emergency quarters in which to sleep for one or two nights.

A great challenge for the community health nurse is the care of the client who lives on the street. If the client stays in a specific area, the nurse may carry the necessary supplies (e.g., a dressing change) and visit the client on the street. As street visits are not reimbursable, their feasibility depends on the criteria of the local community health agency. Most agencies require a specific address in order to accept a referral, and others feel that a street visit is unsafe and will not accept the client for care. Such policies effectively screen the client out of the health care system.

Summary

This chapter has reviewed the components of a home care visit, including planning, making, and recording the visit. Other issues discussed include: travel, safety considerations, communication, goals, priorities, and postvisit procedures and documentation. Universal precautions, hand washing, and necessary equipment, such as the nursing bag and its contents, have also been described. Supervision of HHAs and other unlicensed personnel in the home has been reviewed. Providing care for the homeless is discussed.

KEY WORDS

Planning the visit
Nursing equipment for home visits
Postvisit responsibilities

QUESTIONS

DIRECTIONS: Choose the one *best* response to each of the following questions.

1. The community health nurse calls Mr. Smith in preparation for a home visit. Mr. Smith states, "I still have this chest pain after three doses of nitroglycerine." The nurse should tell Mr. Smith to

   A. call his physician.
   B. phone 911 for emergency assistance.
   C. take another dose of nitroglycerine.
   D. lie down and wait for the nurse to visit.

2. The first visit the nurse should make in the morning would be to

   A. Mrs. Handl, an insulin-dependent diabetic who is learning injection technique.
   B. Mr. Gerale, a lonely, blind person with cancer.
   C. Baby Front, an infant of normal weight who is not eating enough according to the mother.
   D. Ms. O'Mally, a single, pregnant, school dropout.

3. Which of the following clients needs an on-the-spot mental health referral?

   A. Ms. Galy, who is sad about losing her job due to a long hospitalization.
   B. Mr. Smeet, who is talking about ending his life.
   C. Mr. Cammero, who is angry that his wife's surgery was not successful.
   D. Ms. Larop, who is anxious about physical therapy.

4. The community health nurse visits a teenager who is 7 months pregnant and who has made little preparation for the infant's birth. Which statement by the nurse is most appropriate?

   A. "Why did you get pregnant if you did not want a baby?"
   B. "You will have enough time to prepare for the baby if you begin now."
   C. "How did your mother prepare for your birth?"
   D. "Tell me what you think about being pregnant."

5. The community health nurse makes a home visit to a client who has just been diagnosed with diabetes. The client lives with his wife and three adult children and is having difficulty maintaining a diabetic diet. The nurse and client plan for the next visit to be in the evening because

   A. the entire family will be present and can discuss the client's inability to maintain his diet.
   B. it is on the nurse's way home, and it will be the last visit.
   C. the nurse will be able to meet with the family members to assess their needs.
   D. the nurse wants to teach the family about diabetes and a diabetic diet.

ANSWERS

1. *The answer is B.* The progress of the chest pain requires immediate help.

2. *The answer is A.* Routine insulin doses are given in the morning.

3. *The answer is B.* Suicidal ideation requires immediate intervention.

4. *The answer is D.* An open-ended question allows the client to express how she or he is feeling.

5. *The answer is D.* Working with the entire family lends maximum support to the client.

ANNOTATED REFERENCES

American Nurses Association. (1995). *The ANA basic guide to safe delegation.* Washington, DC: Author.

   The guidelines for delegation by the nurse are presented from the professional associations' point of view.

Bates, B., Bickley, L. S., & Hoekelman, R. A. (1995). *A pocket guide to physical examination and history taking* (2d ed.). Philadelphia: J. B. Lippincott.

   The essentials of the physical examination are reviewed in this text.

Community Health Accreditation Program. (1996). *Benchmarks for excellence in home care.* New York: Author.

Outcomes of excellence are identified for home care agencies to track ongoing improvements as well as comparison to other agencies.

Zang, S. A., & Bailey, N. C. (1997). *Home care manual: Making the transition.* Philadelphia: J. B. Lippincott.

This pocket book is an excellent reference for nurses beginning home care practice.

$\mathscr{F}$AMILY HEALTH ASSESSMENT

$\mathscr{D}$EFINING THE FAMILY

Family health is reflected in the health of the community; healthy families mean healthy communities. By promoting and protecting family health, the community health nurse improves and preserves community health. The family, then, is an important client of the community health nurse.

The family is a vital social structure in every community. Definitions of the family tend to include reference to blood relationships and a shared value system, but families are as diverse as the individuals that comprise them. A family may be a single person or consist of an elderly woman and her six dogs and cats. Still other families may be multigenerational networks of persons or include non–blood-related companions or friends. Some use "kin" to refer to the biological family, that is, relatives by blood or ancestry, and "kith" to refer to one's friends, acquaintances, and associates. In these terms, the kith-family is the family one chooses, and the kin-family is the family into which one is born; one can belong simultaneously to both.

The family is a living social system, a source both of great stress and of supportive resources. "The family is the primary and most powerful emotional system that humans belong to and …is the greatest potential resource as well as the greatest source of stress" (Fogarty, personal correspondence, 1997; Fogarty, 1976; Fogarty, 1975). The emotional bonds between family members are among the earliest and most powerful bonds experienced, connecting family members to each other throughout their lives and even beyond their deaths, transcending time, distance, and strife. This emotional connectedness is a basic feature of the family.

Often it is easy to assess the deviant and dysfunctional patterns of a family; problems in many family clients are glaringly obvious to the community health nurse. It may be more difficult to clarify the strengths of a family. Yet it is important to understand the family as a source of actual and potential strengths, which empower the family to cope with its problems and challenges. The strengths of the family are inner resources that can be translated into concrete ways in which the family nurtures, protects, and guides its members. On the other hand, the family is also a source of stress. Indeed, stress is a natural and necessary occurrence in family life.

Stress motivates the family to face its challenges and to mobilize its resources in its own particular coping style. Naturally, if the family's strengths and inner resources are depleted and stress is mounting out of control, family members will resort to defensive behavior in an effort to protect themselves. Generally, however, the family will be able to contend with its stress by relying on the strengths it either possesses already or develops in its efforts to cope with the tasks of everyday life.

$\mathcal{T}$HE FAMILY AS CLIENT

The community health nurse cares for the individual members of the family, for the family as a unit, and for the family within the context of the community (Bomar, 1996; Friedman, 1992; Kirschling, Gilliss, Krentz, Camburn, Clough, Duncan, Hendricks, Howard, Roberts, Smith-Young, Tice, & Young, 1994; Wegner & Alexander, 1993). The community's health is dependent on the health of its members, all of whom, by some definition, are members of families. Therefore, the community health nurse wishes to identify commonalities of need among families in the community to be able to address its family-based health concerns.

Subsystems within Families

Subsystems within Families

Dyad—two people in interaction
Triad—three people in interaction
Generational hierarchies—interactions across generations

The family is a system comprised of individual members who form various constellations with respect to each other. Two members in interaction are referred to as a **dyad**. Three members in interaction are referred to as a **triad**. Interacting groups of members that traverse generations are referred to as **generational hierarchies**. These varied configurations, in addition to the individual members, are the subsystems of the family system.

The position a member holds in the dyadic, triadic, or hierarchical configurations of the family is dynamic; that is, the membership of these configurations is constantly in flux. Family relationships are thus characterized by dynamic change; positions in the family change all the time. Both close and peripheral relationships may change. Transactions between family members are noted by the community health nurse appraising role function and communication patterns in the family. The nurse deciphers the web of family relationships to understand how members relate to each other, how the family functions as a unit, and, finally, how the family relates to the larger community.

The Family as an Open System

A functional *open system*, such as the healthy family, is open to its environment, which is enveloped by semipermeable boundaries that define its limits while allowing for exchange with the larger environment through input and output. *Input* is information coming into a system from the larger environment, and *output* is information contributed to the larger environment by the system. *Throughput* is the processing of information within the system. Such exchange is characteristic of open systems. The functional family is an open system; it exists in an environment with which it interacts, from which it derives input, and to which it contributes output. This openness is necessary for the survival and growth of the system. The family acts as a buffer, filtering information to and from larger systems. Therefore, each family must be viewed within the context of its larger environment.

Goal-Directedness and Families

Functional human systems move purposefully toward goals. Each family has the potential to define its own meaningful goals and choose the steps that it will take to achieve them. A family's sense of purpose and direction gives it the fuel it needs to sustain itself; goal-directedness may provide a core of order for a family in otherwise stressful and chaotic times.

The goals that families strive to attain vary over time and from family to family. For some families living in poverty or constrained by financial stress, the goal of survival itself takes precedence, as other goals, though recognized as desirable, are unreachable. The goals of some families may include education, employment, recreational plans, geographical changes, new housing, and health. Movement toward goals enables the family to become more complex and diverse, characteristics indicative of the family's ability to function more effectively. However, goal-directedness is defined by each family, and achieving goals is an ongoing process. This process of defining and achieving goals is renegotiated by families as they change over time.

Holistic Functioning of Families

The family functions holistically, that is, if one member is ill then the whole family system experiences *dis-ease* or disequilibrium. Thus, the experience of the individual affects that of the family as a whole.

Members are connected to each other through relational bonds (Minuchin, 1974). If one member is depleted or distressed, then the whole family experiences depletion and distress to some degree. The nurse focuses care on individual members in particular need while also caring for the family as a whole. The family is a *unit*, and the community health nurse treats it as such; rather than view an individual member of the family as the client of concern and the others as a support network, the community health nurse views the entire family as the client of concern. Family *dis-ease* requires family-focused intervention. The community health nurse employs skills in group dynamics in working with the family as a group (Clark, 1994).

Family Process

Families operate through actions and transactions. These actions and transactions are called family process. Family process includes each family's particular style of interacting with itself and of accomplishing its tasks. The community health nurse may discern family process through observation of how the family relates to and cares for its members, negotiates with the nurse and the larger community, and meets its own needs.

Family process is frequently automatic. Indeed, the community health nurse may witness family patterns that have repeated themselves for generations. However, the new problems that every generation faces require that each family constellation attempt to find its own solutions; that is, families are not doomed to repeat patterns that may be limiting or depleting. Each family has the capability to become different and to establish its own patterns—to make its own mark. Change is always possible. Healthy families have the ability to change and transform themselves.

FUNCTIONAL AND DYSFUNCTIONAL FAMILY PATTERNS

Looking at how families function helps the community health nurse define the parameters for assessing family wellness. The nurse is skillful in assessing both the functional patterns of well families and those dysfunctional patterns that result when families develop defenses to deal with overwhelming stress. Responding to stress, all families develop defenses to protect their integrity; however, when defenses become ongoing patterns rather than responses to specific episodes, then a pattern of family dysfunction may result. The nurse is mindful that nursing interactions with a family merely sample family exchanges at a particular point in time, much as photography captures a moment of action. It is important for the nurse to determine whether this exchange is indicative of an ongoing pattern of dysfunction in the family's dynamics or if the exchange is related to a new family situation. Families defend themselves to protect their members and their ability to function. Dysfunctional patterns develop when coping skills become exhausted or are no longer effective and defenses are employed repeatedly, rather than episodically, becoming the family's habitual way of interacting.

The community health nurse is concerned not only with the dynamics and issues of each family as a unique entity but also with the patterns that link families to each other and that signal problems and concerns shared by families in the community. The community health nurse is concerned with each family as it grows and deals with health care concerns and adversity and is also concerned with the problems and issues that families share as common strengths, risks, and problems. Identifying commonalities of concern among families enables the nurse to develop a community-based agenda for family health.

Functional Patterns of Family Dynamics

The community health nurse develops knowledge and skill in family assessment to deliver family-based care, identifying family health concerns that require family solutions. She or he seeks to impart knowledge and skills that enable the family to care for itself and to contend with and solve its own problems. The nurse works as a partner with the family sharing knowledge and skills, which the family may then integrate into its own practices. For the nurse to identify family-based health concerns and issues, a thorough family health assessment must be accomplished. The categories of assessment that a community health nurse must examine are identified in the Family Wellness Assessment Guide. This Guide can be used to gather assessment data (Fig. 12-1).

Patterns of Daily Living

Assessment of patterns of daily living provides the community health nurse with clues to the family's ability to carry out routine functions common to all families. This category of assessment can include the nutritional choices of the members, their sleep/wake/rest cycles, their capacity for work and leisure activities, performance of exercise, expressions of sexuality, and educational endeavors. Each of these patterns provides basic nurturance to the family system and enables it to grow and develop, fulfill its functions, and achieve its goals. Frustration of these basic needs results in depletion of the family system.

The *nutritional status* of the family can best be ascertained through 24-h (or longer) recall of dietary intake. Variations for individual members should be considered since not all family members eat all meals together. In addition to an analysis of dietary intake, the community health nurse also considers the meaning of food to the family and how meals are used for family socialization and interaction. Some families may choose to watch television together with their dinner plates on their laps, some will set a table and take the telephone off the hook to avoid interruptions during meal time, and others will expect individual members to prepare their own food or take food from a common pot.

Functional Patterns of Family Dynamics

Patterns of daily living
Multigenerational transmission
Boundaries and differentiation
Family roles
Communication patterns
Norms and values
Decision-making
Power
Conflict and stress
Energy
Change
Environment
Self-care

Patterns of Daily Living

Nutrition
Sleep/wake/rest
Work/leisure
Physical activity
Sexuality
Education

FIGURE 12-1

Family Wellness Assessment
Guide

Name of family_____

Address _____

I.   FAMILY CONSTELLATION
     A. Genogram
     B. Members Living in Household—name, date of birth, sex, occupation
     C. Members Not Living in Household—name, date of birth, sex, occupation, location

II. PATTERNS OF DAILY LIVING
     A. Nutrition—assessment of nutritional status of members, meal preparation, financial considerations, opportunities for socialization
     B. Sleep/Wake/Rest—pattern of sleep-wake cycle, adequacy of sleeping arrangements, safety
     C. Work/Leisure—balance of work with recreation, adequacy of financial support of family, sources of financial support, resources for leisure activities
     D. Physical Activity and Fitness—exercise pattern, types of physical activity, motivation
     E. Sexuality—satisfaction, sexual expression, safety
     F. Education—educational status and goals of members

III. INTRAFAMILY DYNAMICS
     A. Patterns of Communication
         1. Relationships between each dyad
         2. Relationship of family as a unit
         3. Extrafamilial relationships—friends, neighbors, organizations, social activities
     B. Role Functions
         1. Roles assumed by each member
         2. Nature of role functions—flexible, complementary, reciprocal
         3. Identified unmet role functions
     C. Patterns of Decision-making—consensus, accommodation, de facto, unilateral, indecision
     D. Norms and Values—culture, religion, spirituality traditions, priority placed on health
     E. Distribution of Power among Members—personal and shared power
     F. Patterns of Conflict Management—issues of importance and sources of stress, resolution
     G. Energy to Accomplish Tasks and Goals—patterns of flow, blockages, sources of depletion and restoration
     H. Capacity of Family to Change and Grow over Time—identification of goals and resources for achieving goals

IV. ENVIRONMENT
   A. Housing—type, condition, context in community
   B. Resources Available—bathroom, kitchen, refrigeration, water supply, heat
   C. Safety—hazards
   D. Use of Community Resources

V. IMPACT OF ILLNESS ON FAMILY—what happens when illness strikes and when illness is chronic or terminal

VI. ANALYSIS OF FAMILY FUNCTION
   A. Family Health Risks
   B. Family Health Problems
   C. Family Health Strengths

VII. FAMILY SELF-ASSESSMENT—capacity for self-care

FIGURE 12-1 *(continued)*

⬚

Family Wellness Assessment Guide

Appreciation for cultural food patterns is also critical to the nurse's appraisal of nutritional status, for food has different meanings in different cultures. The community health nurse should become familiar with the meaning of food to each particular family. Other considerations include who shops for the food, who prepares the meals, and who cleans up after meals. Further, the nurse should consider the family's financial ability to provide for its nutritional needs. Nurses often teach families to purchase more nutritional food choices, given their financial constraints. Guidance is also offered regarding the relationship of the family's diet to standards like the food pyramid.

Sleep/wake/rest cycles are circadian cycles that provide energy for meeting daily needs. The community health nurse is concerned with each family member's ability to achieve the sleep and rest needed to feel replenished for daily activities and with family member's needs for privacy, quiet, and adequate space for sleeping and resting. Space can be a very precious commodity, and inadequate housing is a serious public health problem. Many families are homeless or live in substandard housing. Problems with heat, ventilation, rodents, and insufficient space or bedding are common problems in the lives of many families. Another consideration is the family's designated sleeping arrangements. Culture is clearly a consideration here, as some members may be accustomed to sleeping on the floor or together in one room. It is within the cultural context that psychosexual development and the need for privacy must be considered. The nurse must weigh familial and cultural considerations against the possibility of thwarted personal growth and safety. Sexual abuse is not uncommon, and the nurse must be alert to signs of possible sexual abuse.

The family's *balance of work and leisure* is another pattern of daily living. Work generally provides some kind of purposeful activity that enables the adult family member to contribute to the family's financial stability.

A members' capability to work may be greatly influenced by health status. The community health nurse is concerned with maximizing each member's personal health status by supporting their search for paid work, volunteer work, and leisure activities that are personally meaningful. The nurse can make referrals for job training, if desired, by becoming familiar with employment training resources in the community and with the mechanism for referral. Leisure is often neglected in families, yet it provides a balance to work and helps in dealing with the stresses of daily life. The community health nurse should be knowledgeable about recreational facilities in the community, including parks, community centers, special programs on parenting, teen centers, scouting, and other opportunities for leisure that the family may enjoy.

Physical activity contributes to enjoyment and personal satisfaction with life. Also, fitness is correlated with health as a risk reduction strategy for a number of diseases conditions. Purposeful exercise is, therefore, an important health consideration for all family members. The community health nurse determines the extent to which members have time for physical activity and the appropriateness of various activities, given their health status. The nurse appraises the types of exercise that members select and teaches members about safety and accident prevention. Motivation is often a limiting factor in this aspect of daily living; the nurse can discuss the individualized health risks associated with little or no physical activity and can assist members with strategies for integrating physical activity into their lives. Some members will benefit from recommended guidelines for daily physical activity regimes while others will need teaching about armchair exercises or progressive physical activity following hospitalization for a depleting health condition.

Sexuality is part of a pattern of daily living. It is a healthy, natural part of life. Every health assessment should include an assessment of sexuality. Sexuality is more than performing sexual activities; it involves attitudes, beliefs, and values that are determined by families and culture, as well as the individual's role function, identity, and thoughts and feelings about relationships. The community health nurse is concerned about whether the sexual needs of individual members are met, the degree to which they feel satisfied with themselves and their sexual lives, and the quality and nature of their relationships.

Health care providers are often uncomfortable and ill equipped to consider sexual history as part of a health assessment—yet it is a vital aspect. The community health nurse becomes adept at including assessment of sexuality as part of a health assessment. Appraisal of satisfaction with one's sexual life and ability to find sexual expression are important components of the assessment. The nurse is nonjudgmental in accepting the choices and experiences of the family members and is particularly conscious of accepting individual differences in sexual orientation. Finally, the nurse is concerned with the safety of all sexual practices (e.g., the correct use of condoms). Sexual health is an important area for health teaching and guidance.

The *educational goals* of family members are also key to health and health assessment. The community health nurse should be alert to the educational opportunities of each family member and, in particular, of the child members. Communication with the school nurse is an important form of nurse-to-nurse collaboration in consulting about the educational and health status of children. School performance is often affected by diminished health, and the nurse can be instrumental in early remediation of health problems via screenings and health assessment.

The community health nurse may encounter children who are not in school for a variety of reasons. Families in transient housing may consider it more traumatic to enter and exit different schools frequently than to stay out of school altogether. Sometimes child members stay at home to assist an ill parent or caretaker. Day care and early childhood programs are also important for working parents and for children considered at-risk for or identified with developmental delays. More generally, the nurse is concerned with connecting members of the family to educational resources in the community regardless of age or circumstance. Education is often a way for members to exceed family expectations; it can provide a way for members to distinguish and empower themselves as members of the family and the community. Educational settings also provide opportunities for socialization and for the identification of learning and health concerns and problems.

Functional patterns of daily living are basic needs of family life. The community health nurse will often encounter families with limited or depleted capability to meet these needs, which, in turn, affects the family's health. The community health nurse is dedicated to helping families to meet the demands of daily living through the restoration and maintenance of these patterns of health.

Multigenerational Transmission The fact that health patterns and practices can be transmitted from one generation to another gives rise to the concept of multigenerational transmission (Bowen, 1978). Health patterns and practices can be transmitted across generations through genetic predisposition, life-style learning, or both. In analyzing a family's multigenerational health patterns, the community health nurse collects assessment data that reveal the health problems, predispositions, and risks not only of the current generation, but also of future generations. This knowledge alerts family members to their own health risks and to the importance of reducing risks for their decendants.

The best tool for uncovering family health patterns that traverse generations is the family **genogram**. The genogram is a diagrammatic representation of family relationships that includes vital data on age, gender, culture, occupation, emotional connections, geographical location, and health data, including occurrences of disease and causes of death.

Genogram is a diagrammatic representation of family relationships; a family heirloom.

To construct the genogram, one begins by assembling information about the family and organizing it into a diagram. Take note of the symbols for constructing the genogram, then examine the sample genogram (Fig. 12-2). A three-generational genogram is illustrated. "At least three generations in the family are necessary as a minimum overview of the (family) emotional system and its climate" (Fogarty, 1973–1978, p. 60).

The genogram is an excellent tool for portraying a wealth of family data in a concise, readable document. Data can be added as it is gathered. Analysis of the genogram also helps to identify those members of the

Sample Family Genogram

Family Name

Date

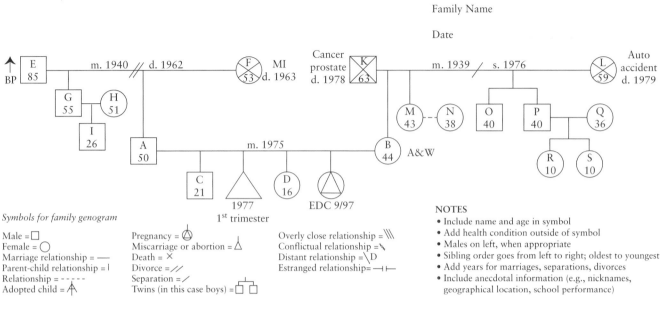

Symbols for family genogram

Male = □
Female = ○
Marriage relationship = —
Parent-child relationship = |
Relationship = - - - - -
Adopted child = ⌒

Pregnancy = △⃝
Miscarriage or abortion = △
Death = ✕
Divorce = //
Separation = /
Twins (in this case boys) = □ □

Overly close relationship = \\\
Conflictual relationship = ⌇
Distant relationship = \D
Estranged relationship= ⊣⊢

NOTES
• Include name and age in symbol
• Add health condition outside of symbol
• Males on left, when appropriate
• Sibling order goes from left to right; oldest to youngest
• Add years for marriages, separations, divorces
• Include anecdotal information (e.g., nicknames, geographical location, school performance)

FIGURE 12-2 Sample family genogram [NOTE: Symbols adapted from "A Guide to the Genogram," by E. G. Pendagast & C. O. Sherman, 1973–1978, *The Family. Compendium I. The Best of the Family* (p. 102), Washington, DC: Georgetown University Family Center.]

FIGURE 12-3

Genographic representation of marriage. (Formation of a non-marital partnership would be represented by a dashed line.)

family about whom little is known and so alert the nurse that the family health assessment may not be complete. A genogram is like a road map; it can be read with accuracy if its symbols are used correctly and consistently. The symbol for males is a square and that for females is a circle. Note that the name and age of each individual is marked inside the symbol. Anecdotal information, especially concerning health, can be added outside and next to the symbol. As a rule, males are put on the left, except in the case of same-sex relationships, or when sibling order places females to the left. Sibling order is always drawn portraying the oldest to the left and the youngest to the right, in descending order. Non–blood-related members of the family can be added to the genogram and are simply placed near the appropriate relationship. Pets can also be added to the genogram, using creative symbols, if desired.

The sample genogram tells us that A and B married in 1975 (Fig. 12-3). Their first child, C, is a male. Sometime after C's birth, A and B experienced a first-trimester miscarriage. After the miscarriage, a daughter, D, was born. A and B are expecting a child (Fig. 12-4) The expected date of confinement (EDC), or due date, can be entered on the genogram.

B is apparently "alive and well" (A & W), and space is available to list the health condition of A and of A and B's children. Note that A and B are placed horizontally on the same generational line and their pregnancies and

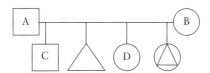

FIGURE 12-4

⬚

Genographic representation of a couple's childbearing history.

children on another generational line. Clarity in depicting generational lines makes it easier to read the genogram and conveys an accurate picture of generational relationships.

Going back a generation to A's and B's families of origin reveals their respective parents, on another generational line, and their respective siblings (see Fig. 12-2). In this genogram, A and B are dropped lower than their respective siblings in order to focus on the family they have created through their marriage. A's father is E, who has hypertension. A's mother is F, who died in 1963 of a myocardial infarction (MI). E and F were married in 1940 and divorced in 1962. Before A was born, a brother, G, was born. G was E and F's first child. G has married H and they have a son, I.

B's family of origin consists of her father, K, who died in 1978 of prostate cancer. B's mother, L, died in 1979 in an automobile accident. K and L were married in 1939 and separated in 1976. K and L had 4 children together. B was their first child and M their second. M has established a same-sex partnership with N. Sometime after M's birth, K and L gave birth to male twins, O and P. P has married Q and they have twin daughters, R and S.

This sample genogram alerts the community health nurse to the importance of cardiovascular risk reduction and screening for A and general cancer-prevention education and screening for B. A and B can be taught about the importance of cardiovascular and cancer risk reduction and education for their children, as well as about the importance of accident prevention and other generic parenting skills. A and B could also benefit from health counseling about over-40 pregnancy. Referrals may be indicated.

Emotional connections can be diagramed once the basic structure of the genogram is constructed (Fig. 12-5). For example, a conflictual relationship between A and E could be symbolized by connecting A and E with a zigzag line, the symbol for conflict. Likewise, if B and E experience an emotionally intense or overclose relationship they could be connected with a triple line, the symbol for intensity of relationship. A and B may be emotionally distant from each other; this relationship could be indicated by the D-labeled single line, the symbol for emotional distance. Note that

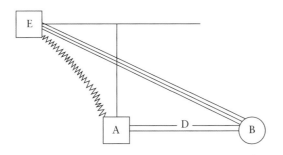

FIGURE 12-5

⬚

Genographic representation of emotional relationships. Note the A and B are connected both by a single, solid line that indicates marriage and by the symbol for emotional distance.

when emotional relationships are diagramed, the interconnectedness of members to each other becomes evident. Later in this chapter the concept of *triangulation* will be covered. Referring back to Fig. 12-5 will then clarify the dysfunctional connections among A, B, and E.

The importance of the genogram is to alert the community health nurse to the impact of multigenerational patterns of disease and to elevated risks for health and emotional problems. The genogram is a ready reference of family health history, risks, and patterns, conveying much information at a glance. The community health nurse can quickly ascertain repeating patterns in a family, giving special attention to patterns of disease and causes of death. The genogram can be enriched with additional information during each family contact. As information is added, the family is able to join with the nurse in identifying strengths, risks, and problems, and the community health nurse becomes aware of gaps in information about individual members that otherwise may have been overlooked. Sometimes a member will provide valuable information about every other member of the family, but the nurse comes to realize that little is known about that particular member. The nurse takes care to observe who knows what and what information is not stated (is suppressed) by the members.

The genogram also provides the family with an aid to reflection on its own dynamics and intergenerational issues and problems. The community health nurse can construct the genogram with the family as a way to encourage family reflection, and members can assist the nurse in filling in gaps of information. Aged members of the family are often great historians and are able to reveal important data about the extended family. The genogram can become a family heirloom—a source of family information that can be passed to future generations.

Boundaries and Differentiation **Boundaries** identify and define the family, providing for the integrity of the family system. The family operates as an open system if its boundaries maintain the integrity of the family as a unit while remaining semipermeable to input and output, that is, selectively allowing input to and output from the family system.

Family boundaries are probably the most crucial means families have of facilitating adaptation to environmental (outside) demands and family (inside) needs. The family may tighten its boundaries when it feels it needs to defend its integrity and may loosen them when it trusts its environment and seeks more input. When faced with illness or death, for instance, families have varying responses. On the one hand, it is not uncommon for a family to tighten its boundaries in the face of an illness or death in the family. The family turns inward to conserve its resources and to deal with the stress of illness and the pain of loss. Thus, self-reliance—an important family capability—is often fostered by tightening the family boundaries in a time of need. On the other hand, when illness or death strikes a family, its members may loosen the family boundaries to admit people who can help. For example, the family may meet with a community health nurse and adopt suggested strategies for dealing with illness and loss. The family may attend counseling sessions with a nurse bereavement therapist and seek the

Boundaries identify and define the family.

assistance of clergy following the death of a family member, opening the family system to professionals who may be able to assist in the time of need.

Family boundaries may change as the family constellation changes. If a new member of the family is added, its boundaries can grow and change to enable the new member to function as a member of the family unit. It is also possible that the family may be unable or unwilling to accept a new member. In this case, the failure to open and grow will have consequences for the new member and the whole family system.

Not only may new members be added, but some members die and their memory continues on as part of the family unit. Members may leave temporarily and rejoin the family, or families can be divided by separation and divorce (i.e., blended and reconstituted with other families). Blended or reconstituted families are created as members from one family join with members of another to form a new family system. It is not uncommon to see reconstituted families created through remarriage as each partner brings children from a previous marriage that ended in divorce.

Differentiation can be thought of as a sense of individuality and separateness among family members (Bowen, 1978). To differentiate means "to be distinct, well defined, and to grow into a special entity that is a self, a person. It means I know where I begin and end, and where others have their self boundaries. It acknowledges that there is always a space between the self and other" (Fogarty, 1985, p. 18). Each member of the family is connected to the family system, yet characteristically separate and individual. Members are thus subsystems in the family system. Each subsystem is distinct and separated by a personal boundary that promotes and protects its integrity.

Individual differentiation can thus be described as "the amount of emotional maturity in an individual within the family system" (Wegner & Alexander, 1993, p. 360). Differentiation is necessary for each person to be separate and for the family to be defined by clear lines on connectedness. The community health nurse is alert to indicators of differentiation, which include a sense of separateness among the members; the toleration and even encouragement of different points of view; and the fostering of emotional maturity. The goal is to separate thinking processes from feelings so that members are able to problem-solve and come up with solutions to concerns.

Differentiation allows for individuality and separateness among family members.

Family Roles Roles are assigned or assumed behaviors in the family. *Assumed roles* are behaviors that a member takes on willingly, while *assigned roles* are behaviors that may come with a title (e.g., mother or father) or are given to a member. Roles permit orderly social interactions and transactions among family members, helping to provide balance and sense of stability. Each member's behavior becomes expected, thus facilitating family functioning.

Even within functional families, the community health nurse witnesses members experiencing role conflict, overload, and confusion. The nurse can assist members by helping them understand that healthy struggle often takes place in assuming and being assigned family roles. Consider the dynamics involved when a member becomes a parent: the new parent may experience role conflict, wondering how to balance work and parenting responsibilities; role overload, when the demands and responsibilities of parenting feel overwhelming; and role confusion when unsure of how to parent and care for the newborn.

In functional families, there is a tendency for roles to be complementary, reciprocal, and flexible. When roles complement each other it means that together they make up for what each may be lacking; complementary roles make up a whole. Thus, if roles are complementary in a given family, then ordinary daily tasks are more easily accomplished. Meals are prepared, laundry is done, and the other household functions that each member expects from the others are performed. Together, the family members are able to accomplish all the roles assigned to them (or which they have come to assume) and so support the functioning of the individual members and the family as a unit.

When roles are reciprocal, it means that they are mutual, that is, assigned or assumed behaviors are mutually beneficial for the members. In most cases, family members are satisfied with the arrangement of role functions. In some cases, they even enjoy their reciprocal role functions and are reluctant to share them, as they feel a sense of pride, expertise, and possession.

When roles are flexible, assigned or assumed behaviors are not rigid. Flexibility implies that roles can bend and yield. Family members may take on each other's roles in times of stress, for example, during an illness or when members are otherwise challenged and unable to fulfill their roles. Willingness to pitch in and take over the responsibilities of another member for the sake of the family as a whole is a sign of flexibility. Role assignments that are always divided evenly may appear egalitarian, but they are often a sign of rigidity. If roles are flexible, they allow for role behaviors to shift asymmetrically so that the family can achieve its functions. The community health nurse must, therefore, keep in mind that in functional families, during times of illness or depleted health of any member, roles will shift to accomplish the tasks and responsibilities of the ill member.

The community health nurse looks for signs of complementarity, mutuality, and flexibility in family roles. The nurse also helps the members cope with role conflict, role overload, and role confusion.

Communication Patterns Human beings are always communicating (Watzlawick, 1978). Communication takes place regardless of whether words are spoken; people may communicate through words, eye contact, body movement, signals, and silence.

The objective of effective communication is for the receiver to get the same message that the sender intends. Ideally, communication is synchronous, that is, the spoken word and all forms of nonverbal communication are in synchrony—there is harmony and consistency among all these forms. Functional communication can be broken down into components that describe the communication process. The sender states his or her case; the receiver and sender may clarify and qualify the message; the sender asks for feedback; the sender is open and receptive to the feedback; and both the sender and receiver are responsible for their own thoughts, feelings, and actions. Effective communication is best described as a dynamic interchange resulting in clarity. Clarity does not mean that the sender and receiver necessarily agree but that the message received is the message intended.

Family members develop patterns of communication over time. For example, members communicate in dyads, triads, across generations, and with the family as a whole. Assessing communication between members of the family as well as between members and the family as a whole are important approaches in understanding how the family communicates. The most effective way to analyze communication within the family is to study the interaction between each set of dyads within the family; thus, the community health nurse is interested in the degree to which communication in the dyads is effective. In a traditional four-member family, consisting of a mother, father, daughter, and son, there are six possible dyads: mother-father; mother-daughter; mother-son; father-daughter; father-son; and son-daughter. Assessment of dyadic communication patterns informs the nurse about the way communication flows within the family and about potential communication blocks.

The community health nurse must be skilled in assessing patterns of communication within the family. Often, in the midst of a crisis precipitated by illness, communication patterns in the family may become splintered and chaotic as each member goes in a different direction while attempting to cope. The community health nurse can facilitate a family meeting to offer members an opportunity to clarify the situation, establish mutual goals, and openly communicate personal needs and concerns about the family and its ability to function.

Since family-based care focuses on the entire family as an interacting unit, the community health nurse may be a catalyst for strengthening the bonds among family members. The community health nurse encourages family members to communicate with each other, clarifies issues and concerns, and defuses areas of emotional intensity so that clear messages can be sent and received. Effective communication can enable the family to identify and achieve its goals.

Norms and Values Norms are rules that guide and regulate the family and provide standards by which the family lives. Norms determine what members should do. Each family has spoken and unspoken norms that guide its internal interactions and transactions and that are influenced by family history, culture, religion, and lifestyle choices. Norms provide a sense of stability because members know what is expected from them and the extent to which their behaviors are acceptable. There are consequences when norms are broken. In caring for a family, it is important for the nurse to appreciate its norms and be aware of consequences when norms are not firmly held. Knowledge of family norms provides a solid foundation for the community health nurse's understanding of family behavior. The nurse also needs to acknowledge family rules as a guide to professional behavior, for the nurse does not want to infringe upon or ignore family rules, thereby jeopardizing a therapeutic relationship with the family.

In assessing family norms, the community health nurse seeks to gauge their flexibility. As a family grows and develops, there is a great deal of change; the family is in flux. Given the dynamic nature of family life, family norms need to be flexible. Norms should also be humane so that no member is subjected to cruel consequences. The community health nurse is mindful of the importance of protecting each member of the family from unhealthy or inappropriate behavior. Norms that are not fitted to the family's situation may hamper family unity and place undue stress on the members. Clarifying family rules is an important community health nursing strategy.

Family values are closely allied to norms. Values are inner convictions about right and wrong, good and bad, and the desirable and the undesirable. A family's values reveal what the family believes to be ethical, moral, and just. Religion and spirituality are important forces in shaping a family's values. Families often socialize with others who share similar beliefs, so the family value system clearly influences socialization patterns. For example, family members may hold values that promote human service and dedication to others; in this case, members may agree that community service is important and encourage each other to engage in service projects that promote and protect the well-being of the community. Other families may value a work ethic and expect their members to hold wage-earning positions of responsibility at an early age and to continue that pattern throughout their lives. Individuals may wish to depart from their family's values if their own beliefs about right and wrong differ from those of the family. For example, if racism is acceptable within a family but an individual member chooses to believe that all people are equal, then the individual's dissent may be instructive to the family. Otherwise, family conflict will arise. If a member of the family resorts to stealing to support a drug habit yet the family finds these behaviors intolerable, perhaps the family's beliefs may eventually serve as a source of strength for the affected member.

Decision-Making The goal of effective family decision-making is agreement followed by commitment to the selected course of action. Agreement can be achieved in a variety of ways.

Consensus is a kind of decision-making in which all members of the family come to agree on a course of action that they believe is the best possible. Consensus takes time and willingness on the part of all members to explore the pros and cons of all possible courses of action. Further, consensus requires that all members listen carefully to each other, especially when there are divergent points of view or differences of opinion. Members are not expected to give up or give in to the others; rather, consensus is usually achieved through lengthy clarifying discussions that continue until each member comes to believe that the selected course of action is the best possible. Consensus may require that members willingly shift their perspectives.

Accommodation is another kind of decision-making. To decide by accommodation means that a family decision is achieved but some members, or maybe even all, have had to compromise. Accommodation may involve sacrifice. Family members may decide to go along with what other family members prefer rather than risk disunity or because of their inability to handle conflict; members accommodate each other for the sake of being able to achieve a family decision.

De facto decision-making is agreement by lack of dissent rather than through active assent. In some cases, an individual's role in de facto decision-making can be characterized as a shrug of the shoulders. A de facto decision is one in which the members let go rather than disagree or invest energy in some other form of decision-making.

Unilateral decision-making describes a situation in which one member of the family decides for the rest. Consultation with other members may or may not occur. The decision-maker takes on this responsibility alone and is generally accountable only to himself or herself.

Indecision may also characterize decision-making. A family may get bogged down in the details of making decisions or be paralyzed by the expected consequences of its possible actions. In a family characterized by indecisiveness, the need for agreement is left unaddressed. Events unfold but the family does not direct them.

Power Power is the ability to reach an end or produce an outcome, and each member of a functional family has some personal power. To learn about the distribution of power in a family is to gain access to the dynamics of its inner functioning. Power may be associated with a member's potential to generate and control the income of the family; it may also be associated with gender, age, or ownership of possessions. In many contemporary families, even the individual controlling the television channel changer may temporarily be regarded as possessing a special form of power. The identification of power relationships is key to uncovering the structure of the family. It is thus important for the community health nurse to understand the possession and use of power in each family.

Some families have been identified as child-focused; that is, the children possess an unbalanced distribution of power compared to their parents. The children dictate to the parents, and the parents fulfill their demands. In more authoritarian families, the power may reside primarily with one adult member, often the breadwinner.

As two-career families come to predominate, power distribution tends to become more egalitarian. Cultures tend to assign power in varying ways, such as to the family elders or even to deceased members responsible for overseeing the extended family.

Conflict and Stress Conflict is necessary for growth. In families, conflict situations involve "issues of power, use of resources, relationship needs, and differing value systems.... Whatever the cause, the result is usually increased stress until the conflict is resolved" (Mealey, Richardson, & Dimico, 1996, p. 236). Participation in decisions is a healthy way to deal with conflict. Conflict can also promote other open and healthy forms of communication; without conflict in family relationships, there would be no disagreement. Without disagreement, one member might become too submissive, giving in to another, or harbor unshared feelings, hurts, and disappointments. When conflict is ignored, it does not disappear but is tucked away, only to reappear in other forms that can cause dysfunction in the family. Conflict can be characterized on a behavioral scale from benign arguing to quarreling to outright aggression. Resolving conflict within the family requires that each member own his or her piece of the conflict rather than blaming other members. Careful listening and therapeutic communication are key to facilitating discussion (and even nonviolent fighting) over a disagreement, for underneath conflictual issues are feelings that need to be brought forth and addressed. Trust and commitment to the family and its structure are essential if underlying feelings are to be shared. Members also learn negotiation skills when managing conflict, skills that are readily transferred to extrafamilial situations and become life skills to foster each person's ability to participate in decisions that affect them.

The community health nurse can help the family understand that conflict and stress are a normal part of growth. He or she can teach the family about effective communication skills and help the family examine its internal discords. The nurse also helps identify sources of stress within the family and define healthful ways to manage stress, ways that are appropriate and acceptable to the family.

Energy   Family energy can be thought of as the family's collective attitude. Energy is needed to maintain family unity and integrity. In a healthy family, energy flows and is channeled in ways that support the family and its capacity to carry out its functions. When problems or stress arise that drain energy from the family system, the family is able to replenish itself by taking in information or resources that can assist the family or by reorganizing itself to meet the challenges it faces. Depleted energy can be restored if input and output are channeled effectively.

The community health nurse attempts to sense the family energy level when entering a home; the family may appear lifeless and its members unable to express their needs or to consider possible solutions because they lack the energy required to engage in need-identification and problem-solving. If energy is blocked, the nurse may sense an undirected abundance of energy that is not being used productively and might be channeled more effectively. Other families may appear depressed, still others chaotic. Productive use of energy to maintain family unity and integrity is indicative of a functional family.

Illness and other family crises tend to deplete family energy. Members can assist in the refueling process by contributing their positive and constructive attitudes and desires to protecting the strengths of the family. Clearly, if the family expends its available energy without refueling, it can become depleted and depressed, but if there is constant fueling and infusion of energy not used for growth, then the family can suffer overload and frustration. Balanced use and replenishment of energy maintains the family's integrity and empowers the family to respond to its needs and to evolve.

Change   All human systems are in flux; change is inherent to the human condition. The family, too, is in continual flux. Change is thus a continuous process—the tendency of the family to become different.

The community health nurse is sensitized to those gains and losses in the family that characterize its capacity for change. Gains and losses are celebrated and grieved in order to integrate such changes into family life.

The nurse especially appreciates the dynamics of the grieving process as they relate to family change. A wide array of emotions characterize human grief, including shock, disbelief, anger, depression, confusion, and feelings of worthlessness. The family may be grieving losses yet not realize that it is doing so. The community health nurse can translate these expressions of grief into an understandable process that the family undergoes as it deals with change.

Death, illness, moving, members leaving home, the arrival of new members, marital separation, divorce, changes in employment, and changes in financial status are among the wide range of possible changes that occur in family life. Change may be welcomed, unexpected, or resisted, but the family grows and becomes different regardless. The family is never static. The community health nurse may assist the family by legitimizing the inevitability of change and placing it in a developmental context. He or she may also enable the family to view change within the context of the grieving process and help its members understand the holistic nature of grief and the impact it has on each member and on patterns of family functioning. The nurse can also assist the family that is overwhelmed by change and lacking the skills to move forward. Helping the family break down the task at hand into smaller, more manageable tasks enables the family to cope with change.

Environment The community health nurse is always cognizant of the impact of the environment on family health and functioning. A family's environment is the entire context in which it lives: housing, immediate community, and wider community. Environmental factors are critical to the health and safety of family members and of the family as a whole. The community health nurse assesses environmental conditions and the family's use of the environment and its resources.

Household conditions are paramount and provide clues about the family's ability to function. On first inspection, the community health nurse ascertains the level of household hygiene. Household cleanliness reflects the ability of the members to care for the home, that is, to clean it and to maintain the safety of the household by making minor repairs and keeping up the physical structure. The mere number and quality of objects in the home is not important; functionality is the primary concern. For example, a baby can comfortably and safely sleep in a dresser drawer (removed from the dresser) just as well as in a designer crib. The walls may be enhanced in appearance by painting, but if they are clean that is all that really matters.

An environmental assessment and safety check are part of the home assessment. The community health nurse strives to be astute in appraising the household environment, recognizing the importance of reducing safety risks and the importance of a plan for household emergencies. The nurse assesses with the family the conditions of the household, including space for all the members to sleep and have some degree of privacy, cleanliness, proper lighting, adequate ventilation, heat, bathroom and kitchen facilities, availability of hot and cold water, electrical safety, treatment for roaches, mice, rats, and other forms of infestation, awareness of fire hazards, fire safety precautions such as smoke sensors and fire extinguishers, window guards and locks, proper security in the building and at the entrances to the household, the availability of a telephone or plan for emergency calls, and removal of scatter rugs and other obstacles that might cause falls.

The community health nurse is also concerned about conditions in the immediate community insofar as they may enhance or threaten individual and family health. The presence or absence of community resources and the family's pattern of using such resources are important to the assessment of the immediate environment. The question of whether the immediate community can provide the family with the resources it needs to function on a day-to-day basis must be answered. The community health nurse, therefore, scans the immediate community to determine the availability of food, stores, pharmacies and equipment vendors, clothing shops, police and fire departments, parks and recreational facilities, schools and day care centers, health resources, and religious and cultural resources for spiritual support. The nurse employs the knowledge derived from a thorough community assessment to connect the family to community resources and to assist in the utilization of resources, drawing ever widening circles around the family to ascertain available resources. Some resources will be local while access to others will require travel. The home and community environments are both important to family functioning.

Self-Care The goal of family-based health care is that each family should care for itself as much as possible. Community health nursing care is directed toward identifying and supporting family strengths and capabilities so that the family can care for itself. Therefore, the community health nurse assesses the family's ability to maintain autonomy by meeting its own needs. The nurse wishes to transfer to the family knowledge and skills that empower it to care for itself, to utilize its inner strengths and resources, and to access community resources as needed. To this end, the community health nurse views the family from the perspective of its strengths. All families have strengths, even troubled, depleted families.

The best way for the community health nurse to recognize the actual and potential strengths of a family is to identify the strengths of each family member; of the relationships among family members (i.e., among dyads and triads, as well as the family as a whole); of the household environment; and of the surrounding community and the family's connections to it. If a family member is currently unemployed, the nurse assesses the individual's employment pattern; it may be learned, for example, that this member has held a responsible job for the past 25 years but was recently laid off. Such an individual is clearly a viable breadwinner, and the community health nurse may assist this person in taking an inventory of her or his employable characteristics and becoming motivated to re-tool for another form of employment, while also helping the family to obtain temporary entitlements during this rough financial period. The nurse trusts that the family and its members will be able to care for themselves by negotiating for needed assistance during such periods.

Dysfunctional Patterns of Family Dynamics

The family is an *emotional system* (Bowen, 1978; Heiney, 1993). The emotional relationships in a healthy family facilitate growth and personal development of the members, and such a family adjusts to change by exhibiting flexibility. In families exhibiting dysfunctional patterns, difficulties with conflict management and problem-solving loom repeatedly.

Conflict and stress are inevitably part of family life. However, when a family cannot cope with stressful changes, then anxiety and conflict increase, and the family may not be able to fulfill its functions and develop defenses. All families possess defenses to protect the integrity of the family system. In functional families, a defense is used sporadically and then let-go as the family relies on its ability to problem-solve and as situations change. However, when families are unable to cope with their challenges and their defenses become chronic patterns, then these may become dysfunctional patterns. The family may thus come to rely on dysfunctional patterns that inhibit its growth and development. Some of these dysfunctional patterns will be introduced below. Therapeutic work with families whose patterns are dysfunctional is the domain of the advanced practice nurse; however, an introductory knowledge of dysfunctional family patterns aids the community health nurse in making referrals to the advanced practice nurse or other therapist. The community health nurse needs a thorough understanding of the patterns of family wellness and must establish, through assessment, if the family's defenses are episodic or if they have become long-standing patterns of dysfunction. When the community health nurse understands the functional patterns of family life then he or she will be able to assist the family in finding healthier ways of coping. Movement from dysfunctional patterns to functional patterns is possible.

Tight Family Boundaries Tight family boundaries are those that prevent outsiders from seeing what is inside the family. Tightening boundaries is a way of keeping insiders (i.e., family members) inside and preventing outsiders from entering. Tight boundaries are thus used as a wall of defense. However, when boundaries are pulled in they constrict input and output. Eventually, a system with excessively tight boundaries suffers from lack of exchange with its environment and moves toward disorder and collapse. The family needs energy exchange to live and grow; tight boundaries, over time, prevent this free exchange.

Loose Family Boundaries Boundaries that are excessively loose signify a loss of integrity of the family system. Loose boundaries mean that the family suffers from dispersion and members are emotionally cut off from each other; the family is emotionally scattered rather than whole. Loose boundaries may be illustrated by a family in which the adult children only make ritualized and infrequent visits, there being no strong emotional bonds to hold them together. Loose boundaries can also be illustrated through emotional distancing.

Dysfunctional Patterns of Family Dynamics

Tight family boundaries
Loose family boundaries
Defensive alliances
Scapegoating
Family healer
Withdrawal of affect
Temporary riddance
Negative compromise
Double bind
Pseudomutuality
Silence
Mystification
Violence

In some situations, the family may suffer from system overload as it indiscriminately admits others to assist with its problems. The family may have a community health nurse, a social worker, a welfare worker, an ambulatory care physician, and clergy all involved with family problems, yet without productive use of these resources. Duplication of services, lack of communication among the helpers, and confusion may result because the family has turned over the control of its problems to anyone and everyone that enters the family system. Such a family lacks the capability to screen offers of assistance selectively. Instead, input flows across a loosely connected boundary.

Defensive Alliances Defensive alliances come in a variety of forms but in all cases, members of the family join to form one or more subgroups that undermine the sense of the family unity.

One form of defensive alliance is the *split*. A split is simply a division in the family. For example, a split occurs when a mother and son do not communicate with each other. Other members of the family may also become divided, with some allied to the son and some to the mother.

A *coalition* is another kind of defensive alliance. A coalition occurs when several members team up against one. If three daughters and a mother in a traditional nuclear family team up against the father, the females in the family formed a coalition against the father. In this situation, the underlying pathology may have resulted from disharmony in the mother-father relationship in response to which the mother forms an alliance with her daughters to alienate the father further. In essence, the daughters are manipulated by the mother, who is creating distance between the daughters and their father to strengthen her position against her spouse.

Triangulation is another form of defensive alliance (see Fig. 12-5) (Bowen, 1978; Fogarty, 1975, 1976). Triangulation can become a rigid pattern of emotional interaction among family members, formed in response to stress, in which two people are emotionally very close and a third member is emotionally very distant. When two family members are engaged in an unstable dyadic relationship they may bring in a third to stabilize their relationship. The unstable dyad may use the third member or object to relate *through*, since the dyad's members are unable or unwilling to relate satisfactorily to each other. Such triangulation may occur due to the active efforts of one or both dyad members to involve a third member or by the third member being caught up in the anxiety of the unstable dyad and pulled into its emotional process as a stabilizer. The community health nurse must not be pulled in or choose sides in a dyadic conflict, thereby becoming the third point of a triangle. Unfortunately for all involved, triangulation can cause a closed subsystem within the family. Its dysfunctional or undesirable aspect is that it prevents the emotional process of the dyad from being worked through.

Key to all of these dysfunctional defensive alliances—the split, the coalition, and triangulation—is the dyad, the basic unit of the family. Each dyad is an important relationship and must assume the responsibility of working on its own problems. The community health nurse can best contend with defensive alliances by not supporting them and by encouraging dyads to work on their own relationship problems. A dyad may or may not work on its issues, but the community health nurse should fulfill his or her responsibility by not participating in the conflict and by not supporting the continuation of defensive alliances.

Scapegoating To scapegoat is to deposit or project all responsibility for a problem on one person. A family member may be scapegoated as a way of dealing with a family problem; that is, the other members of the family project responsibility on that member so that they do not have to tolerate the discomfort of being accountable for their behavior in a family problem. For example, children may get anger directed at them by their parents who have not worked through their angry feelings toward each other.

Usually a member is scapegoated as an expression of the family's own confusion, anger, or sense of insecurity. If all members assume responsibility for their own roles, it is not necessary to scapegoat.

Family Healer Like the scapegoat, only voluntarily (although not usually consciously), the family healer is an assigned role. In this case, the family deposits responsibility for its problems with a member who assumes the role of caretaker. In relying on just one of its members to deal with its problems, the family abdicates its shared responsibility for problem-solving and limits its capacity to come up with creative possibilities that may benefit the family and encourage its growth.

As the family healer is relied upon to solve each problem, the other members becomes less involved in and capable of problem-solving and more dependent on the healer. Meanwhile, the family healer may be exhausted by the scope and number of family problems that must be reconciled.

It is not unusual to find that nurses and other members of the helping professions were family healers in their families of origin; thus, professional caregiving may have its roots in family role assignment. It may be an automatic response to assume a professional role grounded in one's own family casting. If this is the case, the helping professional may exceed the boundaries of needed intervention and render the client family dependent on the caregiver. However, the community health nurse should seek to balance the family's needs with strategies that foster the family's ability to care for itself rather than rendering the family dependent on others.

Withdrawal of Affect Emotionality, or affect, is necessary in families. When affect is removed from the family, the community health nurse is challenged to assist the family to relocate its ability to respond appropriately to its joys, losses, and other experiences.

There are several varieties of withdrawal of affect. *Puppetry* is signaled by joylessness. Family members go through the motions of their experiences but do so without expression, robotically. *Passivity* is manifested by the exhibition of little or no response to experiences. Remaining calm is an effort to keep emotions under control and to appear as though the situation does not warrant worry or concern. *Denial* is a declaration that the family does not experience problems—"not our family." Each of these family defenses is a means of withdrawing affect and dealing with emotionally laden experiences by removing their emotionality. In families defended by such means, emotion is not authentic or appropriate.

Temporary Riddance Temporary riddance is the pattern of impulsively removing a problem or problematic family member. The front door to the home of a family that practices temporary riddance may be imagined as a revolving door. When a problem occurs, the family sends it through this door, out of the family system; yet it has a tendency to come right back in. The problem is removed, but the relief is temporary; the family is not effectively solving anything.

However, asking a member of the family to leave may be necessary to preserve the integrity of the family. In a functional family dealing with intractable problems, an eventual decision to bar a member may be life-saving. Consider the family that has been robbed and manipulated by a member with a serious drug addiction. Years of efforts to support and save this member have been unsuccessful. The rest of the family comes to believe, after faithful effort, that this member must no longer continue to be destructive to the family and so this member is told to leave the family and to return when the drug addiction is treated successfully. In this case, removal of a member is a particular episode rather than a pattern of temporary riddance.

Negative Compromise Negative compromise is a distortion of power in the family. As one member asserts himself or herself, another renounces, or gives up, his or her rights to the other. This results in one member gaining power while the other loses it. This subjugation to another is often a frightening and enraging experience for the person who is rendered powerless. Powerlessness depletes the member's sense of personal integrity and can result in depression, anomie, repressed hostility, and other emotional harm. Each person needs power to feel that they can affect the course of their own life and to exert an influence on the family's functioning.

Double Bind The double bind involves conflict in the delivery of a message within the family. The overt content of the message is accompanied by a conflicting, nonverbal message; the verbal component of communication conflicts with the nonverbal component. This conflicted communication leaves the recipient confused and unable to decipher the intended message, making responsiveness impossible since the message in not clear. The receiver of a double-bind message experiences confusion, anxiety, and mistrust, producing the feelings conjured by a no-win situation.

Pseudomutuality Pseudomutuality is false togetherness. In practicing pseudomutuality, family members fuse together based on false assumptions that all members apparently agree to support. Members bind with each other at the expense of differentiation. Families take refuge in pseudomutuality when members dread conflict within the family and seek to avoid it by establishing a facade of harmony (Simon, 1985). The modus operandi of a pseudomutual family is to view differences as a threat; each member maintains relatedness regardless of the cost to personal identity.

The community health nurse reflects on the significance of the developmental process, recognizing that human growth moves from dependence to independence and to interdependence. In the pseudomutual family, excessive mutual dependence is maintained, and differentiation is viewed as a threat.

Silence Silence can limit effective communication. Silence creates a block in communication when used as a family defense. Silence may signify that there are topics that cannot be discussed or history that has not been revealed. Silence is, of course, itself a way of communicating, since it is impossible not to communicate (Watzlawick, 1978). The placement of silence during an interchange may be especially revealing. The silence of one member may enable another to gather thoughts and explore feelings. However, when silence is used defensively, it shuts out the other, creating a blockade in the communication pattern. Silence shuts the door to an area that family members will not allow to be explored. Silence can leave some members feeling alienated and cut off, since communication is the lifeblood of a family.

Mystification Talking a lot without illuminating the issue at hand is a way of mystifying, of detouring members around issues of significance. Questions may be articulated, but the answers are never fully or clearly expressed. Answers are derailed as a flutter of communication, often contradictory or unrelated, consumes space and time. Functional communication, in contrast, is purposeful, allowing give and take. Mystification creates confusion, defending information that will not be revealed because it is being kept from the family. Maintaining confusion meets some family need not being met and meets the family's need to not clarify issues.

Violence Violence, whether threatened or actual, is intolerable yet commonplace. Family violence is usually preceded by a family history of violence; violence is probably learned and transmitted from generation to generation. Violence can be physical, emotional, mental, or sexual. However, families can break away from violence. It is important to report violence.

Violence is often, paradoxically, self-protective in motivation. The underlying emotions are often deeply hidden but often may include a deep sense of powerlessness or impotence, feelings that are relieved by power gained through the subjugation of another.

Summary

Each family is both a human system and a significant unit of care for the community health nurse. Keys to family care are recognition of the family's strengths and capabilities; understanding its problems and concerns and its ability to mobilize its strengths to deal with its problems; and appreciation of its unique relationship to the community of which it is a subsystem. The family must also be considered from the perspectives of its individual members, who are subsystems of the family system.

The community health nurse engages in family health assessment and determines the functional patterns of the family to ascertain its capacity for self-care and for utilization of the community and its resources, which can assist it in dealing with its challenges.

Functional family patterns indicate the presence of particular family strengths. Defensive dysfunctional patterns develop in families subjected to undue stress or unable to contend with the change and conflicts inherent in family life.

The community health nurse is a provider of family-based care, and cares for individuals within the context of their family and of their surrounding community. She or he also cares for the family as a whole; the family is the client. Appreciation of the interrelatedness of family members to each other and to the family as a unit, and of the family to the larger community, is essential. The community health nurse develops knowledge and skills in family dynamics to implement a family-based plan of care.

KEY WORDS

Dyad	Environment
Patterns of daily living	Self-care
Genogram	Dysfunction
Boundaries	Split, coalition, triangulation
Differentiation	Scapegoating
Roles	Family healer
Norms	Withdrawal of affect
Values	Temporary riddance
Decision-making	Negative compromise
Power	Double bind
Conflict	Pseudomutuality
Stress	Silence
Energy	Mystification
Change	Violence

QUESTIONS

Directions: Choose the one *best* response to each of the following questions.

1. Which of the following family constellations can be illustrated in a genogram?

    A. Blended family
    B. Same-sex couple
    C. Single-parent family
    D. All of the above

2. Functional families have which of the following characteristics?

    A. They operate without conflicts and disharmony.
    B. They define behavioral limits and adhere to them.
    C. They suppress disagreements to maintain harmony in the family.
    D. They focus on one member at a time.

3. The family is an important client system in the care of communities. Which of the following statements provides the rationale for the family as a client of community health nurses?

   A. Health can be conceptualized along a continuum.
   B. Health is the absence of disease and infirmity.
   C. Health means adaptation and effective coping.
   D. Health of families determines the health of communities.

4. When one enters a home in the role of community health nurse and refuses a cup of tea offered in a family that feels one should serve and share refreshments, you may be violating an important family

   A. boundary.
   B. norm.
   C. role.
   D. theme.

5. The M. family considers their 7-year-old daughter difficult to manage. When they socialize they say to a friend, "Oh, we would love to go out to dinner with you, but we can't because our daughter throws a temper tantrum if we leave her." They are practicing what family defense?

   A. Scapegoating
   B. Double bind
   C. Puppetry
   D. Mystification

6. According to family systems theory, a family with a son who is severely handicapped would be functioning as an open system if the parents

   A. refuse to acknowledge that anything is wrong with the child.
   B. protect this child from negative contacts with neighborhood children.
   C. seek help to gain a better understanding of their child's needs.
   D. focus much of their time and attention on meeting their son's needs.

ANSWERS

1. *The answer is D.* All family constellations can be diagramed in a genogram.

2. *The answer is B.* Functional families define limits (boundaries) that provide system integrity.

3. *The answer is D.* Community health nurses can improve the health of the community by improving the health of families in the community.

4. *The answer is B.* Norms are rules that guide family interactions.

5. *The answer is A.* Scapegoating is depositing responsibility for a family problem on one member.

6. *The answer is C.* Allowing interchange across the boundaries is signified by reaching outside of the family system for help in understanding the child's needs.

ANNOTATED REFERENCES

Bomar, P. J. (Ed.). (1996). *Nurses and family health promotion: Concepts, assessment, and interventions* (2nd ed.). Philadelphia: W. B. Saunders.

An outstanding text on family health nursing, this collection includes units on family health nursing and family health promotion; concepts and frameworks for family health nursing practice; and family health nursing process.

Bowen, M. (1978). *Family therapy in clinical practice.* New York: Jason Aronson.

This classic introduction to Bowen's family theory is based on his earlier works dealing with families affected with schizophrenia and their treatment. It is a collection of papers from 1957–1977, which develop his concepts of triangulation, intergenerational conflict, societal regression, and differentiation of self in one's family of origin.

Clark, C. C. (1994). *The nurse as group leader* (3rd ed.). New York: Springer Publishing.

This text serves as a valuable guide to group work, including basic group concepts and process. It includes groupwork with the elderly and with focal groups for a variety of aggregates, including people with eating disorders, depression, and co-dependency; rape survivors; domestic violence offenders; and parents.

Fogarty, T. F. (1985). On stress. *The Family,* 12 (2), 15–19.

This article describes stress as a significant force (or group of forces) imposing strain on an individual, affecting personal life as well as interactions within the family and group.

Fogarty, T. F. (1976). System concepts and the dimensions of self. In P. J. Guerin (Ed.), *Family therapy: Theory and practice.* New York: Gardner Press, pp. 144–153.

This chapter explores systems theory as it relates to the family as a unit and the individual person as a member of the family. Closeness, fusion, and triangulation are discussed as well as the forces of togetherness and individuality. Systems theory provides the model for understanding family functioning, what it is to have a functional family, and what it is to be a functional person in such a family.

Fogarty, T. F. (1975). The family emotional self system. *Family Therapy,* 2 (1), 79–97.

This articles clarifies the meaning, definition, and practical implications of 'systems' related to understanding emotional problems within the family. Three types of systems are defined within the family; thinking system; feeling or emotional system; and operating system. The concepts of fusion and triangulation are discussed, including their emotional consequences.

Fogarty, T. F. (1973–1978). Emotional climate in the family and therapy. *The Family. Compendium I: The Best of the Family 1973–1978.* Washington, DC: Georgetown University Family Center, pp. 60–69.

This article describes the emotional systems in the family. Elements in a functional emotional climate, including space; optimism; positive and negative feedback; respect for the "I" position; correcting emotional overloads; expectations and roles; the creation of bridges to maintain connectedness; continual identification, differentiation, and connectedness; real versus verbal positions; humor; and others.

Friedman, M. M. (1992). *Family nursing: Theory and practice* (3rd ed.). Norwalk, CT: Appleton & Lange.

This well-respected family text covers introductory family concepts and processes; theoretical foundations; family nursing practice (theory, assessment, diagnosis, and intervention); general family nursing interventions; and cultural differences among families.

Heiney, S. P. (1993). Assessing and intervening with dysfunctional families. In G. D. Wegner & R. J. Alexander (Eds.), *Readings in family nursing.* Philadelphia: J. B. Lippincott, pp. 357–367.

Heiney uses Bowen's theory of family functioning to assist the pediatric oncology nurse in differentiating families with significant psychopathology from families experiencing situational stress related to the impact of illness. This chapter provides a helpful review of Bowen's framework, including the family as an emotional system, differentiation, and triangulation. Tables differentiating functional from dysfunctional family characteristics are particularly helpful.

Kirschling, J. M., Gilliss, C. L., Krentz, L., Camburn, C. D., Clough, R. S., Duncan, M. T., Hendricks, J., Howard, J. K. H., Roberts, C., Smith-Young, J., Tice, K. S., & Young, T. (1994). "Success" in family nursing: Experts describe phenomena. *Nursing & Health Care, 15* (4), 186–189.

Funded by a U. S. Public Health Service, Department of Health and Human Services, Division of Nursing grant, this group studied the views of family nurses about their practices. The intent was to categorize successful outcomes of nursing interventions to serve as the basis for developing a typology of family nursing care.

Mealey, A. R., Richardson, H., & Dimico, G. (1996) Family stress management. In P. J. Bomar (Ed.), *Nurses and family health promotion: Concepts, assessment, and interventions* (2nd ed.). Philadelphia: W. B. Saunders, pp. 227–244.

Mealey et al. recognize stress as inevitable but surmountable. They define family stress, adaptation, and coping; discuss the role of the nurse in family coping, how the family copes with stress, and use of the nursing process in developing nursing diagnoses related to family stress and coping; and conclude with strategies for adaptation and coping with family stress.

Minuchin, S. (1974). *Families and family therapy.* Cambridge, MA: Harvard University Press.

This classic text on family therapy combines vivid clinical examples, specific details of technique, and sage perspectives on both effectively functioning families and those seeking therapy.

Pendagast, E. G., & Sherman, C. O. (1973–1978). A guide to the geno-gram. *The Family. Compendium I: The Best of the Family 1973–1978*. Washington, DC: Georgetown University Family Center, pp. 101–112.

This article offers a complete guide to the development of the genogram. The genogram is a structural framework that enables one to diagram in concrete and easily understood terms general and complex information about a family.

Simon, F. B., Stierlin, H., & Wynne, L. C. (1985). *The language of family therapy: A systematic vocabulary and sourcebook*. New York: Family Process Press.

This is a handbook of family psychotherapy language and terminology, translated from German.

Watzlawick, P. (1978). *The language of change: Elements of therapeutic communication*. New York: Basic Books.

This path-breaking book by a world authority on human communication and communication therapy helps therapists to grasp the essence of the special language of the unconscious and to use it for the benefit of patients.

Wegner, G. D., & Alexander, R. J. (Eds.). (1993). *Readings in family nursing*. Philadelphia: J. B. Lippincott.

This family text extensively covers family health nursing theory development, family health nursing research, family health nursing clinical practice, and family health nursing education.

⌘

NURSING INTERVENTIONS AND CLIENT OUTCOMES IN A TECHNOLOGICAL AGE

Nurses provide care to people in the community in a variety of ways; nursing care can be given to individuals as well as constellations of people in families and groups. Care provided to individuals, groups, and families in the community is provided by many different nurses, including community health nurses, home care nurses, and school nurses. Some nurses have general responsibilities while others are more specialized. The title "community health nurse" applies to the nurse educated to provide the most comprehensive services to the community.

Community health nurses complete the nursing process when they provide care to individuals, families, and groups as well as to the community as a whole. High-technology home care nurses and school nurses have more limited responsibilities; they each care for a specific subset of the population. Home care nurses focus on acute care needs in the home whereas school nurses focus on the needs of groups of schoolchildren. Home care and school nurses are expected to work with the community health nurse in order to meet the needs of their clients; the community health nurse is the generalist practitioner, concerned for the entire community.

This chapter examines examples of nursing care given to families and groups and the identification of effective care outcomes. Nursing interventions are defined as being high- or low-technology in character and may be provided by nurses in different roles. Care of the community as a whole is discussed in Chaps. 7 to 10.

High-technology care involves the use of complex equipment like intravenous infusion pumps and transcutaneous electronic nerve stimulation (TENS) for pain control. High-technology nursing care is often associated with invasive techniques like intravenous administration of chemotherapy, antibiotics, or total parenteral nutrition (TPN). High-technology care is

Low-Technology Care. Low-technology care is the essence of nursing because of the physical and emotional bond that it establishes between the client and the nurse.

criticized by some because the technology may require more attention and seem more important than the client.

In contrast, **low-technology care** is administered by the nurse without special equipment. Some examples of low-technology care include visual assessment of skin color, verbal instructions to change the dose of a medication, and meditating or sitting quietly with a client who is in spiritual distress. Low-technology care also includes manual tasks like dressing changes, colostomy care, and Foley catheter insertion. Health promotion activities, the cornerstone of public health, are low-technology interventions as well.

The intensity level of a technology (high or low) is not synonymous with the skill level of an intervention. Some low-technology interventions, such as therapeutic communication, require great skill. Many aspects of physical care, although simple in nature, require skill to implement correctly. For example, a bed bath given at a particular time may comfort the client but at another time have little therapeutic value. Fulfilling the various roles and responsibilities of the nurse will most likely require skill in both low- and high-technology interventions.

Nurses must often decide which level of care is most appropriate to the needs of the client. Working closely with the interdisciplinary team assures that changes in the plan of care, as directed by the client's physician, reflect the expertise of the entire team. Continuous reassessment gives the nurse and other team members confidence that their interventions are appropriate.

High- and low-technology care may be viewed as having equal but different importance. Clients' needs are the guideposts that should direct the type of care that the nurse provides. For example, with the diagnosis of advanced cancer, some clients choose surgery while others refuse treatment and select hospice services. The needs and wishes of the client should be respected when planning and providing care.

CARE PROVIDED TO INDIVIDUALS

Today, clients may work, play, and convalesce at home with continuous oxygen therapy, intravenous infusions, mechanical respirators, and dialyzers as part of their lives. Nurses monitor complex medication regimens, administer insulin, and change dressings, all while teaching, nurturing, and comforting people in the community. Table 13-1 provides examples that clarify the distinction between high- and low-technology care.

In Table 13-1, high- and low-technology interventions are categorized as preventive, curative, or restorative. This classification is intended to distinguish the various levels of care that nurses may provide in the community. Nurses may provide more than one level of care at a time. While teaching the essentials of a low-fat diet (preventive care), for example, the nurse may also demonstrate postmastectomy range-of-motion exercises (restorative care).

High- and low-technology nursing interventions are often provided together. Nurses can monitor response to pain medication administered by

◙

TABLE 13-1

CATEGORIES OF HIGH- AND LOW-TECHNOLOGY CARE

Categories	High-Technology Care	Low-Technology Care
Preventive	Interactive computer-assisted teaching	Reviewing instructions verbally
Curative	Chemotherapy via intravenous access device	Massage to decrease pain
Restorative	Mechanical nerve stimulation to increase range of motion	Counseling to resolve grief from loss

infusion pump (high-technology care) while comforting the person with a massage and soothing conversation (low-technology care). Nurses are expected to obtain vital signs and perform a neurological assessment (low-technology care) while adjusting oxygen flow on a respirator in the home (high-technology care). Below, high-technology and low-technology interventions are discussed in more detail.

High-Technology Nursing Care

The volume of high-technology cases referred for home care is increasing as the home becomes the preferred site for care in many situations. Many providers believe that if it is possible to provide care in the home, it should be provided there. Home care is considered attractive, in part, because it is sometimes less expensive than institutionalized care. The hospital is coming to be a care delivery site for only the most critically ill people or for those without a suitable home in which to provide care.

More and more complex care can be provided in the home as long as skilled supportive services are available. However, one problem with high-technology home care is the stress that it imposes on caregivers such as family and friends (Ruppert, 1996). Concern about the emotional and economic toll that caregiving has on family and friends is increasing. Many of the technical aspects of home care are easy to cost out because they are related to discrete tasks or interventions, but the costs to family and friends of caring for a loved one with inadequate or no support cannot be quantified. Such costs include loss of work, decreased productivity, and emotional exhaustion.

There are other barriers to home care. Some family members and friends do not want or are not able to provide safe care. Some lay caregivers are not comfortable with the increased responsibilities professionals encourage them to assume. Occasionally, homes are not physically adequate for client care due to lack of electricity, heat, or water. Some spaces are not large enough to permit placement and movement of equipment.

The lack of respite services also makes assuming responsibility for care difficult. Some family members and friends fear that once they assume care for their loved one, they will not be able to give back responsibility to professional caregivers. Even as cost containment becomes a critical issue, family members and friends are re-evaluating their willingness to provide primary care.

Low-Technology Nursing Care

Low-technology care like teaching and counseling is continuously given by community health and home care nurses, although it is rarely reimbursable as an isolated service unless it is specifically related to a medical diagnosis. Although some level of low-technology care is always necessary, government and third-party reimbursement systems seem uninterested in paying for it. The United States' health care system prefers to fund discrete high- or low-technology medical procedures or tasks like wound care or administration of intravenous antibiotics over health promotion and illness prevention activities.

Low-technology care related to emotional support or teaching and counseling is thought by many people to be a nonessential add-on service. Families expect to receive drug interaction teaching from the nurse but do not expect to pay for it separately. In meeting the nursing needs of the client within the constraints of reimbursement, creativity on the part of the community health nurse is, therefore, essential in contemporary practice. Community health nurses might participate in town meetings or group discussions to help people who may need services in the future (e.g., the frail elderly) and to learn about the limits of the reimbursement system. Community health nurses could be instrumental in organizing groups to explore changes in reimbursement and schedules for payment for services.

Measuring Outcomes of Care Interventions

Community health nurses have the responsibility to identify the expected outcomes of care in cooperation with their clients to meet their comprehensive needs. An expected outcome is the yardstick by which to measure progress in healing. In the following client situations, health-related needs are reviewed, and important observable outcomes are identified. Outcomes that are met suggest that the care provided is appropriate for the client. Outcomes must be reevaluated on an ongoing basis as clients may experience neurological changes, lose dexterity, and experience changes in support networks and in their own self-care ability.

Mastery in planning for expected outcomes allows the nurse to note unexpected changes in the care situation that may or may not be benign. Outcomes change as the client regains health or develops additional problems.

CASE STUDY: OUTCOME: PREVENTION OF INFECTION

Melissa Bran is an 8-year-old, long-term client of home care. She had a tracheostomy placed at 7 months of age due to bilateral vocal cord paralysis. Melissa has been cared for at home with 24-h nursing care provided by a home care agency. Melissa's family, including two older siblings, is involved with her tracheostomy care. It has been noted on several occasions that one of the older siblings uses poor technique while suctioning Melissa's tracheostomy.

The community health nurse working with Melissa's family decides to review tracheostomy care and suctioning with the entire family. In this case, one person needing re-evaluation of technique provides the nurse with an opportunity to re-evaluate this skill with all the caregivers. The goal is to improve the family's skill level, using aseptic technique to prevent infection. The critical *outcome* for Melissa is to *remain infection free*.

To achieve this outcome, the nurse and family agree to participate in a teaching project that requires: (1) handwashing before and after suctioning; (2) keeping the suction catheter in its sterile sheath until just before suctioning; (3) brief, intermittent suctioning with adjuvant oxygen therapy; and (4) reminding other family members of proper technique when violations in asepsis occur.

The nurse and family are working together to keep Melissa healthy. This is the focus of all nursing interventions. As Melissa progresses, other activities may be added to the plan to maintain the outcome of avoiding infection. Some interventions may well be removed from the plan of care over time as they cease to be necessary.

CASE STUDY: OUTCOMES: PREVENTING SKIN BREAKDOWN AND CONTRACTURES OF THE EXTREMITIES

Kim Zen is a 9-year-old, long-term, ventilator-dependent home care client. She was diagnosed with early-onset Parkinson's disease at age 4. Due to the nature of this rare pediatric illness, she has become immobile and wheelchair-dependent. Positioning, skin care, and passive range-of-motion exercises are imperative to prevent severe contractures and skin breakdown.

The home care nurse should be instrumental in achieving the desired outcomes of *preventing skin breakdown* and *preventing contractures of the extremities* for this client. The community health nurse reviews proper positioning and exercise with the home health aides and family members who participate in Kim's care.

Required components of a plan to realize the outcomes of care include, in this situation: (1) changing position every few hours;

(2) observing the bony prominences where breakdown is likely to occur; (3) lubricating and moisturizing skin areas twice daily; (4) daily bathing; and (5) receiving passive range-of-motion exercises of both arms and legs three times a day to minimize or avoid contractures.

It is important to remember that such nursing interventions vary from client to client. Some clients need bathing every other day. Some clients need to have their skin areas inspected and massaged more frequently, or less. The key to successful interventions is individuation of the plan of care. The commonalities of care include the universal need to inspect, clean, massage, and exercise to prevent skin breakdown and contractures. As mentioned before, desired outcomes change to reflect expected client behaviors that are matched to appropriate levels of human development and functional ability.

CASE STUDY: OUTCOME: TOLERATION OF HOME CHEMOTHERAPY WITH MINIMAL SIDE EFFECTS

Nicholas Corte is a 12-year-old who has been diagnosed with acute lymphocytic leukemia (ALL). After an induction (i.e., first) phase of chemotherapy in the hospital, the client was discharged to home. Nicholas and his family live in a rural town 75 miles away from the nearest medical center, making daily hospital visits for chemotherapy inconvenient and difficult.

Home care was planned for Nicholas to provide home chemotherapy while encouraging adjustment to his chronic illness. Nicholas has a double lumen Broviac catheter to facilitate chemotherapy administration.

As part of Nicholas's treatment protocol, he will receive an infusion of cyclophosphamide (Cytoxan) with adjuvant antiemetic administration. The global outcome is to *tolerate chemotherapy with minimal side effects*.

Nursing interventions employed to meet the outcome in this example include: (1) an antiemetic and hydration therapy 1 to 2 h before chemotherapy; (2) maintaining a normal urine output and a low urine specific gravity; (3) tolerating a Cytoxan intravenous drip over a 2-h period; (4) remaining free from nausea and emesis; (5) remaining negative for blood in the urine; and (6) remaining infection-free at the Broviac catheter insertion site.

Nicholas (and his family) will also have outcomes that relate to *coping with cancer*. Nicholas will have needs related to safety and security as well as the need to regain physiological integrity. The community health nurse reviews growth and development concerns with individuals and families and groups as appropriate. Outcomes should be set to reflect expected behaviors for the client.

In this situation, the nurse might expect "coping with cancer" to translate to verbalization of fears about treatments or side effects. Clients entering adolescence have concerns about the influence of peer groups and opportunities to date. Nicholas will identify other outcomes with the community health nurse as he learns how to cope with the experiences of sickness, his fears about death, and his hope to live as long as possible.

CASE STUDY: OUTCOME: NO ACCIDENTS IN THE HOME

Albert Nicoelli, 55 years old, is recovering from a cerebral vascular accident at home. He is experiencing some right-sided hemiparesis and a problem with speaking clearly. His previous health history includes treatment for depression and suicidal ideation with medication and group therapy.

Assessment by the community health nurse identifies the outcome of *no accidents in the home.*

In this situation, the nurse wants Mr. Nicoelli to be able to: (1) personally dial 911 to activate the emergency medical team; (2) open medication bottles and medicate himself correctly; (3) ambulate safely in his residence with a walker or cane; and (4) communicate changes in his mood and negative feelings about himself.

The community health nurse periodically reviews the plan for personal safety in the home because this need is always present in clients like Mr. Nicoelli. Other outcomes would include behaviors related to activities of daily living (ADLs) and communication because they are expected areas of concern following a cerebral vascular accident.

*C*ARE PROVIDED TO FAMILIES AND GROUPS

Care provided to families and groups can also be characterized as being of a high- or low-technology type. Nursing interventions are administered to the family or group as a whole or provided to an individual member to keep the family or group functioning properly. For example, teaching a class on nutrition to expectant parents is an intervention given to the group as a whole, although each individual will experience the class in a unique way.

An individual intervention (i.e., relaxation techniques) may be given to one parent in the group who is experiencing anxiety during the group meetings. The intervention decreases anxiety, enabling the parent to return to the group on a weekly basis. In this situation, the individual intervention also benefits the parenting group as a whole by keeping it intact and by enabling the anxious parent to participate in the functioning of the group.

High-Technology Nursing Care

Families may encounter high technology in care given to family members. For example, blood screening for genetic disorders is performed on individuals but can also be viewed as a family intervention because the results affect the ongoing functioning of the total family.

Immune globulin administration to contacts of an individual resident after the diagnosis of hepatitis in a dormitory can be viewed as a group intervention. This is because efforts are made to prevent or decrease the severity of illness among the students living in the dormitory, which is a social collective.

Low-Technology Nursing Care

Crisis intervention activities applied to dysfunctional families and groups are common low-technology interventions. Such interventions may be used with a family with a history of mental illness or with a group of child abuse survivors. Another example is the setting of limits in a group discussion where anger and frustration are increasing. This intervention has the purpose of keeping the group or family operating in a healthy way. Low-technology interventions like those identified above require great skill. Crisis intervention is one such highly skilled, low-technology intervention.

Family counseling related to birth control or genetic illnesses is provided to support family decision-making related to birth control, which helps the family to function as a unit. Counseling and teaching are performed with families and groups so individuals see themselves as a part of a larger constellation. Proper teaching and counseling, providing useful and accurate information, can be handed down from generation to generation.

Measuring Outcomes of Care Interventions

Families and groups are the recipients of nursing care when the community health nurse intervenes with more than one person at a time. The outcome would be an improvement in group functioning.

CASE STUDY:
OUTCOME: DECREASE DEPRESSION AMONG A GROUP OF FRIENDS

Ed Smith and three of his friends are being considered for admission to the Ambulatory Care Mental Health Clinic for group therapy. The counselor thinks this may help decrease the long-term depression of this group related to the death of their college roommate.

Ed blames himself for the death of his friend because a group of his classmates left his house "a little drunk." Ed says that if he had asked his friends not to drive, "his roommate would be alive and the other friends not hurt." Ed and his friends have been showing signs of more severe depression as the 1-year anniversary of the classmate's death approaches.

Nursing intervention for Ed and his friends will include support for the members as they enter group and individual counseling. The outcome for this group is *a decrease in depression.*

Progress in the health of this group of friends can be evidenced by: (1) expression of fewer episodes of sadness and crying; (2) increased participation in extracurricular activities; (3) participation in an anti–drunk-driving program; and (4) ability to think about the dead roommate without untoward feelings of sadness or depression.

Outcomes for groups are not always as specific as outcomes for individuals, but the nurse and group can identify those behaviors that will signify a movement toward health. In the above-mentioned situation, the nurse, Ed, and his friends together identify the desired outcomes that reflect a movement toward health.

In the following situation, an entire family is the client; each member is trying to adjust to one member's diagnosis of diabetes.

CASE STUDY: OUTCOME: REALISTIC RESPONSE TO DISEASE

Tony Samone is an 18-year-old client being followed by the staff in the Diabetic Clinic. He has missed his last four clinic appointments. During the nursing assessment, Tony expresses concern about "body changes that will make me look like a freak." He has not told his girlfriend about his diagnosis and is very concerned that he will not get a football scholarship if he "doesn't hurry up and get over this disease." Tony's mother does not feel comfortable discussing diabetes because she is afraid she may develop it.

The community health nurse decides that a family meeting might help Tony, his girlfriend, and his mother, to focus as a family unit, on the outcome of *viewing the limitations of diabetes more realistically.*

The community health nurse can help the family to understand the disease better and to cope individually and as a family unit. Family behaviors should include: (1) describing the body in a way that reflects a healthy body image; (2) discussing future plans for participating in self-care and disease management; (3) discussing proper wound care and care of the feet; and (4) accurately describing the potential progression of the disease of diabetes. Although individuals would be responsible for the actual behaviors, their proper support and monitoring and the acceptance of collective responsibility to comply with the plan made by the family with the nurse are family outcomes.

Sometimes the community health nurse has an extended time to prevent particular problems or at least explore them more fully. The time before birth is often used to support the family experiencing pregnancy, as long as the referral is made early in pregnancy. The community health nurse in these situations focuses on the outcomes of *family acceptance of the new member* and *adapting to the new demands of a newborn*.

CASE STUDY: OUTCOME: PREPARATION FOR BIRTH

Mary Cathine is pregnant for the first time and is very concerned about how to prepare for the birth of her child. She is 7½ months pregnant and has done very little physical preparation of her studio apartment for the infant's arrival.

Ms. Cathine, a single parent, has not had prenatal care and was referred to the nurse by her employer. During the first appointment with the visiting nurse, Mary faces her television and answers the nurse in few words. She says, "I can't wait till my baby is born. I hope it is not too much trouble. I want to be a good mother!"

The community health nurse can intervene in the family unit being created by assisting Mary to focus on the outcomes of *accepting her pregnancy* and *preparing for the birth*.

For Mary, behaviors suggesting progress with the outcomes include: (1) listing the items she will need to prepare for the birth; (2) talking to a knowledgeable family member or friend about the experience of birth; (3) making weekly prenatal care visits; (4) attending childbirth preparation classes; and (5) discussing the challenges of motherhood in a weekly support group or parenting class.

The nurse negotiates with the client to identify outcomes that are both desirable and feasible. She or he may suggest some outcomes of which the client may not be aware, while the client may explain that some outcomes are unrealistic from his or her perspective. Patterns of successful outcomes can be used to show how well nurses and other providers meet client needs.

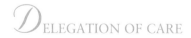

DELEGATION OF CARE

Community health nurses do not provide all the care needed in the community. Home attendants, personal care workers, home health aides, and people with no formal training may assist with care in the home. Proper delegation of tasks from the nurse to other persons requires verification that it is safe to do so. Stable clients who are not medically fragile are candidates for having someone with little or no formal health-related education [i.e., unlicensed assistive personnel (UAP)] to assist with their care.

If the nurse delegates care, he or she must follow up to make sure that the delegation of responsibility is proceeding without problems. Every nurse must consult the specific Nurse Practice Act under which he or she practices; there is wide variation in what constitutes "delegation" among the states and territories. The five essential criteria for delegation are, however, the same in every situation. They are: (1) right task, (2) right circumstances, (3) right person, (4) right communication or instruction, and (5) right supervision (National Council of State Boards of Nursing, 1995). Every community health nurse fulfilling these five criteria for delegation increases the probability of safe delegation.

Delegation, when used properly, allows laypeople or those with minimal training to provide safe supportive care. The benefits of delegation are especially obvious in the care of stable, physically disabled clients. For example, a technician, as an unlicensed person working in the community, may be delegated the tasks of clean catheterization and clean tracheal suctioning after proper training and under proper supervision. Agency policy regulates the frequency of supervision for UAPs working in community settings.

Delegation of Care. Nurses can only delegate care activities that a UAP can complete safely. The nurse can never delegate the supervision of one UAP to another and is responsible for regular reassessment to verify that the UAP is providing care safely.

$\mathcal{A}$GENCY REPORT CARDS

The types of interventions that nurses and other professionals perform are routinely evaluated for effectiveness. The results of such an evaluation can be used, for example, to inform the public about the quality of services. The variables ranked in a report card may influence the licensure decisions of a government agency or the funding decisions of a private organization. Some funders want to know who is eligible for care, how efficient the candidate agency is, and what health care providers think about the agency before they will support its programs.

It is not surprising that an organization might prefer to publicize only those variables that put it in a favorable light. However, a broad list of variables should be made available to allow for public confidence in the delivery of services by a health care organization. Voluntary accreditation, discussed in Chap. 16, requires self-assessment in the areas of (1) structure and function to support a consumer-oriented philosophy; (2) consistent high-quality services; (3) adequate human, financial, and physical resources to do the organization's work; and (4) positioning for long-term survival (Community Health Accreditation Program, 1993).

Variables can also be developed that reflect issues of interest to the community. One community might ask about length of service for the elderly, while another might be more interested in how long a new mother has to wait for a postpartum home visit. One interest group may want to know about nurse-to-client ratios or staff turnover; others might want information on clients' satisfaction.

Some consumers may want report card measurements in categories that are not routinely measured. Consumers might ask: What percent of diabetic clients inject insulin correctly after two home visits? How many

Agency Report Card. Agency report cards are made up of quality indicators that ideally reflect an accurate picture of the agency services.

nurses working in a Latino community speak Spanish? What percent of homebound clients have developed pressure sores since hospitalization? As consumers' influence continues to expand in the home care arena, nurses will be asked to monitor increasingly complex indicators of quality care.

Community health nurses have a great opportunity to identify the quality indicators that are important to the practice of community health nursing. These nurses should help set up quality assurance committees within and among agencies so their voices are heard as evaluation programs are established.

Summary

The technical aspects of providing nursing care vary, as does the intensity of care. Care is generally either high- or low- technology in nature, and nurses provide a mixture of both types of care to individuals, families, and groups.

Client outcomes are the key to measuring the success of nursing (and other professional) interventions. The goal of setting up interdisciplinary care teams is to find out which provider is best suited to provide services to the client. Nurses at times delegate care but must do so with every effort to ensure the client's safety. Nurses have the responsibility to delegate care to others only in stable situations where back-up support and supervision are readily available.

Consumers are increasing their influence by monitoring the quality of home care services, while agencies and service providers are developing report cards to assure the public that they provide quality services. Community health nurses must participate fully in establishing quality indicators so that the public and administrative personnel continue to value community health nursing services.

KEY WORDS

Delegation of care   Low-technology care
Agency report card   Measurable outcomes
High-technology care

QUESTIONS

DIRECTIONS: Choose the one *best* response to each of the following questions.

1. An example of a high-technology nursing intervention in the community would be

    A. facilitating group crisis counseling.
    B. regulating intravenous-pump chemotherapy.
    C. performing therapeutic touch therapy.
    D. teaching acid-base balance content.

2. An example of a measurable outcome related to the plan of care would be
   A. the client demonstrates proper wound care technique.
   B. the nurse completes a certification course.
   C. the hospital institutes evening and weekend clinic hours.
   D. the legislature funds a child development program.

3. Which behavior most clearly reflects the outcome of remaining infection free?
   A. Core body temperature of 37° centigrade
   B. Tenderness at a wound site
   C. Periodic diaphoresis
   D. Decreased range of motion near the wound

4. An example of a family-based outcome would be
   A. each member explains the restrictions of a diet individually.
   B. three-fourths of the family members complete a task correctly.
   C. interventions by the nurse are kept secret from some members.
   D. members make time for a family meeting to discuss problems together.

5. Outcomes for a group are measures of how well the group is working. Which behavior should the community health nurse foster in the group?
   A. The women in the group only talk to women.
   B. Group members often stay late for a subgroup meeting.
   C. Members monitor their input so every group member can participate.
   D. Starting time for the group varies because of different work schedules.

6. Which characteristic would probably not be placed on an agency-generated report card?
   A. People unable to pay full price for parenting class use a sliding scale for payment.
   B. Clients relate that 90 percent of new mothers are pleased with the care they receive.
   C. The agency was unable to meet accreditation criteria in all of the required areas.
   D. The orthopedic clinic remains open on weekends and evenings.

7. Which of the following clients would be a candidate for delegation?
   A. An 84-year-old man with no change in health status for 5 years
   B. A newborn with an increased bilirubin level
   C. A 35-year-old woman recently diagnosed with diabetes
   D. A slightly disoriented person with vague symptoms and complaints

ANSWERS

1. *The answer is B.* Intravenous-pump chemotherapy in the home is a high-technology intervention.

2. *The answer is A.* Measurable outcomes in the plan of care refer to the actions of the client.

3. *The answer is A.* Normal core body temperature reflects an absence of infection.

4. *The answer is D.* Making time for a family conference suggests that the family is working as a unit.

5. *The answer is C.* Individual members who are concerned for other group members show respect for the work of the group.

6. *The answer is C.* Agency-generated report cards tend to report only the most positive information about the agency.

7. *The answer is A.* Although older, the 84-year-old man is the most stable client and, therefore, is eligible to be cared for by someone with little or no formal training.

REFERENCES

Community Health Accreditation Program. (1996). *Benchmarks for excellence in home care: User's guide.* New York: Author.

This computer program allows for the collection of data to create an ongoing quality improvement project. Benchmarks focus on consumer, clinical, organizational, financial, and risk management.

Community Health Accreditation Program. (1993). *Standards of excellence for home care organizations.* New York: Author.

These standards, in ongoing development since 1965, are divided into the following categories: core, professional, paraprofessional, hospice, infusion therapy, home medical equipment, and pharmacy. The major themes of the accreditation program are quality, rights of consumers, long-term viability of services, and integration of community-based services into the total sum of health care services. (More information on accreditation can be obtained by calling 800-669-9656.)

National Council of State Boards of Nursing. (1995). *Delegation: Concepts and decision-making process.* Chicago: Author.

Guidelines for delegation in decision-making are reviewed to facilitate the provision of quality health care by appropriate persons in all health care settings.

Ruppert, R. A. (1996). Caring for the lay caregiver. *American Journal of Nursing, 96*(3), 40–46.

The problems lay caregivers experience are covered in detail in this continuing education article.

Stanhope, M., & Knollmueller, R. N. (1996). *Handbook of community and home health nursing* (2nd ed.). St. Louis, MO: C. V. Mosby.

This pocket-sized text gives examples of many assessment, intervention, and education tools the community health nurse could use in the care of people across the life span.

CONTINUITY OF CARE: ATTEMPTS AT MANAGING CARE SEAMLESSLY

ᚱ𝒫ROBLEMS IN PROVIDING CONTINUITY OF CARE IN A MULTITIERED HEALTH CARE SYSTEM

The watchwords for survival in the ever-changing health care delivery system are continuity of care and care (case) management. Nurses and other care providers who manage care in a continuous way, while conserving resources, are players in current and future health care decision-making (Cohen, 1996; Cohen & Cesta, 1993). Nurses unwilling to accept the challenge of creating innovative care systems will no longer be considered productive professionals.

The economic realities of the various care systems are forcing all care providers to demonstrate a certain level of business savvy and competence in customer satisfaction (Hicks, Stallmeyer, & Coleman, 1993; Newell, 1996). Buyers of nursing services (clients) have moved from the role of passive participant in health care decision-making to the role of involved health care consumer.

The insurance industry and resource utilization committees are closely supervising how care is provided and how much it costs (Landers, 1995). The essentials of continuity of care require nurses to consider their 24-h responsibilities to clients. As members of an interdisciplinary care management team, nurses are expected to assume full responsibility for a segment of the overall case load of clients.

Each member of the team has a specific responsibility to oversee part of the total complement of client needs. For example, a nurse case manager in a hospital may supervise the care on a specific unit while the community health nurse would supervise care in a designated geographic area. Nurse members of the case management team are not shift workers who end their day at 7 A.M., 3 P.M., or 11 P.M. Their responsibilities are as continuous as the care they provide.

𝒜LLOCATION OF RESOURCES

Nurses are accountable to their clients and their colleagues for the welfare of a number of clients on a microlevel and all clients on a more comprehensive macrolevel. For example, nurses in the community are responsible for teaching technical procedures to a diabetic client (microlevel) as well as participating in health planning with the entire community (macrolevel). Daily work assignments of the nurse may focus on caring for new mothers, fathers, and infants (microlevel) as well as educating the community on the need for prenatal care (macrolevel).

Nurses in the community have the unique opportunity to develop special relationships with other health care providers as well as a variety of consumer groups in creating new systems of care. Figure 14-1 identifies examples of the range of therapeutic interventions on the micro- and macrolevel that nurses can use to improve care delivery to individuals, families, groups, and the community as a whole.

Comprehensive nursing care requires services to individuals and families or groups on a microlevel as well as to aggregates and communities on a macrolevel. Nursing has a parallel responsibility to the individual client and the collective society. Nurses have the ethical responsibility to assist clients in getting the care they need (Woodstock Theological Center, 1995).

To provide 24-h care management and establish the appropriate relationships to meet the health care needs of the public, professional nurses should be able to complete many diverse tasks. To that end, this chapter will: (1) identify the problems of providing continuity of care in a multitiered health care system and (2) define the concept of care provider turf conflicts and describe how nurses can work to resolve them.

FIGURE 14-1

⌾

Microlevel and macrolevel therapeutic nursing interventions

MACROLEVEL: Population Focus

- Political activism
  - Petitioning for a safer environment
    - Voting
      - Writing letters of support for health care services needed in an under-served neighborhood

- Teaching a class on infant care
- Leading a cancer survival group
- Dressing change and antibiotic administration
- Administering insulin and monitoring glucose

Focus on Individuals and Families/Groups: MICROLEVEL

$\mathcal{D}$EFINING CONTINUITY OF CARE

Continuity of care suggests an ongoing, uninterrupted provision of services. The idea of seamless care management, at present, is a myth. Such an image of a continuous system of care is not realistic. Except in situations such as chronic, long-term care, continuity of care is actually a continuum of intermittent services varying in intensity. Continuity of care allows for resource conservation because reassessment of the client builds on the existing database; it does not recreate it.

Health care and nursing services need to be carefully developed to match client needs. A key aspect of the concept of continuity of care is the role of surveillance. This role is necessary to modulate the intensity of services that are delivered by various providers. The following story reflects the role of surveillance in continuity of care.

CASE STUDY:
Mr. Smeet Needs Frequent Changes in His Level of Care

Mr. Smeet recently was moved out of the Intensive Care Unit (ICU) to a medical-surgical floor after the stabilization of transient ischemic attacks (TIAs). After an additional 5 days of hospitalization, Mr. Smeet went home where a visiting nurse made daily assessment visits. After 1 week of visiting, the nurse case manager and the primary home care nurse developed a 3-day-a-week visit schedule.

After 1 month, the nurse was visiting only once every other week but calling the client every other week. During one of those calls, the nurse noted that Mr. Smeet was slurring his speech. The nurse could not make an emergency visit so she called 911, activating the emergency response system.

Mr. Smeet was admitted to the Neurological Stepdown Unit for observation for a possible cerebral vascular accident. He was discharged 1 week later with a 4-h-a-day home health aide after a thorough assessment by the nurse in the home. The visiting nurse made the judgment that it was appropriate to make weekly visits for ongoing observation for the next month.

In the situation described above, surveillance allowed the nursing staff to increase or decrease the intensity of services according to the needs of the client. The reason that Mr. Smeet was able to get the care he needed was because the nurse listened to him and did not assume to understand the meaning of his actions. Sometimes surveillance does not work because the client is alienated from the conversation. Some professionals provide the care they only assume or guess meets the needs of their clients.

In the following example, the client is upset because the staff has not included him in the management of his care.

CASE STUDY:

MR. ROBERTS IS UNABLE TO MASTER THE CARE SYSTEM

"It was devastating to get sick. I don't mean the cancer . . . that was the manageable part. The nurses and doctors just didn't listen. They kept saying 'do this . . . do that,' and when I didn't do things the way they suggested, they said I wasn't compliant! What does that mean? I was doing the best I could. I thought I was seeking support and services from people who would listen. The fact that the nurses and doctors did not listen to me was not my fault! How can I get better when I don't know what to do?"

It is unlikely that Mr. Roberts will call the doctors or nurses when he has questions about his care in the future. Mr. Roberts is taking himself out of the communication loop that could have assisted with continuity of care. In this situation, the doctors and nurses were responsible for this communication failure.

The meaning of continuity of care varies according to the types of clients who need care. Examples of the type of care systems that need to be developed include: care for people who are living in poverty and who are under- or uninsured, care for women and children, and care for people living with human immunodeficiency virus (HIV). The myth that continuity of care exists for men will be explored.

It is important to reflect on the idea that the amount of services available to people is a different problem from the lack of continuity of care. Additional, uncoordinated services may not be helpful to populations who have unmet health care needs. An extra dental clinic might be needed by the community more than a hypertension screening program. Adding services that a community does not need is actually an impediment to continuity of care. Unnecessary services lack a purpose for the community.

Continuity of Care for the People Who Are Living in Poverty or Who Are Under- or Uninsured

People living in poverty are especially disadvantaged in the process of experiencing continuity of care. They may have many basic unmet needs, which may make seeking preventive or early treatment health care a low priority. Services may be unobtainable because of monetary, emotional, or practical concerns (Center for Health Economics Research, 1993). People cannot always participate in care when they are hungry, do not have transportation to services, or are not conveniently scheduled for services.

It is impossible for clients to participate in care when they cannot afford copayments or have a restricted menu of services from which to choose. If the $5.00 copayment means that children will not be fed, care will probably be postponed. If the only mammography service available to an uninsured woman is in a dangerous part of town, she may not go for an evaluation.

Continuity of Care for Women and Children

Women may not experience continuity of care as they are busy securing health care for others. Social expectations of women's roles suggest that care for children and spouses or partners may take precedence over their own care. Therefore, society needs to assume responsibility for the poorly developed and fragmented level of care women receive.

Making health services available when women can obtain them is critical. Having women's and children's health services integrated so the whole family can get health care within one setting is one necessary accommodation for health care planning and delivery. Providing services that are sensitive to the needs of a single parent, for example, will allow these parents to care for themselves as well as their children.

Some women cannot care for themselves because they cannot afford to miss work. Social services are often not available at times that allow women to obtain respite from their caregiving responsibilities if it becomes necessary. Some women find themselves on public assistance because they cannot find a work schedule that can accommodate their other responsibilities to family or friends who need them. Other women may find advancement in work settings blocked because of unscheduled absences due to child care responsibilities. Lack of advancement becomes an economic issue, which may make buying health care impossible.

Deficiencies in the care of children, due to a lack of continuity of care is magnified, for example, when infant mortality, infant immunization, and child abuse rates are examined. The prevalence of these problems suggests that they are more complex than issues that would be resolved simply with better parenting skills. The whole community has responsibility for providing for the safety of its children (Clinton, 1996).

Continuity of Care for People Living with HIV

Since HIV is the number one public health problem in the United States, issues related to continuity of care and HIV need to be explored. Health care services vary widely for people living with HIV, according to geographic location, progression of disease, and gender. People living with HIV across the United States get different levels of government (state-level) medical assistance.

Few, if any, states provide the same Medicaid services to people infected with HIV (Jefferys, Fornataro, & Fornataro, 1995). Clients with advanced disease use greater amounts of resources due to recurring and harder-to-treat opportunistic infections. Also, much more is known about the care men should receive; women are still excluded from some basic research protocols that would help define the care they need (Hall, 1995; Kelly, Holman, Rothenberg, & Holzemer, 1995).

In addition to the general fear and concern people show with any communicable disease, continuity of care is also affected by the public's judgment about how the particular disease is transmitted. Americans seem especially averse to diseases that are sexually transmitted and related to the injection of drugs. Some people living with HIV infection do not experience continuity of care because of the negative value judgments and feelings of fear by care providers. These providers might avoid caring for people infected with HIV.

A number of health care providers are unwilling to care for people living with HIV. When assigned to care for people infected with HIV, they provide substandard care or, in some situations, refuse to provide care altogether. Nursing needs to expose prejudicial care when it impacts on the continuity of care, since this is a clear violation of nursing's professional code of ethics.

Continuity of Care for Men

Calls for continuity of care often suggest that women, people of color, and others do not get the same level of health care as that provided to men. The development of distinct women's health services and health services with a strong cultural emphasis suggests that men as a group are able to get their health care needs met more efficiently than other groups. Special services are set up for women and people from different cultural and racial groups because providers need to learn how to care for them properly.

Although it is hard to ignore that many health services like coronary care and sports medicine were developed primarily for men, they, as a group, may not get their health care needs met better than other groups. More health care services may exist tailored to the health care needs of men, but a comprehensive blueprint representing continuity of care for men is not evident.

CONTINUITY OF CARE AND PROVIDER TURF CONFLICTS

Turf Conflicts. These conflicts relate to disagreements among professionals regarding who should provide care. They often have economic underpinnings.

Professions stake out health care turf to protect their influence and role in health care decision making. Each professional group has its vested interest in the way that health care resource allocation decisions are made. Obstetricians and nurse midwives, for example, see their roles and responsibilities differently. Nurse midwives focus on the holistic experience of natural birth, whereas obstetricians focus more on high-risk deliveries.

Health professionals must, however, work together to make client-centered decisions collaboratively. Nurses, physicians, and all other health care providers have an important role in assisting and supporting continuity of care. Professionals must take the time to learn how other professionals approach and solve problems in order to work with them.

The growing consumer movement is calling into question the meaning of professional control over how health care decisions are made. Health care professionals must seek out consumers to develop services that are meaningful to the public. The role of the public is to validate that the services provided in the community are appropriate. Validation is needed to establish that care is meeting the expectations of the public and having an impact on their health.

At times, professionals need to inform the community of the importance of certain services. Public awareness campaigns to increase immunization rates or decrease cigarette smoking behavior are examples of informing the community of the importance of services. The public validates the service, for example, by making funds available for vaccines and smoking cessation groups.

The following discussion focuses on turf conflicts experienced by medicine, nursing, social service, lay community workers, and clients who are participating in deciding how resources are used. Insurance companies are also participants in turf conflicts and are an increasing force in the emerging health care debates about how health care resources will be allocated.

Medical Turf

At one time, physicians made nearly all resource allocation decisions. Whatever care the physician wanted was provided upon request. Hospital and other agency administrators began to share decision making with medicine as the complexity of care and the complexity of delivery systems created the need for more input into decisions.

Attempts at cost control have accelerated the process of decentralizing decision making among professionals. Health-related outcomes, the byproduct of therapeutic interventions, are the shared responsibility of the multidisciplinary team. Physicians are rightfully the directors of medical care as nurses and other care providers guide their respective practices. Each member of the team has responsibilities to their practice as well as to the team.

Nursing Turf

Nurses have always experienced a schizophrenic allegiance to the doctor and employer (e.g., hospital) on the one hand and the client on the other. Nurses often spend the most time providing direct care to clients and, in some settings, have the least influence over deciding what care clients should receive. The growing numbers of nurse practitioners and other advanced practice nurses are changing nursing's role in how resources are being allocated. Advanced practice nurses with admission and discharge privileges in hospitals, for example, have a direct influence on care allocation decisions.

Clinical nurse specialists, certified nurse midwives, nurse anesthetists, and nurse practitioners, representing the advanced practice arm of nursing, many times serve as primary care providers. These practitioners are more likely to make influential resource allocation decisions because they function as case managers. Table 14-1 identifies the many role functions of the clinical nurse specialist/case manager.

❧

TABLE 14-1

CRITERIA-BASED PERFORMANCE EVALUATION

Clinical practice component
- Demonstrates clinical expertise through participation in direct patient care activities for a selected population of clients
- Demonstrates clinical expertise by coordinating managed care to target populations
- Communicates effectually with members of the interdisciplinary team to use critical pathways effectively.

Education component
- Participates in the assessment, development, implementation, and evaluation of educational programs designed to enhance the delivery of nursing care services by staff

Consultation component
- Acts as a consultant to all disciplines regarding issues related to quality patient care
- Acts as a consultant to all disciplines regarding issues specific to managed care/case management

Research component
- Participates in or conducts nursing research related to quality patient care issues

---

NOTE: This performance evaluation was developed by The Long Island College Hospital, Division of Nursing, to evaluate the clinical nurse specialist/case manager.

Increasingly, nurse managers are directing the care of people in the hospital as well as the community where people get care in their homes or other settings like day-care facilities. Nurses in various positions are using each other, as well as people from other disciplines, as consultants in health care planning to provide comprehensive nursing care.

Social Service Turf

The complex relationship between people's health-related problems and the social systems of support has increased the influence of social service in identifying what services people need to get well or stay healthy. Social service systems have been developed to assist families and others to support the needs of the client. Professional social workers monitor social conditions and situations for signs of erosion and intervene to maintain the integrity of social networks. Certified social workers (CSW) or master's prepared social workers (MSW) are educated and credentialed to supervise complex family negotiations, supervise support groups, and use community resources fully.

Increasingly, social workers are creating what may be considered the virtual family. Social workers set up networks of care that might include family and friends living geographically close to and far away from the client. Today, calling together an extended family for a meeting in a short time might involve a multiparty conference call connecting relatives from many locations. Social workers often work with family members that they never meet face-to-face.

A social phenomenon is developing where lay caregivers who are also strangers are increasingly becoming the only caregiver in many situations; however, strangers providing short bursts of care can hardly be considered primary caregivers. For example, when a client outlives family and friends or when multigenerational deaths have occurred as a result of HIV, clients are often supported by individuals previously unknown to them.

Many social service or community-based organizations have formal volunteer programs to provide assistance in the home. Supervision is needed so that volunteers are not providing skilled health-related services in the home. Use of volunteers in providing support services will be discussed at the end of the chapter.

Turf of Lay Community Health Workers

People from the community who are not formally educated in a health care field are increasingly being called upon to contribute to the health of the public. Lay outreach, lay health educator, and companion roles are developing where there is a shortage of health care personnel and when the cost of using professionals in these roles is prohibitive. Not surprisingly, lay workers are more accepted where there are shortages of trained personnel.

The nursing profession has always been concerned about the growth of **unlicensed assistive personnel (UAP)** or technicians in care delivery settings. Part of the concern relates to the quantity and quality of the education they receive to become technicians. It makes business sense to have workers cross-trained in many tasks as long as their education is sufficient to keep the technicians from performing skills that are beyond their abilities. Currently, the majority of UAPs are trained for acute care hospital positions.

The successful history of using UAPs in the military as corpsmen and medics supports the idea that technicians can be used safely in many settings. The people who are wary of using technicians suggest that the potential lack of adequate supervision makes the use of UAPs potentially disastrous. Nurses in both community and acute care settings should actively confront the employment of UAPs in health care and supervise their assignments for appropriateness and safety.

When working with UAPs, the community health nurse should be careful to give exact instructions that can be evaluated easily. Table 14-2 is an example of a schedule of activities that a UAP might complete. The UAP is collecting information guided by the community health nurse.

The activities the UAP would complete in this example are telephone calls to clients needing follow-up. Depending on the results of the calls, the nurse will make additional calls to certain clients.

Unlicensed Assistive Personnel (UAPs). Concerns with the use of UAPs relate to the fact that without licensure and the related guidelines for education, nonprofessionals may not be adequately prepared for the complex tasks of health care delivery.

▒

TABLE 14-2
SCHEDULE OF ACTIVITIES FOR UNLICENSED ASSISTIVE PERSONNEL (UAPs)

Client	Phone/Fax #	Activity to Verify/Remind
Calls for 10 A.M.—Please call your team nurse with questions. Call 911 for an emergency.		
Terry Berry	567-3456	Ask if he went to the M.D. yesterday. Call his sister (123) 456-7891 if he is not home.
Betty Urich	567-7654	Ask her about her medication at 10 A.M. Does she have an appointment yet for clinic?
Faith Alpert	324-0989	Did she report the drainage on her dressing to the nurse at the clinic? Is she having any trouble taking her insulin in the morning? How often does the visiting nurse see her?
Calls for 2 P.M.—Please call your team nurse with questions. Call 911 for an emergency.		
Marie Stuler	555-1027	Hard of hearing. Ask her if she had lunch and if she is having any pain while walking. Did she make another appointment with the chiropractor?
Kevin Erbork	676-7878	Remind Kevin about his 4 P.M. visit to the M.D. Remind him to take bus fare for both trips.

Emerging Client-Controlled Turf

Consumers are getting increasingly more involved in health care decision making. Appropriately, empowering consumers to identify health care proxies, for example, allows the locus of decision making to remain client-centered. A health care proxy is a person who carries out the specific wishes of a client after the client is no longer competent to direct his or her health care. The health care proxy acts for the client as if the client could still decide what health-related services they want.

The legal role of a proxy assures that the wishes and requirements for care will not be ignored when the client can no longer communicate with the health care team. Nurses have a special opportunity to encourage their clients to identify a health care proxy well before a grave physiological or psychological problem develops that would impair their decision-making ability.

Insurance Carrier as Payer and Player

In the past, insurance companies were fairly passive participants in the allocation of health care resources. Sick people were often prohibited from obtaining insurance as obvious risks to the plan. The healthy people in the insurance pool often had claims paid on demand. Fee-for-service, paying for whatever services, tests, or procedures were completed, gave way to increasing restrictions on what services would be covered by the insurance plan. Now, insurance carriers are monitoring all decisions about how people get their health care needs met.

$\mathcal{S}$UMMARY

It is difficult to provide any continuity of care in a multitiered system of care. It is problematic to allocate resources when different people or groups of people have more success getting their needs met. In this chapter, examples of people with problems in getting the care they need are people living in poverty, those with HIV infection, and those who are under- and uninsured. Although men as a group have access to more health care services, it is not clear if they experience an improved level of continuity of care.

Providing continuity of care is made more difficult because of the professional turf conflicts that occur in the health care system. Nurses, physicians, social workers, lay health workers, clients, and insurance companies are all fighting over who will provide care and thereby allocate resources. A spirit of cooperation is needed so that health care needs are met appropriately and ethically (Woodstock Theological Center, 1995).

KEY WORDS

Turf conflict   Unlicensed assistive personnel (UAP)

QUESTIONS

DIRECTIONS: Choose the one *best* response to each of the following questions.

1. Many problems in providing continuity of care relate to the balance between cost and
   A. difficulty of tasks.
   B. quality of services.
   C. economic stability.
   D. care provider availability.

2. An example of a macrolevel therapeutic intervention is a

   A. vitamin K injection.
   B. back massage.
   C. health-related radio program.
   D. gastric lavage.

3. Which of the following statements by the client suggests continuity of care?

   A. "Sometimes I do not see my physical therapist for months, but I know how to contact him."
   B. "They change pharmacist's every 6 months at my drugstore. I have to keep explaining my health history."
   C. "My physician is always busy; it takes 72 hours for her to call back!"
   D. "My favorite nurse works in different areas of the city. I wait to tell him my symptoms the next time he visits."

4. Sometimes women have problems getting the care they need because of their

   A. multiple caregiving roles.
   B. complicated work schedules.
   C. need to ask for second opinions.
   D. unwillingness to follow directions.

5. Validation of services for acceptability and cultural appropriateness should be completed by the

   A. professional psychologist.
   B. social service department.
   C. client using the service.
   D. the patient service representative.

6. The core of meaning of turf conflicts with various professions often relates to

   A. ethical responsibility.
   B. legal regulation of practice.
   C. clinical experience.
   D. financial security.

7. The community health nurse should refer a client who is speaking incoherently about suicide to the

   A. client's psychiatrist for a next day appointment.
   B. social worker for group intervention.
   C. emergency medical system by calling 911.
   D. Evening Visiting Program nursing administrator.

8. Which of the following statements about the use of lay community health workers is true?

   A. They usually know more about the community needs and wants.
   B. They are involved in more malpractice suits.
   C. They can function as nurses with the proper training.
   D. They never continue with formal professional education.

ANSWERS

1. *The answer is B.* Decreased costs often suggest a decrease in quality of services.

2. *The answer is C.* Macrolevel interventions are directed to groups or aggregates of clients.

3. *The answer is A.* Continuity of care does not mean that there are no variations in the pattern of care, but that care is monitored overall.

4. *The answer is A.* Women traditionally care for all other members of the family or group in almost every culture.

5. *The answer is C.* Clients should validate services. Assumptions about what is appropriate for a group is stereotyping.

6. *The answer is D.* Financial security often underlies conflicts about who can or cannot perform certain tasks.

7. *The answer is C.* The immediate nature of the problem (i.e., suicide) requires emergency intervention.

8. *The answer is A.* Lay workers are selected because of their knowledge about a community.

ANNOTATED REFERENCES

Center for Health Economics Research. (1993). *Access to health care: Key indicators for policy.* Princeton, NJ: The Robert Wood Johnson Foundation.

This document explores three barriers to access to health care: economic barriers, supply and distribution barriers, and sociocultural barriers. Of particular interest in this important document is the connection between poverty and lacking access to health care.

Clinton, H. R. (1996). *It takes a village: And other lessons children teach us.* New York: Simon & Schuster.

This book reviews the concept of social responsibility in caring for others, especially children.

Cohen, E. L. (1996). *Nurse case management in the 21st century.* Philadelphia: C. V. Mosby.

This book is a summary of the many issues nurses face in case management. It predicts the types of activities with which nurses will be involved in the future.

Cohen, E. L., & Cesta, T. G. (1993). *Nursing case management: From concept to evaluation.* Philadelphia: C. V. Mosby.

This text provides a basic yet comprehensive overview of the many complexities of case management. Every step of setting up a quality case management program is covered completely.

Jefferys, R., Fornataro, N., & Fornataro, K. (1995). *The access project.* New York: AIDS Treatment Data Network.

This document explains the variation in the medications that are available to people living with HIV through state medical assistance.

Hall, J. K. (1995). Exclusion of pregnant women from research protocols: Unethical and illegal. *IRB: A Review of Human Subjects Research,* 17(2), 1–3.

Omitting women from research protocols has an effect on what is known about women's health and how they respond to treatments and get well.

Hicks, L. L., Stallmeyer, J. M., & Coleman, J. R. (1993). *Role of the nurse in managed care.* Washington, DC: American Nurses Association.

Some of the topics covered in this comprehensive text include: structure of health maintenance organizations (HMOs), characteristics of plan enrollees, financial incentives with managed care, and the emerging roles of the nurse in these programs.

Kelly, P., Holman, S., Rothenberg, R., & Holzemer, S. P. (1995). *Primary care of women and children with HIV infection: A multidisciplinary approach.* Boston: Jones and Bartlett.

This book identifies the many problems women and children with HIV face in obtaining health care and social services.

Landers, T. (1995). Medicaid managed care: A brief analysis. *Journal of the New York State Nurses Association,* 26(3), 7–11.

This article discusses the many concerns of Medicaid-managed care. Areas discussed include fiscal incentives, the role of market forces, and quality assurance. The risks and potentials of managed care are examined.

Newell, M. (1996). *Using nursing case management to improve health outcomes.* Gaithersberg, MD: Aspen Publications.

This book uses many case studies to examine the business and quality of care issues related to case management.

Woodstock Theological Center. (1995). *Ethical considerations in the business aspects of health care.* Washington, DC: Georgetown University Press.

The framework for making ethical decisions includes: compassion and respect for human dignity, commitment to professional competence, commitment to a spirit of service, honesty, confidentiality, good stewardship, and careful administration.

THE INFRASTRUCTURE FOR CARE DELIVERY AND THE ROLES OF THE COMMUNITY HEALTH NURSE

This chapter explores how the infrastructure of the health care delivery system relates to the type of care that is available to the public. Learning about the various health care systems provides insight into which systems need improvement or development. In addition, the key roles nurses assume in health care systems—such as that of care provider, educator, screener, advocate, planner, coordinator of care, and supervisor of ancillary personnel—are examined.

Nurses in community-based practice frequently assume multiple roles; thus, they need the flexibility to assume these roles and to make referrals when they are unable to meet the needs of certain clients. Few if any community health nurses work in only one capacity. The skills necessary for community health nurses include critical thinking, computer literacy, creativity, a facility with group interactions, and especially therapeutic communication skills. An appreciation of the growth and development of individuals, families, groups, and communities is also necessary. The role of the nurse researcher is discussed separately in Chap. 17.

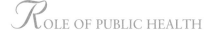

ROLE OF PUBLIC HEALTH

The primary and essential role of the entire medical-industrial complex is to protect and promote the health of the public. All preventive, curative, and restorative nursing interventions must be related to the health needs of the entire population. Since the beginning of organized health care, public health has focused on aggregate-level interventions—that is, services directed at whole age groups or populations-at-risk.

Immunizations, sexually transmitted disease screening, sanitation, monitoring for communicable disease, and violence prevention programs are all examples of public health interventions. These interventions protect, detect illness, and promote health for the general public. These services have traditionally been provided by official or government-managed agencies. The state department of health, for example, has the legal mandate to meet the overall public health needs of the people who live in that state.

In order to meet the public health needs of the United States, consensus has been reached on the core functions of public health for this country. The three **core functions of public health**—assessment, policy development, and assurance that services are available—are global; that is, they are intended to serve the entire population of the United States (National Association of County Health Officials, 1993).

Assessment is critical because it reveals health care problems and resources to remediate them. *Policy development* is crucial to assure that health promotion is a priority for society. *Assurance* that needed services are available is necessary so that health-related problems can be solved.

The cornerstone of public health is prevention of illness (Anderson & McFarlane, 1996; U.S. Department of Health and Human Services, 1994). Preventive interventions are in the public's interest and are qualitatively different than illness care. For example, providing classes to promote healthy parenting is a very different public health intervention than caring for children who have been abused at the hands of their parents. Table 15-1 identifies a number of preventive interventions and the associated diseases that could be avoided by implementing these preventive interventions.

Though no one argues against the benefits of prevention, there is great conflict about which services should be available to the public. The benefits

Core Functions of Public Health

- *Assessment* of community health status and available resources

- *Policy development* resulting in proposals to support and encourage better health

- *Assurance* that needed services are available

⬚

TABLE 15-1

EFFORTS TO PREVENT DISEASE AND DISABILITY

Preventive Nursing Actions	Disease/Disability/Condition Avoided by Preventive Nursing Action
Teaching proper use of condoms	Human immunodeficiency virus (HIV) and other sexually transmitted diseases Avoiding pregnancy or an unwanted, medically, or emotionally at-risk pregnancy
Child safety classes for new parents	Accidents, permanent neurological damage, or death
Reviewing "Right to Know" guidelines for a safe working environment	Exposure to toxic chemicals or radiation, which could cause birth defects, sterility, and neoplasms
Counseling children on how to interact with their grandparents with Alzheimer's disease	Dysfunctional family dynamics or stereotypic views about aging

of preventive services take time to manifest. For example, classes that teach children to eat healthful foods may help prevent heart disease and stroke 40 years after they are taught. However, heart surgery often extends life in a way that can be measured immediately because a progressive decrease in cardiac symptoms is obvious within a few hours or days.

Since the outcome of preventive services are not as immediate as curative interventions, they are less tangible and, therefore, seem less important. Thus, because preventive services may take generations to show health benefits, they may be delayed for interventions with more immediate results. An extended life without disease or disability is not appreciated until old age.

Role of hospitals and acute care centers

Hospitals and acute care centers were developed in part to promote the centralization of resources and expensive equipment, decrease the duplication of services, and add convenience for health care providers. Centralization also enabled nurses to care for more patients at a time.

The dramatic explosion of technology in health care increased the number of hospitals and acute care centers. Hospitals specializing in heart surgery, orthopedic procedures, and cancer care were established, for example, because of the technological developments in specialized care.

The ways of treating clients quickly outgrew the skills of lay people and many health care generalists. Clients were moved into central facilities where professionals had the latest high-technology skills to care for them. The role of the specialist emerged as the public increasingly made demands for high-technology care.

As health care enters the 21st century, hospitals and acute care centers are drastically downsizing and radically reorganizing their approach to care delivery. Care is now moving to community-based sites where professionals predict that quality care can be provided less expensively, more comprehensively, and with fewer disruptions in a client's pattern of living. In the future, hospital resources will be available for only the most acutely ill who cannot be cared for safely in the community.

Role of community-based organizations

The proliferation of community-based organizations (CBOs), sites for nonacute care or short-term care located where clients live, has had a major impact on the decentralization of care in many areas of the country. A child, for example, may get his or her immunizations from a school health office, emotional counseling at a neighborhood clinic, and sutures for a laceration at a local free-standing emergency center. In each situation, the child uses community-based services, not hospital-based services.

Many community-based services are linked to specific diseases or specific clients' needs. They may be national organizations with local chapters (e.g., American Cancer Society), or facilities very specific to the needs of an aggregate (e.g., Coalition for the Homeless in Washington, D.C.). One benefit of community-based organizations is that they ideally provide services that are appropriate to the needs of that community because they are developed within and by the community.

SHIFT IN RESPONSIBILITY FOR CARE DELIVERY BY FAMILY MEMBERS, FRIENDS, VOLUNTEERS, AND STRANGERS

Increasingly, family members are asked to intensify their care responsibilities in the home and other health care settings. Often, family members provide very complex care in these settings. In situations where family members are absent or not helpful, friends, volunteers, or strangers are asked to provide care. Although nonprofessional caregivers have limited supervision in the home, it is difficult not to rely on lay caregivers when no care would be administered otherwise. A particular concern for the community health nurse relates to the number of lay caregivers who provide skilled care beyond their abilities.

In the United States, the aging of the population and the pandemic of acquired immune deficiency syndrome (AIDS) provide two examples where the idea of the virtual family is created. The elderly who outlive their families may be forced to join group homes for protected or supervised living. People living with human immunodeficiency virus (HIV) may outlive their support systems and require group living with people they do not know.

Support for Lay Caregivers

Community health nurses are faced with the challenge of establishing support networks for lay caregivers. Volunteers are often eager to assume assistive roles; however, family members are not given the luxury of volunteering for a caregiving role. The community health nurse needs to be aware that while the client may cope better in the home environment, this same environment may overwhelm the caregiver. The lay caregivers may resist increased responsibilities because they do not have adequate support systems.

Nursing can support lay caregivers by working to anticipate problems and by encouraging the lay caregiver to seek support through counseling or group work. Lay caregivers often work full-time jobs to support themselves while working a second "full-time job" caring for a loved one. The emotional and financial toll is an issue that must be addressed by professionals to support the lay caregiver.

One area of support for lay caregivers is to provide education so they can provide unskilled care safely. Classes in a number of health-related activities can help lay caregivers provide care and not enter the realm of professional practice (Ripple & Holzemer, 1995). Three common areas where education by professionals can support the role of caregivers are: **communication, body mechanics, and universal precautions/infection control.**

These three service areas are important because they represent areas where volunteers may have problems providing care. Volunteers need information on communication so they can assist clients in getting their needs met. They need information on body mechanics to protect themselves while assisting others with ambulation or changing position. Finally, volunteers need information on universal precautions and infection control so they can be comfortable providing assistance. Other educational supports for volunteers may be necessary according to their roles and responsibilities.

CONTEMPORARY ROLES OF THE NURSE IN THE COMMUNITY

Care Provider

Nurses provide care in increasingly complex and innovative settings. Traditional community-based roles are found in schools, home care departments, visiting nurse associations, and public health agencies. Additional care settings provide more employment opportunities for nurses, such as community-based research facilities, parish nursing settings, corporate wellness and occupational sites, and neighborhood community centers.

Nurse entrepreneurs are developing and managing community nursing centers that provide primary, secondary, and tertiary levels of nursing care. Advanced practice nurses work in all traditional and evolving care settings. The most critical skill in care provision is assessment. Ongoing expectations for all health care personnel relate to the development of excellent assessment skills.

Employers expect health care providers to make assessments quickly and resolve problems in ways that conserve resources. It is also expected that the new employees bring these skills with them as opposed to expecting the agency to provide the related training. Although new graduates will not have the same assessment skills that seasoned practitioners have, strong basic assessment skills will be expected by employers.

Educator

Nurses may educate individual clients or families and groups of clients in various health and illness situations. Nurses may also educate one another through continuing and inservice programs so they maintain competence in care delivery. Nurses have a primary role in educating the public about the changing role of the nursing profession that may potentially improve the public's health. Education involves informing oneself and others about the potential for change to improve levels of well-being.

Sample Basic Volunteer Services

- *Communication*
  Interpersonal
  Negotiating with the health
     care team
  Confidentiality

- *Body Mechanics*
  Assisting with lifting
  Assisting with ambulating
  Assisting with transfer to
     bed or chair

- *Universal Precautions and
  Infection Control*
  First aid
  Basic food preparation and
     storage

Care Provider. Nurses are among the many care providers who make up the interdisciplinary team. The nursing profession sets the standard for providing care in the community.

Educator. Community health nurses educate clients, other nurses, and the public about the health-related problems they discover and the roles of nurses who work to resolve these problems, thereby improving health.

Health- and illness-related education allows clients to improve their health and to accept the limits of their physical or emotional state. Nurses teach clients how to prepare for death and grieve the loss of family or friends and may also have a role in helping communities cope or recover from natural disasters and civil unrest through crisis counseling.

Nurses educate other nurses through continuing education, which provides an update for clinical competencies. Continuing education may involve a short seminar or a week-long refresher course on a variety of topics from high-technology home care to crisis intervention with a family. The nurse educator makes a diagnosis of a learning deficit among a group of nurses and then provides the continuing education that should improve clinical practice. Continuing education is often approved by state-level nursing organizations so that continuing education units (CEUs) can be awarded.

Inservice education is a more narrowly focused intervention; it is often focused on a single topic. Staff nurses may be required to attend yearly classes that reinforce previously taught material. Different state regulatory, accreditation, and funding sources require updating education in such areas as fire safety cardiopulmonary resuscitation, universal precautions for infection control, and confidentiality of client information. Education may also be conducted on a variety of agency-specific policies and procedures. Instruction on how to use new record forms and changes in use of equipment may need to be repeated, as necessary, to assure a standard of care. Participants in inservice education programs are not usually awarded CEUs.

Nurses also educate the public about changing nursing roles. The public is broadening its view of and appreciation of professional nursing. Once restricted to the hospital and nursing home, nurses are increasingly associated with the role of primary care provider or adjunct to primary care services.

Screener

Screener. When health problems are known to exist, care providers can screen populations at risk for early warning signs. Community health nurses also observe for patterns of symptoms that could represent a previously unknown health problem.

Nurses screen individuals, families, and groups (clients) for problems such as lack of knowledge, inadequate immunization, prevalence of sexually transmitted disease, and malnutrition. Nurses can screen families as clients for the presence of domestic violence, elder abuse, and for how family members respond to the birth of a new member.

Screening functions are the core of secondary prevention activities. Screening is used to identify problems early and ameliorate them. Screening is a special role because it does not involve treating obvious problems but rather searches for warning signs of a problem. Screening assumes that there are warning signs that a problem exists like an antigen marker, a tissue lump, or a decrease in visual acuity. Screening is the link between successful prevention and full-scale disease; it attempts to prevent the spread of physical or emotional problems before more resources are needed to correct them.

Community health nurses may screen individual clients for bleeding gums and tooth pain, both of which suggest dental caries. Referral to a dentist would be appropriate because the problem needs the expertise of another care provider. Nurses with expertise in care of families with emotional problems would screen families for signs of decreased communication between members and a history of physical or emotional violence within the family, suggesting dysfunction. The nurse could treat these families if she or he had the proper credentials to do so.

Screening for previously unknown diseases is not possible because the nurse or other care provider cannot identify the new pattern of related symptoms or illness-related warning signs. The community health nurse is, however, observant for unusual patterns of symptoms in general that could foretell an emerging (and previously unknown) problem or a resurgence of a previously controlled problem.

Advocate

Advocacy is a complex role that involves acting for another person who cannot navigate the health care system to get his or her needs met. People need advocates when they cannot get services because they lack knowledge; when they are unable to see, speak, or hear; or when they are confused about what services are available. Some people become depressed when they are sick and may need a temporary advocate until they feel better. The role of nursing is to act as an advocate for clients until they can care for themselves.

Vulnerable populations like prisoners, children, people with neurological conditions, and elders often need advocates for the rest of their lives or until their circumstances allow for more freedom of choice and independence. Nursing has the responsibility for promoting advocacy in part because of the frequency of ongoing long-term therapeutic relationships. The community health nurse may follow the same family as infants are born, children grow, and older members die.

Advocate. The role of advocate is filled when a person acts for another person in a way that is reasonable and prudent. Acting for another is necessary when the person cannot get her or his own health care needs met independently; for example, nurses act as advocates for children, prisoners, and clients who do not speak English.

Planner

Looking ahead to make some prediction about what health care resources will be needed to meet client needs is the core of health care planning. Planning for the health of the community requires the cooperation of clients as well as professionals. The importance of sound planning relates to the fact that generations of people may benefit or be limited by the careful or careless nature of planning.

The emergence of high-technology equipment and services has made planning even more imperative. Expensive equipment and high-technology services may be in demand for different groups, making organized health planning difficult. Providers from different specialties with different skills each define planning as it relates to their various needs.

Planning for future needs is difficult because existing problems take precedence. A disturbing trend in the United States society is a preference

Planner. Community health nurses are involved in health planning in an effort to meet the needs of the community. Health planning should include the client whenever possible so that health care services are relevant to client needs.

for the immediate resolution of problems even at the risk of creating greater future problems. For example, the decreased funding for Headstart programs for children is tolerated even though children without this type of education may not be as likely to succeed in school. Shifting money from this program to another program or cutting funds to contain costs may result in devastating long-term results for an entire generation of children.

Coordinator of Care

Coordinator of Care. Community health nurses coordinate the care of clients to conserve resources as well as to provide appropriate services. Care must be coordinated to avoid the duplication of services.

Coordination of services is the major underpinning for a cost-effective and efficient health care delivery system. Community health nurses are active in the coordination of care in order to meet client needs appropriately. The role of the nurse in coordination of care is especially important in multigenerational diseases like HIV (Kelly, Holman, Rothenberg, & Holzemer, 1996). The community health nurse coordinates complex care needs between professionals of many disciplines and among clients, families, friends, volunteers, and strangers.

Coordination of care is especially challenging because of the volume of care that is being shifted to community settings. Much of the care that was provided in the hospital was not expected to shift to community-based settings. It used to be said that people needing high-technology support were too sick to go home for care. Today almost any level of care can be provided in the home as long as support systems are in place.

The infrastructure for care delivery discussed earlier in this chapter has not been designed for the great influx of care moving into the community. Formerly, a mother and infant might have a 3-day hospitalization to learn the new roles of parenting; more recently, discharges have been encouraged 24 to 36 h after delivery. Community-based services are not in place to provide the additional services necessary for the new family, even if they were covered by insurance.

Supervisor of Ancillary Personnel

Supervisor of Ancillary Personnel. An expanding role for nursing is supervision of ancillary personnel. Many people who provide care at an assistant level need direction and guidance by the nurse; for example, supervision of UAPs is necessary because of their limited training.

Community health nurses supervise many people in the home, ambulatory care, and various community-based organization (CBO) settings. Increasingly, the business aspects of home care and community health require close supervision of ancillary personnel that may work for an organization or are subcontractors from a second agency.

Cost-effective care delivery by professionals and ancillary personnel is a requisite for survival in emerging settings (Newell, 1996), especially as they relate to managed care. Community health nurses usually have very little preparation in leadership, management, and supervision of ancillary personnel in their undergraduate programs. Increasing skills in this area are needed, especially with the growth of the use of unlicensed assistive personnel (UAPs) in all health care settings (Cohen & Cesta, 1993; Cohen, 1996). Community health nurses need to expand their competence in working with and evaluating the care provided by people in the role of UAP or health care technician.

$\mathcal{S}$UMMARY

The soundness of the health care infrastructure and the roles of the nurse intended to improve the public's health are both important concerns for the community health nurse. The infrastructure for the delivery of health care is made up of public health facilities, hospitals and medical centers, and CBOs. Health care is becoming more decentralized; service delivery is moving into the communities where people live. Increases in community-based care can be seen, for example, in the growth of school-based and occupation-based health care services.

Care delivery is augmented by lay people in many situations. Care is provided by family members, friends, volunteers, and strangers. Community health nurses need to accept the complex role of supporting the care networks as they develop. Community health nurses, knowing that each support network is unique, assist the group to provide care to the client needing services.

Community health nurses assume many roles in their practice. They work as care providers, educators, screeners, advocates, planners, coordinators of care, and supervisors of ancillary personnel. All nursing roles are being examined for their cost-effectiveness and success in improving care. Community health nurses are increasingly being asked to demonstrate that the outcomes of acting in various roles is improving care to clients in a cost-effective way.

KEY WORDS

Advocate
Care provider
Coordinator of care
Educator

Planner
Screener
Supervisor of ancillary personnel

QUESTIONS

DIRECTIONS: Choose the one *best* response to each of the following questions.

1. The action that relates most directly to the role of public health includes

   A. monitoring the spread of sexually transmitted disease.
   B. supervising the individuals working in the sanitation department.
   C. electing government officials with platforms including animal protection rights.
   D. responding to a plane crash in a remote location.

2. The community health nurse who performs yearly scoliosis assessments in grade school is acting in the role of

    A. provider of care.
    B. screener.
    C. advocate.
    D. coordinator of care.

3. The community health nurse who triages clients, changes visit schedules, and discharges clients from services is acting in the role of

    A. provider of care.
    B. screener.
    C. advocate.
    D. coordinator of care.

4. The community health nurse working with a deaf client makes ambulatory care appointments only when a sign language interpreter is present. This nurse is acting in the role of

    A. provider of care.
    B. screener.
    C. advocate.
    D. coordinator of care.

5. Which action by the nurse reflects the role of supervisor of ancillary personnel?

    A. Calling the pharmacist to clarify a drug side effect.
    B. Mailing laboratory reports to the primary care provider.
    C. Instructing the home care assistant on proper home safety practices.
    D. Ordering necessary supplies from the medical equipment company.

ANSWERS

1. *The answer is A.* Monitoring for sexually transmitted disease is a population-focused activity related to public health.

2. *The answer is B.* Assessment for scoliosis is a screening activity.

3. *The answer is D.* Coordination of care involves the changes needed in meeting the needs of a group of clients. Nursing interventions change with the needs of the clients.

4. *The answer is C.* Providing for client needs is the goal of advocacy. The nurse intervenes to assist the client in getting health care needs met.

5. *The answer is C.* Instructing ancillary personnel to assist them provide care is part of the supervisory role of the community health nurse.

ANNOTATED REFERENCES

Anderson, E. T., & McFarlane, J. M. (1996). *Community as partner: Theory and practice in nursing* (2nd ed.). Philadelphia: J. B. Lippincott.

This textbook examines the potential relationships between nurses and clients as partners in creating solutions to health-related problems.

Cohen, E. L. (1996). *Nurse case management in the 21st century.* Philadelphia: C. V. Mosby.

This book is a summary of the many issues nurses face in case management. It predicts the types of activities with which nurses will be involved in the future.

Cohen, E. L., & Cesta, T. G. (1993). *Nursing case management: From concept to evaluation.* Philadelphia: C. V. Mosby.

This text provides a basic yet comprehensive overview of the many complexities of case management. Every step of setting up a quality case management program is covered completely.

Kelly, P., Holman, S., Rothenberg, R., & Holzemer, S. P. (1995). *Primary care of women and children with HIV infection: A multidisciplinary approach.* Boston: Jones and Bartlett.

This book identifies the many problems women and children with HIV face in obtaining health care and social services.

National Association of County Health Officials. (1993). *Core public health functions.* Washington, DC: Author.

This document identifies the core functions of public health as: assessment of community health status and available resources; policy development, resulting in proposals to support and encourage better health; and assurance that needed services are available.

Newell, M. (1996). *Using nursing case management to improve health outcomes.* Gaithersberg, MD: Aspen Publications.

This book uses many case studies to examine the business and quality of care issues related to case management.

Ripple, J. L., & Holzemer, S. P. (1995, June). *Managed care, volunteers and the new political and financial reality.* Paper presented at the meeting of The National Community Service Conference. Kansas City, MO.

This paper examines the expanded role of volunteer caregivers in the era of managed care. Special methods for supervising volunteers are discussed.

U.S. Department of Health and Human Services. (1994). *Prevention '93/'94: Federal programs and progress.* Washington, DC: Author.

This document explains the national effort: Healthy People 2000. Existing services and proposed solutions to problems are identified for all units of the Public Health Service, Administration on Aging, Administration for Children and Families, and the Health Care Financing Administration.

THE EFFECT OF ACCREDITATION AND PROFESSIONAL CERTIFICATION ON CONTINUITY OF CARE

To foster continuity of care, nurses can become credentialed (certification) and participate in the accreditation of organizations. Certification and accreditation are activities in which nurses and other members of the interdisciplinary team can participate to improve the quality of systems of care; they are processes that denote excellence in how client care needs are met.

This chapter relates the benefits of agency accreditation and care provider certification to continuity of care. Care provider certification and agency accreditation are both marks of excellence that are not considered mandatory activities. These voluntary actions are completed by professionals to increase consumer confidence in the various services provided by the organization or individual nurse.

COMMUNITY HEALTH ACCREDITATION PROGRAM

The Community Health Accreditation Program (CHAP), a subsidiary of the National League for Nursing (NLN), has been accrediting home care and community health organizations since 1965. Accreditation status represents a level of excellence in management and care delivery beyond state regulations or Medicare certification. Accredited organizations can bill for services given to clients receiving Medicare services without undergoing a separate state regulatory visit to assess the quality of services.

Fundamental to the CHAP accreditation philosophy is the belief that voluntary participation in self-evaluation and ongoing quality improvement is the best way to insure high quality health care in the home and community setting. As a result, the first and most important step in the accreditation process requires that the institution enter a period of self-study. Through self-study, the organization profiles its own operations and services, using CHAP standards, which are set by peers in the industry from accredited agencies. The organization issues a report stating how it measures up to national standards.

Organizations seeking accreditation must be committed to the process of change. If the organization does not meet all of the accreditation standards, the staff needs to create a detailed plan for improvement. After corrections are made and the self-study document or report is written, the organization is ready for a site visit for performance evaluation. Site visitors are representatives from similar agencies who verify information detailed in the self-study document for accuracy—that is, the visitors seek evidence that the self-study report correctly reflects the work of the organization.

The key principles of the accreditation process are to evaluate that the organization: (1) has a structure and function that supports its consumer-oriented philosophy and purpose; (2) consistently provides high-quality services and products; (3) has adequate human, financial, and physical resources to do its work; and (4) is positioned for long-term viability.

Site visitors evaluate the facility by reviewing documents, interviewing staff, and meeting with consumers to elicit their opinion on how the organization is meeting their health care needs. Accreditation site visitors also evaluate the organization in terms of the actual care given to clients, monitoring how staff members work together to provide comprehensive interdisciplinary health care. Finally, CHAP site visitors evaluate an organization's financial planning and risk management measures to identify potential threats to fiscal stability and the ability to maintain services.

Organizations receive a full site visit every 3 years when all standards for accreditation are reviewed. Interim unannounced site visits occur every 9 to 15 months to evaluate ongoing compliance with accreditation requirements. These visits may generate the need for progress reports if problems are identified in providing quality care or maintaining the organization's mission.

Final decisions about granting accreditation status is made by a Board of Review. This board, made up of representatives from accredited agencies, reviews observations of site visitors as well as any clarifying material submitted by organizations seeking accreditation. The Board of Review can grant initial or continued accreditation status or decide to defer an accreditation decision. The board can deny accreditation or revoke accreditation status if the agency no longer meets accreditation requirements.

ACCREDITATION AND CONTINUITY OF CARE

Accreditation by CHAP fosters continuity of care because the standards cannot be met adequately without frequent and thorough evaluation of the client services. Quality care is defined holistically by CHAP; it includes all aspects of services and operations from consumer satisfaction and clinical services to long-term financial management and strategic planning.

The process of accreditation fosters interpersonal cooperation within and among disciplines. Entering the self-study process of accreditation shows the staff and administration where work must be coordinated throughout the organization to improve products and services. Managers are able to identify potential problem areas within the agency that need improvement and strengths that need to be reinforced.

Teamwork and respect for other departments or caregivers are fostered because the contributions made by staff, in the process of self-study, are made clear to all participants. Instead of competing for the organization's resources, the employee group learns to work together to conserve resources. Each team member learns the complexities of each program and service and has the opportunity to broaden their perspective. Staff members can develop a feeling of ownership for programs and services outside their area of expertise. Staff see the organization's individual services as a unified complement of services.

In order for the accreditation process to be uniform across the nation, CHAP bases all activities and accreditation decisions on adherence to a set of outcome-based standards. All organizations must complete core standards as well as standards that reflect their services and products.

Successfully accredited organizations, in turn, participate in the regular revision and updating of the standards, thereby defining quality for the industry. For every accreditation cycle, the organization must meet the standards that reflect the services they provide. If an organization has added services since the last site visit, the focus of the next site visit expands to review the added service.

*P*ROGRAM DEVELOPMENT

The accreditation standards of excellence can also be used to develop new services. The situation described below illustrates how a nonaccredited organization can use the outcome-based standards of CHAP to create services that will eventually qualify for the CHAP designation of excellence. The standards are used in program development so that the accreditation process, when the organization seeks it, unfolds smoothly. Staff support the accreditation process because they are familiar with the standards and how to meet them with measurable outcomes. If standards change in the future, the organization makes the necessary changes in their services to meet new requirements.

CASE STUDY: NURSE MANAGERS PLAN FOR EXPANDING SERVICES

Michael Giff, M.A., R.N., Vice President for Nursing and Consumer Relations, meets with nurse managers to plan the addition of home infusion therapy services to their home care business. Mr. Giff uses the CHAP home care standards to orient the other nurse managers to their duties as they accept responsibility for the new service.

Service-Specific Standards

- Professional services
- Paraprofessional services
- Hospice care
- Home infusion therapy
- Home dialysis services
- Home medical equipment (e.g., wheelchairs, infusion pumps)
- Pharmacy services
- Private duty nursing
- Supplemental staffing
- Public health programs
- Community nursing centers

Each manager oversees the development of standards that answer the following questions: How will this service support the consumer-oriented philosophy and purpose of the organization? What effect will this service have on overall quality of care? How are organization resources impacted by this new service? Is long-term viability promoted by adding this service?

As the infusion therapy program is put into place, the nurse managers value the use of the accreditation standards because they keep the staff work groups focused, give different disciplines a common language, assure that the service is client friendly, and provide ongoing feedback to group members about their strengths and limitations in creating a new service.

Accreditation Standards:

- Keep staff focused
- Create a common language among disciplines
- Assure client-friendly services
- Provide staff with ongoing feedback about care delivery

In the scenario above, Nurse Giff decides to plan the addition of home infusion therapy services carefully, using accreditation standards. Table 16-1 identifies the list of standards for home infusion therapy that the organization must adopt to meet the requirements for accreditation. Mr. Giff has prepared the organization to meet all essential criteria when the organization seeks accreditation.

✦

TABLE 16-1

HOME INFUSION THERAPY STANDARDS

The Home Infusion Therapy Program's structure and function consistently support the organization's philosophy and purpose.

- The stated purpose of the Home Infusion Therapy Program supports the overall philosophy and purpose of the organization.
- The Home Infusion Therapy Program is organized to promote its stated purpose.
- A qualified professional is responsible for the direction, coordination, and general supervision of the program.
- The Home Infusion Therapy Program activities reflect the program purpose.

The Home Infusion Therapy Program consistently provides high-quality services and products.

- Infusion therapy services and products are provided, in accordance with program policies, to clients in their place of residence.
- Necessary care is available 24 h a day, 7 days a week, with the ability to respond to clients as follows:
  1. Telephone response within 30 min
  2. On-site response as required within 2 h
  3. Medication and equipment delivery at least 30 min before scheduled use
- Services to clients are coordinated.
- Program-specific policies and procedures covering the scope of services are written and implemented.

(continued)

▧

TABLE 16-1 *(continued)*

- Clinical records contain the following:
    1. Reason for service
    2. Referral source
    3. Diagnosis and prognosis
    4. Appropriateness of the plan of care
    5. Individual(s) to contact in emergency or death
    6. Safety measures
    7. Functional limitations
    8. Physician's name
    9. Client's family database, including physical, psychosocial, and environmental data
    10. Identification of client's problems, plan of treatment, and long- and short-term goals
    11. Medication profile and intravenous procedures performed
    12. Prescribed nursing intervention
    13. Complications
    14. Consent and authorization forms
    15. Identification of and evaluation measure of individual client outcomes
    16. Written indications of any client advance directive
    17. Laboratory results
    18. Pharmacy assessment and reports
    19. Appropriate, current, signed medical orders
    20. Copies of summary reports sent to physician
    21. Timely progress notes, dated and signed by the individual providing the services
- The quality of the infusion therapy services provided is assessed routinely.
- Infection control and safety measures are established and implemented and are a part of every infusion procedure.

The Home Infusion Therapy Program has adequate human, financial, and physical resources effectively organized to accomplish its purpose.
- The Home Infusion Therapy program has adequate, qualified, and experienced intravenous staff.
- The Home Infusion Therapy program has adequate financial resources to support its purpose.

The Home Infusion Therapy Program is positioned for long-term viability.
- The Home Infusion Therapy Program reflects the organizational and program purpose and is integrated into the overall organizational plan (when appropriate).
- The Home Infusion Therapy Program fosters a climate and direction of innovation.

NOTE: From *Standards of Excellence for Infusion Therapy Programs*, by Community Health Accreditation Program, Inc., 1993, New York: Author. Reprinted with permission.

Accreditation is one way for nursing and interdisciplinary care delivery organizations to maintain their social contract with society. Accreditation means that the providers are listening to clients and providing services that people value. The accreditation process also infers that the personnel of the organization accept responsibility for a long-term commitment to providing health care to the community it serves. In times of constrained finances, accreditation is a wise investment for organizations to include in their strategic plan for survival.

In preparation for deciding about entering the accreditation process, the interdisciplinary team must perform a readiness check to see if they have the working skills to be successful in the accreditation process. This assessment relates closely to how well the team functions successfully with case management of clients. Figure 16-1 links the concepts that must be considered prior to entering the accreditation process.

The interdisciplinary team must evaluate how it measures up to these components of case management, accepting responsibility for remediation of its practice if there are deficiencies. Nurse administrators might consider placing these types of behaviors in the job descriptions and annual review assessments of employees to mold a staff that is able to support program goals. Increasingly, case management activities are becoming the core of professional nursing and interdisciplinary practice. The CHAP accreditation process gives care providers a valuable tool to keep their case management services well developed and at a national level of excellence.

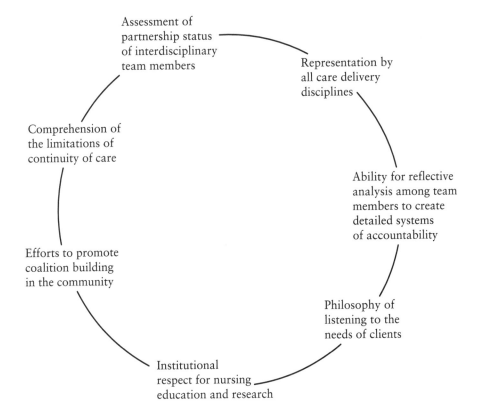

FIGURE 16-1

◙

Critical components of case management as they relate to readiness for accreditation.

CONTINUOUS QUALITY IMPROVEMENT
AND CONTINUITY OF CARE

The Benchmarks Program evaluates:

- Consumer empowerment
- Relationship between consumers and caregivers
- Knowledge or information needed by the consumer
- Family support
- Consumer expectations of the provider

Community-based organizations frequently are looking for ways to document the quality of their services. Competition makes sharing of information at times unlikely. The Benchmarks Program entitled *Benchmarks for Excellence in Home Care* developed by CHAP (1996) allows organizations to track the outcomes of their services and thereby assess their strengths and weaknesses on an ongoing basis. The Benchmarks Program directs administration and staff to the areas where quality improvement efforts need ongoing development and improvement.

Continuous quality improvement programs are important to organizations because they generate feedback from every department within the organization and tie them all to the quality of the service delivery. All members of the organization own the services that are provided to the public. Provision of quality services becomes more important because the services are reviewed in part from the consumers' perspective.

The Benchmarks Program monitors aspects of consumer satisfaction through a series of carefully tested questionnaires designed in response to the unique nature of home care. These questionnaires track elements of a consumer's experience of satisfaction with clinical, educational, and general psychosocial exchanges between the consumer and the clinician(s). Results of the questionnaires also reflect other aspects of the organization's operations, which are necessary to support quality consumer services.

In addition to evaluation of consumer satisfaction, the Benchmarks Program also includes questionnaires and data collection protocols to cap-

◙

TABLE 16-2

BENCHMARK VARIABLES

Clinical Services Includes the recording of vital signs, personal care, provision of activities of daily living (ADLs), and other behavioral outcomes. Comparisons will show the effects of clinical interventions by measuring the health status on admission and any changes that have occurred at the time of discharge.

Empirical Indicators of Consumer's Functional Ability Includes whether consumers are able to carry out their ADLs to the extent they are capable and/or to the extent that these activities are consistent with their goals.

Physiological Indicators of Consumer's Functional Ability Includes whether consumers attain the physical health status (physiological functioning) of which they are capable.

Organizational Dynamics Measures team building, staff-wide commitment to quality, and coordination of care.

Financial Management Includes liquidity ratios and calculations, profitability ratios and calculations, viability-score calculation (V-score), efficiency ratings, productivity ratios, cost, and utilization comparisons.

Risk Management Includes infection rate monitoring, claims management and recognition, injury occurrence, incident reporting, potential malpractice issues, financial management, contract execution and review, adverse drug reactions, and medication errors.

ture the outcomes of other services throughout the organization. These data collectors are specific enough to provide detailed maps of all organizational divisions, and interrelated enough to provide a whole picture of the organization as a single entity. The Benchmark Program evaluates the relationship between consumers and caregivers, through an extensive review of clinical services, organizational functioning, financial management, and risk management as indicated in Table 16-2.

The Benchmark Program is different from the CHAP accreditation process. Although both address quality of services, an organization might participate in the Benchmark Program prior to accreditation or between accreditation cycles. The Benchmark Program offers more frequent quality checks and assurance that services are meeting client needs on an ongoing basis.

PROFESSIONAL CERTIFICATION

Professional nurses working in the community are registered in the state in which they practice as basic safe care providers. In actuality, the nurse is a basic safe practitioner, as measured by the National Council Licensure Exam (NCLEX-RN), on the day the exam is administered. In many states without mandatory continuing education regulations, it is possible that a nurse will never be required to update his or her knowledge base after graduation.

Professional certification is a measure of personal expertise and is sought by the professional nurse voluntarily. Certification is available from various professional organizations and in different clinical specialties. Some of the certifications accomplished by nurses are identified below.

The American Nurses Credentialing Center, a subsidiary of the American Nurses Association (ANA) is the largest credentialing organization for nursing. Nurses are certified initially and then are recertified every 5 years. Certification reflects an ongoing effort by the nurse to stay competent at an expert level of practice.

Nurses with bachelor's preparation in nursing can be certified as a community health nurse (generalist). These nurses demonstrate an understanding of public health and nursing problems as they relate to the community. Nurses with graduate preparation in nursing or public health can be certified as a clinical specialist in community health nursing. Clinical specialists are considered experts in community health practice as well as the research and education needed to resolve community health problems. The American Academy of Nurse Practitioners (1996) credentials adult and family nurse practitioners, also called advanced practice nurses; these nurses frequently work with community health nurses in many settings.

Nurses can also be credentialed as certified case managers. The Commission for Case Manager Certification (1992) recognizes nurses in their independent practice of assessment, planning, implementing, coordination, monitoring, and evaluation of health care services. Nurses seeking credentialing must demonstrate that they are directly involved in coordination

---

TABLE 16-3

EXAMPLES OF CASE MANAGEMENT CORE AREAS
FOR CERTIFICATION

Coordination and Service Delivery
- Understands restrictions on the release of confidential information
- Assesses clinical information to develop treatment plans

Physical and Psychological Factors
- Acts as an advocate for an individual's health care needs
- Assists individuals with the development of short- and long-term health goals

Benefit Systems and Cost-Benefit Analysis
- Understands requirements for prior approval by payer
- Understands home health resources

Case Management Concepts
- Documents case management activities
- Develops case management plans that address the individual's needs

Community Resources
- Understands the Americans with Disabilities Act
- Knows how to establish a client's support system

NOTE: From *CCM Certification Guide: Certified Case Manager* (pp. 5, 6), by Commission for Case Manager Certification, 1992, Rolling Meadows, IL: Author. Reprinted with permission.

and service delivery, understand physical and psychological aspects of care, have explored benefit systems and cost-benefit analysis, apply case management concepts, and accurately use community resources.

SUMMARY

Continuity of care is affected by accreditation of organizations as well as professional certification of nurses. In both situations, criteria are met to identify excellence of services in an organization and the excellence of nursing practice. Certification and accreditation are obtained when an organization or an individual meet nationally set standards.

Accreditation is a process of self-study directed at program improvement. Participating organizations meet nationally set standards created by other providers of excellent quality services. Organizations write a self-study report and have qualified visitors verify services and recommend accreditation status. Reaccreditation occurs on cycles for an ongoing review of services.

Continuous quality improvement is another way to demonstrate excellence. The Benchmarks Program entitled *Benchmarks for Excellence in Home Care* developed by CHAP allows organizations to compare their services with other businesses in the areas of consumer satisfaction, clinical services, coordination of staff and management functioning, financial management, and risk management. The Benchmarks Program is used by some organizations to prepare for the accreditation process or assess their quality status between accreditation cycles.

Nurses can be certified in general, specialized, and advanced practice. Certification is a credential that suggests that the standard of practice of the nurse is of highest quality. Recertification is required at time intervals set by the profession. Nursing as a profession has set an example for other care providers in evaluating its practice for excellence and ongoing quality improvement when necessary.

KEY WORDS

Accreditation	Certification
Board of review	Site visitors

QUESTIONS

DIRECTIONS: Choose the one *best* response to each of the following questions.

1. The overall focus of accreditation is to influence improvements in

   A. client outcomes.
   B. organizational politics.
   C. development of standards.
   D. provider skill in care delivery.

2. Professional certification denotes

   A. safe and prudent clinical practice.
   B. adherence to agency policies.
   C. expert care delivery.
   D. completion of an academic degree program.

3. One of the benefits of agency accreditation for the various staff members is

   A. improving competition between departments.
   B. fostering team building.
   C. allowing independent decision-making.
   D. creating objectives for short-term survival.

ANSWERS

1. *The answer is A.* Accreditation is completed with the goal to improve client outcomes.

2. *The answer is C.* Certification denotes expert clinical practice at a generalist or specialist level.

3. *The answer is B.* Team building is a major benefit of accreditation for the staff of the organization.

ANNOTATED REFERENCES

American Academy of Nurse Practitioners. (1996). *National competency-based certification examinations*. Austin, TX: Author.

The Academy certifies graduates by approved master's level adult and family nurse practitioners. Information can be obtained by calling (512) 442-4262.

American Nurses Credentialing Center. (1996). *Certification catalog*. Washington, DC: Author.

The Center credentials nurses in 26 practice areas. Information on certification can be obtained by calling (800) 264-CERT (2378).

Case Management Society of America. (1995). *Standards of practice for care management*. Little Rock, AR: Author.

These standards for care management can be applied to various clinical settings. Standards of practice relate to: case identification and selection, identification of problems, planning, monitoring, evaluating, and outcomes.

Commission for Case Manager Certification. (1992). *CCM certification guide: Certified case manager*. Rolling Meadows, IL: Author.

The process for case manager certification is clearly explained. Applications can be obtained from the Commission by calling (847) 818-0292. The examination covers the knowledge areas of: coordination of service delivery, physical and psychological factors, benefit systems and cost-benefit analysis, case management concepts, and community resources.

Community Health Accreditation Program, Inc. (1996). *Benchmarks for excellence in home care: User's guide*. New York: Author.

This computerized program allows for the collection of data to create an ongoing quality improvement project. Benchmarks focus on consumer, clinical, organizational, financial, and risk management.

Community Health Accreditation Program, Inc. (1993). *Standards of excellence for home care organizations*. New York: Author.

The standards, in ongoing development since 1965, are divided into these categories: core, professional, paraprofessional, hospice, infusion therapy, home medical equipment, and pharmacy. The major themes of the accreditation program are: quality, rights of consumers, long-term viability of services, and integration of community-based services into the total sum of health care services. More information on accreditation can be obtained by calling (800) 669-9656.

Community Health Accreditation Program, Inc. (1993). *Standards of excellence for infusion therapy programs*. New York: Author.

These service-specific standards identify exactly how providers can meet the requirements for accreditation in this area.

Re-ENGINEERING THE NURSING PROFESSION FOR SURVIVAL IN ONGOING CARE DELIVERY SYSTEMS

Economic market forces continue to influence how health professionals do their work (Reinhardt, 1996). Nurses and other providers care for clients with increasingly complex health problems with the same or fewer resources. In addition, most nurses in practice have not been educated in community-based care; this preparation has historically been reserved for nurses with baccalaureate and higher degrees. Nurses must examine their ability to continue in their mission to provide appropriate health care to people (Rawnsley, 1990), where and when they need it (National League for Nursing, 1993).

The focus of this chapter is to plan re-engineering strategies for the future marketability of undergraduate and advanced practice (i.e., graduate, clinical nursing degree) nurses for work in community-based settings. The concepts relate to nurses in practice as well as students of the profession. The focus of re-engineering is to tie education to safe practice so practitioners can do their work safely (American Association of Colleges of Nursing, 1995).

Traditionally, nursing education and nursing care delivery have not always worked closely together. Some argue that for a practice discipline, nursing education has become too theoretical and nursing care delivery too technical. This problematic relationship between the theoretical and the technical orientations to nursing must be resolved so that the nursing profession can continue to meet the needs of clients effectively.

A more reciprocal and cooperative relationship is needed between nursing care delivery and education (Pew Health Professions Commission, 1993), as with all other health-related disciplines. Partnerships are needed in order to conserve resources while still giving appropriate care (Anderson & McFarlane, 1996). The concept of alliances, introduced in Chap. 5, is central to changes in nursing care delivery, research, and education. Alliances suggest a mutual contribution by the client and the nurse in health care decision-making.

ℬASIC NURSING PREPARATION

Changes in Care Delivery and Research

Managed care programs have permeated all aspects of nursing care delivery. These programs present a dilemma for nursing because they are accused of undercutting many aspects of quality assurance in the name of cost containment. Providing services at the lowest cost is a philosophy that is predictably at odds with the idea of comprehensive quality services. In order to maintain quality in managed care and other settings, nurses need theoretical and clinical competence in:

* Health promotion and prevention of illness on an aggregate level of care
* Computer literacy
* Interdisciplinary collaboration and shared decision making
* Philosophy and ethics of managed care
* Management of resources for high-technology care as well as low-technology care
* Supervision of ancillary personnel and proper delegation
* Fiduciary risks and responsibilities of community-based care

[National League for Nursing, 1993; American Nurses Association (ANA), 1995; Hart, 1995; Holzemer, 1995].

Managing groups of people to meet their health needs is a major opportunity for nursing. It is an opportunity for nurses to keep the concepts of quality and safety of care central to any health care discussion about care delivery. Instead of fighting managed care, nurses should embrace the opportunity for creating new systems of care that meet the needs of their clients. In order to enter the debate concerning which health care service will be available to the public, nurses must develop plans of care that are collaborative, outcome-specific, and consumer-friendly.

Recommended reforms to guarantee competence and accountability for health care professionals are reflected in the *SAFE vision* acronym, which translates: "standardized where appropriate; accountable to the public; flexible to support optimal access to a competent work force; and effective and efficient in protecting and promoting the public's health, safety and welfare" (The Center for the Health Professions, 1996, p. 8).

Changes in Education

In many areas, nursing education continues to prepare students for work in a hospital-like setting. Some educators equate legitimate learning experiences with those in a high-technology environment, and unfortunately, some faculty members and graduates see community-based care merely as an add-on to the acute care, hospital-based curriculum. Some faculty also see community-based experiences as detracting from the essential core of nursing as practiced in acute care settings. How will nursing have a future

SAFE Vision

Standardized
Accountable
Flexible
Effective/Efficient

⊠

TABLE 17-1

NECESSARY CHARACTERISTICS OF NURSING CARE

Collaborative

Nursing is expected to work well with other disciplines providing services. Nurses need to examine how they can become team players, collaborating with other care providers.

Outcome-Specific

Nursing needs to connect its services to measurable outcomes that other disciplines and the public understand, like decreased length of stay. Nursing services would be valued more if people could see the impact of services.

Consumer-Friendly

The public views nursing in a positive light but does not really understand what nursing is or does as a discipline. Nursing needs to become more consumer-friendly so the public demands good nursing care.

---

in care delivery if nurses are not educated for the realities of the practice arena? How can we help students of nursing learn (Kohl, 1991)?

Employers in community agencies often require previous medical-surgical experience, which reinforces the primacy of hospital-based care. With hospitals and medical centers downsizing, it is unclear where students are expected to get their medical-surgical experience. What changes are necessary in nursing education so graduate nurses are prepared to move directly into the community arena after graduation? It is safe to assume that every nursing school is examining how it prepares graduates in such a time of turbulent change in health care delivery.

Learning How to Manage Care

One problem in nursing education is that nurses are expected to manage care after graduation, but they do not get sufficient (if any) experience in care management during their formal education. Consideration should be given to having nursing students manage a group of clients with a variety of clinical problems. Nurses need to develop interpersonal rapport with the clients with whom they work to get health care needs met. The following situation explores a significant client-nurse relationship.

CASE STUDY: MARGARET WANTS THE SAME COMMUNITY HEALTH NURSE TO PROVIDE CARE TO HER FAMILY

"I hate calling the Ambulatory Care Department; you could be dying and they act like it is your first time calling. I always ask to speak to Edward, the community health nurse, and go to the clinic when he is on the schedule. It is so important to have a nurse who knows you. . . . Even if I was real sick, I would wait until Ed was back in the clinic. The other nurses are nice enough, but if they do not know you, you might as well not even go to the clinic."

The community health nurse in a similar situation needs to talk to her or his clients to clarify roles so that the clients do not delay getting necessary care when the nurse is not available. Nurses and students need to learn how to work with clients like Margaret and her family in a long-term care experience. They need to learn the parameters of ongoing support that are needed while managing clients, parameters that are very different from those needed for one-day assignments to visit clients or to observe care.

To manage clients safely, at both the basic and advanced levels of practice, nurses should be taught a wide range of skills that will most likely be needed by all practitioners in the future. Two important skills are working in community-based organizations and working with unlicensed assistive personnel.

Community-Based Organizations (CBOs) CBOs, growing providers of physical, emotional, and culturally competent care, are developing rapidly across the country. Students must be educated in these types of agencies to learn how decentralized, consumer-managed health care services are provided. Many schools of nursing limit student experiences in community health to acute, home care experiences supervised by the community health nursing faculty. This is not helpful in providing students with a broad base of exposure to CBOs, the sites where increasingly more wellness and health promoting activities are provided.

Unlicensed Assistive Personnel (UAPs) The movement toward embracing UAPs or technicians in lieu of nurses in the work force is due, in part, to the fact that many nurses are out of step with what the health care system needs. At one time, the health care system rewarded specialization. In response to this situation, nurses focused their time on developing and providing an increasingly narrow list of activities. These specialized services came to represent professional nursing.

Currently, health care employers are seeking flexible, multiskilled workers at a time when some nurses are fixated on providing only those services that are identified in their employment contract. Nursing needs to reclaim a generalist perspective for part of their practice. Nurses can secure a place in future care systems if they are willing to work in teams to provide whatever care is necessary to meet the needs of clients.

Future changes in the practice of nursing can be done without the fear of losing professional integrity. Nurses actively engaged in developing future roles for nurses will secure control over nursing practice. Nurses need to embrace prudent delegation and supervision as a way to stay active in controlling nursing practice in care settings (ANA, 1995). Avoiding or refusing to work within the current economic realities is the greatest threat to nursing's professional status.

Some nurses are stalled in their professional development because they view nursing as a job instead of a profession. These nurses often choose not to continue learning or expanding their practice opportunities. They are not major players in emerging health care systems because they are not major players in their professional development or in the nursing profession.

Pew Health Commission Competencies   The Pew Health Professions Commission (1993) competencies for future practitioners are ideal for curriculum revision in professional schools and staff development departments. These competencies are appealing because they were developed by a multidisciplinary team of health care professionals; they transcend any one clinical specialty or theoretical orientation to nursing. The competencies reflect a common voice spanning disciplines related to the need for future providers.

The competencies are a functional tool for curriculum revision because they give faculty a common language unrelated to the specialty turf conflicts. Educators who value medical-surgical content will not compete for time with faculty teaching developing-family content. All educators look to how they can improve clinical and classroom teaching from a new perspective.

The Pew competencies foster a revolutionary way of looking at what should be taught to students in a constantly changing, relationship-centered health care delivery system. The 17 competencies listed in Table 17-2 can be used to guide faculty dialogue and focus all curricular discussions.

▣

TABLE 17-2

THE PEW COMMISSION COMPETENCIES FOR FUTURE PRACTITIONERS
FOR THE YEAR 2005

The nurse of the future will need to:

1. Care for the community's health
2. Expand access to effective care
3. Provide contemporary clinical care
4. Emphasize primary care
5. Participate in coordinated care
6. Ensure cost-effective and appropriate care
7. Practice prevention
8. Involve patients and families in the decision-making process
9. Promote healthy life styles
10. Assess and use technology appropriately
11. Improve the health care system
12. Manage information
13. Understand the role of the physical environment
14. Provide counseling on ethical issues
15. Accommodate expanded accountability
16. Participate in a racially and culturally diverse society
17. Continue to learn

SOURCE: From *Contemporary Issues of Health Professions Education and Workforce Reform*, by Pew Health Professions Commission, 1993, San Francisco: Author. Reprinted with permission.

Practitioners and educators need to work together to create the appropriate mix of theoretical and practical skills for students in the future. Clinical experts from the clinical arena need to be on curriculum committees to keep them working from a "hands-on" perspective.

𝒜DVANCED NURSING PREPARATION

Changes in Care Delivery and Research

Advanced Nursing Practice Advanced nursing practice is defined by Styles (1996) as expert practice with emphasis on a specific population matrix (e.g., community health or primary care), requiring expanded skills and knowledge. The bottom line in such practice is the two-pronged notion that the advanced practice role requires both *accountability* and *responsibility* in regard to determinations that are made and subsequent clinical actions. More complex clinical issues can be managed because the nurse in the advanced practice role has the knowledge and expertise to make independent, sound clinical judgments and decisions.

The roles of advanced nursing practice include: *nurse practitioner (NP), clinical nurse specialist (CNS), certified registered nurse anesthetist (CRNA),* and *certified nurse midwife* (CNM). The advanced nursing practice roles require educational preparation that includes a master's degree in clinical nursing. Increasingly, the master's degree prepared *case manager* is viewed as an advanced nursing practice role.

Advanced Practice Nurse and **Advanced Nursing Practice.** The advanced practice nurse is educated at the master's level to function as a certified nurse midwife, a nurse practitioner, a clinical nurse specialist, or a certified registered nurse anesthetist. Increasingly, case managers are considered advanced practice nurses. The level of practice responsibilities is called advanced nursing practice.

Advanced Practice Nursing Advanced practice nursing refers to the *occupational niche* of the nurse working in advanced nursing practice. Advanced practice nurses deliver care in a variety of settings from the more traditional avenues of home and hospital to changing environments, including school-based clinics, mobile and stationary clinics, and private as well as public office settings. Just as the location of care delivery has changed, so too has the general mechanism for delivering that care.

Research dealing with care delivery by advanced practice nurses has been key to supporting, and indeed suggesting, these changed locations and mechanisms for care delivery. McGuire and Harwood (1989) assert that research dealing with trends in health care delivery points toward how and where advanced practice nurses practice their skills. Clearly, the evolvement of advanced practice derives from health care outcomes research with the continuing evolvement of advanced practice giving direction to that research.

Largely because of both research and clinical practice demands, the level of expansion of practice differs for each advanced practice nursing specialty. These practice parameters differ from one provincial or state board of nursing regulation to another in Canada and the United States. Research should provide guidelines for clinical practice expectations across state and province boundaries.

Research examining advanced practice outcomes supports validation for the practice domain of each advanced practice nursing specialty. For example, the certified registered nurse anesthetist uses protocols based on sound scientific evidence in managing preoperative and intraoperative anesthesia selection, administration, monitoring, and evaluation as well as immediate postoperative analgesia. This role is quite different from that of the nurse practitioner, whose practice's focus may be either acute care (generally hospital or intensive care) or primary care.

In contrast, the certified nurse midwife diagnoses and manages uncomplicated pregnancies through delivery and the postpartum periods. Many certified nurse midwives also practice in the area of women's health. The case manager may practice in either an institutional or home health setting. This advanced practice nurse coordinates care delivery with the primary goal of providing cost-effective medical, nursing, and other health vendors' services to clients in a timely and humane manner.

The clinical nurse specialist is a skilled and proficient advanced practice nurse whose practice base encompasses clinical specialization in an area (e.g., eating disorders) as well as formalized expertise in education, consultation, and research in nursing and an area of specialization as with other advanced practice nurses.

The clinical nurse specialist functions as a clinical leader, spearheading and facilitating change in many clinical settings. The clinical nurse specialist collaborates with others in these practice endeavors, acting as an advocate for clients, be they patients or nurses. The clinical nurse specialist is, thus, a powerful role model, a nontraditional nurse with expanded boundaries (Hamric & Taylor, 1989).

Many clinical nurse specialists are moving into insurance and reimbursement businesses as case managers because of their specialized skill in understanding the level of care patients need after they leave the hospital. Many clinical nurse specialists use their skills to follow cohorts of patients in and out of multiple care settings.

Focus on Promoting Primary Care Research

Scholars, practitioners, and the public are united in recognizing the need for well-articulated, rigorous research in the areas of health policy, health care needs, as well as in cost containment. More than this research agenda is needed if advanced practice in nursing is to thrive in the health care sector. Multiple studies have been done that support advanced practice nurses as delivering health care, including primary care, at a consistently high level and at substantial cost savings to health care consumers.

With the inevitable onset and projected growth of managed care delivery systems in our society, however, research by advanced practice nurses that focuses on demonstrated improvements in consumers' health care outcomes must occur. Care delivery standards must be set in this evolving managed care system, and it is essential that advanced practice nurses are players in this work. The active involvement of advanced practice nurses in standard settings assures that nursing practice is not unduly influenced by business, managed care systems, or other professional disciplines like medicine.

The questions facing nursing about the ongoing changes in the health care system are too complex for simple answers. The logical solution is to involve all levels of health care providers in undertaking interdisciplinary research. This solution provides all players with a voice in designing and implementing a national research agenda. This approach will more realistically address complex health care delivery challenges for nursing and other disciplines.

An interdisciplinary focus to care and research can better guide the development of standards of care that build on valid and reliable practice competencies. Competencies are created and demonstrated by each practice discipline. They must result in proven, cost-effective health care outcomes, as well as direct the creation of health care services that are capable of meeting the health needs of the public.

Core competencies have developed for advanced practice programs in nursing to provide consistency in program offerings. The Alliance for Health Model, introduced in Chapter 5 suggests that core competencies in advanced practice need to focus on: (1) the needs of the community, (2) systems of care management, (3) the influences on resource allocation, (4) the functioning of the interdisciplinary team, and (5) the validation of services by the client.

Changes in Education

Education for advanced practice in nursing has changed greatly over the last century. The first advanced practice nurse trained in 1877, Sister Mary Bernard, worked as a nurse anesthetist at St. Vincent's Hospital in Erie, Pennsylvania (Bankert, 1989). Nurses in advanced practice roles were commonly "trained" rather than educated up until the 1970s, when graduate education in nursing in the United States and Canada became more readily available to nurses outside of the metropolitan areas.

In the last quarter of the 20th century, it has become increasingly clear that advanced practice cannot occur through "training," nor is the baccalaureate degree sufficient for either the knowledge base or practice credibility required of this role. The nursing profession has designated that the master's degree in nursing be the minimum credential awarded for new advanced practice programs. Graduate preparation in nursing provides the practitioner with the theoretical and scientific basis for undertaking research-based practice.

Focus on Interdisciplinary Education

Education in the advanced practice arena during the 1960s and 1970s was an interdisciplinary endeavor. Medical students attended lectures and participated in patient rounds and clinical learning activities alongside their nurse practitioner student peers. The outcomes of these interdisciplinary education and practice models proved beneficial to all parties involved, namely clients, families, communities served, and the practitioners themselves.

The interdisciplinary endeavor, developed and refined over a 20-year period in the 1960s and 1970s, was abandoned in the spirit of professional isolationism, which arose in the 1980s. Historically, this was a period when health care disciplines "circled the wagons," not out of professional protectionism but, rather, out of a spirit of professional elitism.

Current financial constraints under which nurses have grown used to operating in health care were not concerns during the 1970s and 1980s. In addition, the nation faced a shortage of nurses, physicians, and allied health professionals. The times were right for each discipline's belief that it could justify its role in the duplication of educational efforts. So what had formerly been interdisciplinary in didactic and clinical learning endeavors became separate and isolated for each discipline.

Educational isolation and separation are being revisited in the 1990s. Health care delivery needs to be streamlined in these fiscally constrained times. To avoid waste and duplication, all health care disciplines need to come back together again, as was done in the experimental spirit of the 1960s, to create interdisciplinary educational and clinical practice models. These models will help providers better serve both student constituencies as well as health care consumers. Research is needed in this area to identify the best educational linkages for student learning among and between professions.

Summary

The nursing profession is changing as health care systems enter the third millennium. The historic separation between nursing education and care delivery is ending. Nurses at both the undergraduate and graduate (advanced practice) levels are re-engineering their practices for community-based care settings.

Changes are being made in continuing and formal nursing education programs to augment the learning of contemporary nursing care delivery and discover the type of health care clients' find important (Micozzi, 1996; Pew Health Professions Commission, 1995; Williams & Wold, 1996). Nursing has the opportunity to play a key role in the development of new care delivery systems.

KEY WORDS

Advanced nursing practice
Advanced practice nursing
Primary care research

QUESTIONS

DIRECTIONS: Choose the one *best* response to each of the following questions:

1. The most cost-effective area where nurses need to demonstrate competence is
   A. health promotion.
   B. management of high-technology resources.
   C. supervision of ancillary personnel.
   D. computer record keeping.

2. The major reason the nursing profession should work closely with unlicensed assistive personnel is to
   A. make sure they complete their assignments.
   B. report any acts of malpractice.
   C. protect the professional practice of nursing.
   D. suggest where more responsibilities can be accepted.

3. A multidisciplinary team is one in which
   A. nurses choose with whom they want to work.
   B. physicians make decisions about who is on each team for each client.
   C. the needs of clients dictate who is on the team.
   D. clients who pay privately can create their own teams.

4. An advanced practice nurse specializing in the care of clients receiving agents to cause nerve blocks and numbing of surgical areas is called a(n)
   A. circulating nurse.
   B. surgical physician's assistant.
   C. operating room nurse.
   D. nurse anesthetist.

ANSWERS

1. *The answer is A.* Prevention of health problems is always less expensive than treating illness.

2. *The answer is C.* Professional nursing practice can only be protected by nursing and nurses. People practicing nursing without a license should be reported to the State Board of Nursing in each state.

3. *The answer is C.* The needs of clients dictate the members needed on the interdisciplinary team.

4. *The answer is D.* Nurse anesthetists are advanced practice nurses who monitor sedation and pain relief related to surgery. They work independently yet collaboratively with their physician counterparts, anesthesiologists.

ANNOTATED REFERENCES

American Nurses Association. (1995). *The ANA basic guide to safe delegation*. Washington, DC: Author.

This pamphlet identifies issues of delegation that professionals must consider as they delegate to unlicensed personnel.

American Association of Colleges of Nursing. (1995). *A model for differentiated nursing practice*. Washington, DC: Author.

This text compares the complexity of nursing care with the various programs educating nurses. The model would have associate degree graduates providing the least complex care, the baccalaureate graduates next, and the master's degree graduates providing the most complex care.

Anderson, E. T., & McFarlane, J. M. (1996). *Community as partner: Theory and practice in nursing* (2nd ed.). Philadelphia: J. B. Lippincott.

This textbook examines the potential relationships between nurses and clients as partners in creating solutions to health-related problems.

Bankert, M. (1989). *Watchful care: A history of America's nurse anesthetists*. New York: Continuum.

This book highlights the evolvement of the nurse anesthesia movement from 1877 to the late 20th century.

Hart, S. (1995). *Managed care curriculum for baccalaureate nursing programs*. Washington, DC: American Nurses Publishing.

Key areas of content are identified that should be included in baccalaureate nursing programs.

Hamric, A. B., & Taylor, J. W. (1989). Role development of the clinical nurse specialist. In A. B. Hamric & J. A. Spross (Eds.), *The clinical nurse specialist in theory and practice* (p. 43). Philadelphia: W. B. Saunders.

This text examines the role of the clinical nurse specialist.

Holzemer, S. P. (1995). CCHS confronts issues in community-based and managed care. *NLN Update, 1*(1), 5.

The results of a conference of educators and care providers called for a shift toward a more business approach to nursing care in the community.

Kohl, H. (1991). *I won't learn from you!* Minneapolis: Milkweed Editions.

Failure in education is explored in this text about common problems in the teaching–learning process.

McGuire, D. B. & Harwood, K. V. (1996). Research interpretation, utilization, and conduct. In A. B. Hamric, J. A. Spross, and C. M. Hanson (Eds.), *Advanced nursing practice: An integrative approach*. Philadelphia: W. B. Saunders.

This chapter delineates research competencies needed by advanced practice nurses for use in their many complex clinical roles.

Micozzi, M. S. (1996, August 16). The need to teach alternative medicine. *The Chronicle of Higher Education*, p. A48.

This editorial encourages educators to teach students about alternative medicine because clients are choosing to use this form of healing.

National League for Nursing. (1993). *A vision for nursing education.* New York: Author.

The essential changes necessary for nursing to adapt or mold to emerging nursing systems are identified.

Pew Health Professions Commission. (1993). *Contemporary issues of health professions education and workforce reform.* San Francisco: Author.

This report discusses 13 issues facing the health professions in contemporary practice.

Pew Health Professions Commission, California Primary Care Consortium. (1995). *Interdisciplinary collaborative teams in primary care: A model curriculum and resource guide.* San Francisco: Author.

A variety of concerns that relate to interdisciplinary collaborative teams are discussed in this reference. Of special interest are the case studies for interdisciplinary problem-solving.

Rawnsley, M. (1990). Of human bonding: The context of nursing as caring. *Advances in Nursing Science*, 13(1),41–48.

This article examines the meaning of the construct of nursing as a professional prerogative. The metaphor and meaning of caring are examined as they relate to nursing care delivery in the lived experience.

Reinhardt, U. E. (1996). Economics. *Journal of the American Medical Association*, 275(23), 1802–1804.

Health care markets as with other markets ration by price and ability to pay. The article questions the "choice" in many care programs when clients are not able to negotiate for the care they want.

Styles, M. M. (1996). Conceptualizations of Advanced Nursing Practice. In A. B. Hamric, J. A. Spross, & C. M. Hanson (Eds.), *Advanced nursing practice*. Philadelphia: W. B. Saunders.

This book describes the semantics of advanced practice nursing versus advanced nursing practice.

The Center for Health Professions. (1996). What's the fuss? Front & Center, 1(1), 8.

The Center for Health Professions at the University of California, San Francisco was created to assist health care professionals cope with changes in education and the health care work force. For more information about the services of the center call (414) 476-8181.

Williams, A., & Wold, J. L. (1996). Healthcare for the future: Caring for populations in alternative settings. *Nurse Educator*, 21(2), 23–26.

The shift to community-based settings for student learning is the focus of this article. The use of alternative settings is suggested to support the goals of Healthy People 2000.

THE BUSINESS AND POLITICS OF COMMUNITY HEALTH NURSING

❧

ℬUSINESS OF COMMUNITY HEALTH

One of the most difficult concepts for nurses to grasp is the concept that health care is a business. For many nurses, health care and business are contradictory terms. Nurses view health care as a giving, caring, nurturing fundamental right of those clients with whom they come in contact. Business, on the other hand, is viewed as a cold, calculating, profit-driven, dollars and cents enterprise.

Most nurses in the United States are salaried employees. They report to work, care for their clients, and collect the same pay check regardless of the number of clients they have seen. They rarely get involved in the business side of care. However, today, as more nurses are affected by the business of re-engineering, downsizing, and issues of reimbursement (e.g., preauthorization from insurance companies), they have been forced to examine the business side of health care.

Some of the questions that nurses should be posing today are: Who should be looking at the business side of health care? Who is the largest group of professionals in the health care delivery system? Who understands how care should be delivered? Who knows where the waste is in the system? Who advocates for clients' rights? Who explains the health care system to clients? Who knows how, when, and where care should be delivered? Who sees what effects re-engineering and downsizing are having on the delivery of care? Nurses have always been strong client advocates, and they have always been concerned about the quality and access to care. Thus, why is it that nurses do not have more of a say about how our health care system is run, about who is running it, and how the profits are being spent?

The largest industry in the United States is the health care industry. It serves the greatest portion of the population and represents 14 percent of the gross national product (GNP). The Bureau of Labor Statistics (BLS) reports that the health care industry employs the most workers (8,871,000). The American Nurses Association (ANA) reports that nurses form the largest group of professionals employed in this industry (ANA, *Nursing Facts*, 1995).

The fastest growing segment of the health care industry is community health, and nursing has been the cornerstone of community health since the late 1800s. In this chapter, the business of community health is examined, including the different forms a business can take and the differences between "for-profit" and "not-for-profit" organizations. This chapter discusses what community health is, and how, where, and by whom health care is delivered in the community. It also focuses on home care, the fastest growing segment of the community health business. This chapter identifies the major players in the health care field, the largest industry in America, the profits of this industry, and the major recipients of these profits. Finally, the business of community health is examined from an entrepreneurial perspective complete with "how-to" steps.

*B*USINESS: WHAT IS IT?

Enterprise a term often applied to a newly formed venture.

Barron's Business Guide defines business as "a commercial **enterprise**, profession, or trade operated for the purpose of earning a profit by providing a product or service" (Friedman, 1987, p. 193). Businesses are created by entrepreneurs who put money at risk to promote a particular venture for the purpose of earning a profit. They vary in size from a single-person proprietorship to an international corporation with billions of dollars in assets and thousand of employees. *Webster's* defines business as "an activity engaged in as normal, logical, or inevitable, usually over a considerable amount of time, directed toward some end. It can be a commercial activity engaged in as a means of livelihood and typically involving some independence of judgment and decision-making" (Gove, 1976, p. 302). Perhaps with this definition in mind, nursing can be viewed as a business. For nurses, delivering care is the normal, logical, and usually inevitable activity in which they engage when someone needs their services. For most nurses, it is a means of livelihood, and nursing care typically involves some independence of judgment and the need to make decisions. Some nurses have taken the business of caring to the next level; they have put money at risk to promote a particular venture for the purpose of earning a living.

Types of Businesses

Businesses may be classified as unincorporated (e.g., a sole proprietorship) or a partnership (e.g., general or limited), or incorporated (e.g., not-for-profit or for-profit).

Sole Proprietorship Sole proprietorship is the simplest form of organization because it is a business that is owned and operated by one person. It is easy to form and just as easy to sell or dissolve. A sole proprietor pays a personal income tax on all business income (i.e., the business does not pay taxes) and is allowed to set up an individual retirement account (IRA). The sole proprietor has complete control over the business or practice. Many private nursing practices are set up as sole proprietorships (e.g., psychotherapists, nurse practitioners). There are disadvantages, however. The sole proprietor is personally responsible for all debts. Personal assets, such as a home, bank accounts, stocks, bonds, boats, and cars may be seized in lieu of payment of debts. Also, after a sale of the business or practice, profits are not considered **capital gains** but ordinary income and are taxed as such.

Capital Gains. This is a profit on a securities or capital transaction when the interval between purchase and sale is longer than 6 months.

Partnership A partnership is defined as an organization of two or more persons who pool some or all of their money, abilities, and skills in a business and divide the profit or loss in predetermined proportions. This organization is a legal relationship. The two most common kinds of partnerships are general and limited.

General Partnership In a general partnership, the liability of a partner is unlimited. Each partner is liable for the business's debts and for the actions of the other partners. In this type of partnership, each partner is involved in the day-to-day operations of the company. Many professionals, such as nurse practitioners, clinical nurse specialists, physicians, physical therapists, and attorneys set up their practices as general partnerships.

Limited Partnership In a limited partnership, the liability is limited to the amount of the limited partners' investment, and typically, a limited or "silent partner" receives a share of the business profits in return for the investment. Limited partners have no right to participate in the management and operation of the business. A limited partnership is often used in real estate ownership because of favorable tax treatment that allows no double taxation of income and the **pass-through** of losses.

Pass-Through. This is a term used to refer to income that passes from debtors through intermediaries to investors. The most common form is a mortgage-backed security in which the principal and interest payments from homeowners are passed from the banks to investors.

Corporation A corporation is defined as a legal entity, chartered by a state or the federal government, which is separate and distinct from the persons who own it. It may own property, incur debts, sue, or be sued. It is a body formed and organized by law to act as a single person, and it is endowed by the law with the capacity of succession. Liability in corporations is limited to the assets of the business. A corporation is easily transferable through the sale of shares of stock. The two most common types of corporations are the not-for-profit and the for-profit corporations. Both types of corporations require a board of directors and bylaws. While a professional corporation extends benefits to licensed professionals, it does not protect them from liability or malpractice. For-profit business owners who incorporate as a **subchapter S corporation** avoid double taxation on their shareholders' dividends and corporate incomes and can offset corporate losses against their income.

Subchapter S Corporation. This is a corporation with a limited number of stockholders (35 or fewer) that elects not to be taxed as a regular corporation and meets certain other requirements. Shareholders include in their personal tax returns their pro-rata share of the capital gains, ordinary income, tax preference items, and so on. It avoids corporate double taxation while providing legal liability protection to shareholders of a corporation.

Many nurses may work for organizations that are either for-profit or not-for-profit. However, many nurses often do not understand the meaning of either term or the difference between the two; thus each will be examined here.

For-Profit Corporation This is a business that has incorporated within the state in which it exists to deliver a service or a product for a profit. This type of corporation is required to have a board of directors and by-laws. Liability for the corporate officers in a for-profit corporation is limited. If a corporation is a subchapter S corporation, taxation is regulated under subchapter S of the Internal Revenue Service (IRS) code. This corporation has shareholders and has the ability to transfer interest, sell equity, and retain earnings. It is considered a separate taxable entity and may allow its business owners to avoid double taxation, once on corporate earnings and then again on shareholders' dividends. An example of this type of corporation would be Metropolitan Life Insurance Co., one of the nation's largest health insurers.

Not-for-Profit Corporation This is a business that must submit articles for incorporation to the state in which it does business. In this type of organization, no stockholder or trustee shares in the profits or losses since such a business usually exists to accomplish some charitable, humanitarian, or educational purpose; it is also called "nonprofit." Such groups are exempt from corporate income taxes, and donations to these groups are tax deductible for the donor. A not-for-profit business has limited liability. It is required to have a board of directors and bylaws. It is tax exempt under section 501 (c) (3) of the IRS code, and grant monies are available. Such businesses are exempt from sales tax, corporation fee, and federal unemployment tax. An example of this type of corporation would be the Visiting Nurse Service of New York.

Business of Community Health

Community Health: What Is It?
Community health is an extremely broad term used to identify the wellness or illness of a population in a certain geographical area. The World Health Organization (WHO) defines community as a social group determined by geographical boundaries or common values and interests. It functions within a particular social structure, exhibits and creates norms and values, and establishes social institutions.

The ANA defines community health nursing by the scope of its practice. "Community health nursing practice promotes and preserves the health of populations by integrating the skills and knowledge relevant to both nursing and public health. The practice is comprehensive and general and is not limited to a particular age or diagnostic group; it is continual and is not limited to episodic care" (ANA, *Standards*, 1995, p. 17). The primary responsibility of community health nursing practice is to the population as a whole not just the individual, family, or group. The "population as a whole" is a very large target audience for the business of community health!

The business of community health, simply put, is to supply health-related services or products to a person, family, group, organization, village, town, county, state, country, or nation. To get a better understanding of the scope of the community health field, consider the following case and identify the many different businesses that are involved.

CASE HISTORY: THE CASE OF JESSICA PHILLIPS

Have you ever seen the commercial in which a senior citizen is shown lying on the floor and crying, "I've fallen and I can't get up"? In this scenario, the woman simply pushes the button on the emergency response unit that she is wearing around her neck, the paramedics are summoned, her physician is notified, and her emergency contact person is called. Let us now accompany Mrs. Phillips on her journey through the health care system, which illustrates the many different businesses that are involved.

The ambulance arrives. It appears to the paramedics that Mrs. Phillips has fractured her hip, so they take all of the necessary precautions and transfer her to a hospital where she can be admitted to the orthopedic unit. The next day, Mrs. Phillips undergoes surgery for an open reduction of the fractured head of the left femur. She is up and out of bed the next day and begins physical therapy. On day 7, she is discharged and transported home by an ambulette. Since Mrs. Phillips has no family or significant other, the discharge planner has made arrangements with a home care agency to coordinate her care at home. The agency contacts the physician, obtains orders for the home care services, and arranges for a nurse, Virginia Suarez, to visit Mrs. Phillips the afternoon she comes home. Ms. Suarez, the visiting nurse, finds Mrs. Phillips in pain, very anxious, and depressed. Mrs. Phillip's neighbor is with her. After completing the assessment, Ms. Suarez calls the physician to report and discuss the findings and receives orders for the requested services. Ms. Suarez then calls the appropriate home care agencies and arranges for a physical therapist, a social worker, and a home health aid to visit. Ms. Suarez also orders a walker and a commode. Ms. Suarez then calls the pharmacist to arrange for the delivery of the medications that the physician has ordered.

Can you guess how many different businesses were involved in this scenario? The answer is 18. Did you miss one? Did you miss a few? The first business is the company that supplied Mrs. Phillips with the personal response unit (1). This company, in turn, contracted with the manufacturer of the unit (2) and the company that supplied the telephone service access lines (3) that its operator response service uses. The ambulance company (4) (e.g., private or public service) took Mrs. Phillips to the hospital, and the ambulette company (5) took Mrs. Phillips home. The hospital (6) is one of the largest businesses with its numerous components and services. The home care agency (7) subcontracted with the nurse (8) and the physical therapist (9), who is either a private practitioner or from a physical therapist company. The home care agency may also have subcontracted for the social worker's services (10) and the home health aide's services (11). The durable medical equipment company (12) subcontracted with the manufacturers of the individual pieces of equipment (13) and possibly with a trucking company (14) for their deliveries. The local pharmacy (15) was involved, which may have been a **mom and pop business** or part of a major chain that contracts with the many pharmaceutical supply companies (16) that, in turn, contract with the pharmaceutical companies (17) that manufacture the drug that Mrs. Philips' provider has ordered. Last but not least, there is the insurance company (18) that influences every business mentioned because it controls the reimbursement for these services and products.

The businesses mentioned above are just a few of the different types that provide our communities with health-related services or products. Community health includes a variety of business venues, each of them replete with roles for nurses.

Nurses can be employed by a business organization, can contract their services, or can be self-employed: self-employment may encompass a private practice or an ownership, partnership, or the position of corporate officer of a business that services the community or provides services or products for one of the agencies or organizations servicing the community. Some of the areas in which nurses are employed in the community are in outpatient clinics, ambulatory care facilities, departments of health, public health clinics, school-based clinics, **community nursing organizations** (**CNOs**), home care agencies, insurance companies, urgent care centers, rural health centers, health planning agencies, community-based organizations (CBOs), correctional facilities, hospices, day care, community mental health centers, nursing homes, retirement centers, neighborhood health centers, **managed care organizations** (**MCOs**), private physicians' offices, private practices, and nurse-owned health-related businesses.

In 1992, the U.S. Department of Health and Human Service (DHHS), Division of Nursing, Health Resources and Services Administration, reported that there were approximately 333,000 nurses (18 percent of the 1,853,024 active registered nurses) employed in ambulatory or community settings (ANA, *Nursing Facts*, 1995). This is an increase from 237,000 in 1988. The breakdown of where these nurses are employed is shown in Table 18-1. It has been estimated that there will continue to be an increase of such employed nurses from 1992 to 2000. These nurses have been educated at many levels and hold a variety of degrees (ANA, *Nursing Facts*, 1995). Table 18-2 shows the distribution of nurses according to degrees.

Mom and Pop Business. This is a small retail store with limited capital that principally employs family members.

CNOs. This is one of four pilot projects selected by the HCFA of the DHHS in 1992 and is a form of nurse-managed health care delivery system in the community

MCOs. These are companies that have been formed to provide high-quality, cost-effective health care to its enrollees (e.g., HMO, PPO, point of service).

◙

TABLE 18-1

WHERE NURSES ARE EMPLOYED

Place	Percent of Nurses
Hospitals	66.3
Community and public health	10
Ambulatory	8
Nursing home/extended care facilities	7
Nurse education	2
Student health	2.7
Occupation health	1
Miscellaneous	3

NOTE: Adapted from "Today's Registered Nurse—Numbers and Demographics" (pp. 1–5), by the American Nurses Association, 1995, *Nursing Facts*, Washington, DC: Author. Reprinted with permission.

◙

TABLE 18-2

EDUCATIONAL LEVELS OF NURSES EMPLOYED IN AMBULATORY CARE

Level of Education	Percent of Nurses
Baccalaureate degree	37
Master's degrees	10
Advanced practice nurses	12

NOTE: Adapted from "Today's Registered Nurses—Numbers and Demographics" (p. 2), by American Nurses Association, 1995, *Nursing Facts*, Washington, DC: Author. Reprinted with permission.

Factors That Influence the Rapid Growth of the Community Health Care Business

Increased Life Expectancy According to the City of New York, Department of Health, Summary of Vital Statistics and Epidemiology (1980 to 1993), the average life expectancy for men in the United States increased from 70.0 in 1980 to 71.8 in 1990. The average life expectancy for women increased from 77.5 years to 78.8 years (United Hospital Fund, 1996).

Aging of Americans The increase in the number of people over 65 in the last 10 years has been significant. However, this is viewed as "the tip of the iceberg," since the "baby boomers," those people born in the years following World War II (i.e., 1945, 1946, 1947), will start to retire in 2010 as demonstrated in Fig. 18-1.

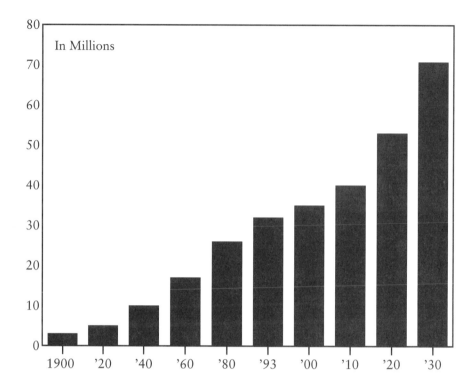

FIGURE 18-1

Number of Americans 65 years of age and older. [NOTE: From "Saving Medicare for the Boomers" (p. 30), by S. Rich, February 12–18, 1996, *The Washington Post* (National Weekly Edition). Reprinted with permission.]

Advances in Health Care Technology These advances now allow people to receive highly technological care in their home, such as intravenous therapy and kidney dialysis. For example, antibiotic therapy can be administered intravenously by a registered nurse in the client's home. This therapy traditionally was only available for clients in a hospital setting.

U. S. Bureau of the Census. This is an agency of the U. S. Department of Commerce best known for its publication of population and housing statistics.

Changing Makeup of the Nuclear Family According to the **U. S. Bureau of the Census (1992)**, 24 percent of households in the United States with children under the age of 18 have single heads of households: 20.4 percent are women and 3.6 percent are men (ANA, *Nursing Facts*, 1995). The geographical location of family members has also changed. Children no longer live in the same home with their aging parents or in the same town. Instead, they live hundreds or even thousands of miles away, creating a need that community churches, senior centers, and other organizations are left to meet. These long-distance family relationships have also created a new reliance by people on their community as their virtual family.

DRGs are a reimbursement system by which reimbursement is determined by diagnosis.

Impact of the Diagnosis Related Groups (DRGs) Since the inception of DRGs, a reimbursement system that limits a client's hospital stay, clients have been discharged "quicker and sicker" to homes where there is no significant other to care for them. They are also sent home with wounds or conditions that require the skills of a registered nurse or other member of the interdisciplinary team. For example, a client with a fractured hip before DRGs were instituted would have been hospitalized for 3 to 6 weeks. With the DRG system, clients are discharged home after 6 days where a nurse, physical therapist, and home health aid (the interdisciplinary team) will assist the client back to her or his optimal level of functioning.

Where Care Is Delivered By far the greatest factor influencing the rapid growth in community health nursing is the shift in where care is delivered. Health care delivery has shifted from the acute care setting to the community or ambulatory setting.

Shift from Acute Care Settings to Community and Ambulatory Care Settings

The shift in where people receive health care directly correlates with the most notable shift in health care itself: the shift from a system designed to treat and cure people after they become ill to a system that focuses on preventing people from becoming ill in the first place. It is believed that this shift will reduce the national expenditures for personal health care, which the Congressional Budget Office (CBO) reported were approximately $1.069 trillion dollars in 1995. These expenditures provoked a loud outcry from the taxpayers. The United States government responded by directing its efforts to controlling the rapidly escalating costs of health care. During the early 1990s, health care reform was number one on its agenda [National Association for Home Care (NAHC), *Home Care*, 1995].

In addition to health care reform, a national program called "Healthy People 2000" has defined a prevention agenda for the nation to pursue. Healthy People 2000 is a decade-long plan for reducing preventable deaths, disabilities, and diseases. This plan sees prevention as the foundation of health. This preventive health initiative helped move health care from acute care settings to community settings. One of the major premises of the initiative is that if preventive health care services were offered to people at local community health care centers and if prevention outreach programs and projects could be presented to people in their "own backyards," then they would be more likely to take advantage of these services. A major portion of the Healthy People 2000 agenda is to come through three functions of public health: assessment, policy development, and assurance. Leadership for this process comes from a cross section of people in American communities working through a Healthy People 2000 consortium of more than 300 organizations.

Community health prevention programs include immunization programs, prenatal care programs, Smoke Enders programs, parenting classes, exercise classes, nutrition programs, abuse prevention programs, drug and alcohol abuse prevention programs, and flu shot programs. In addition, there are screening programs, such as lead screenings, sickle cell screenings, mammography screenings, and cervical cancer screenings. Other important tools are asthma prevention programs for both adults and children, blood pressure screenings, cholesterol screenings, stress management programs, human immunodeficiency virus (HIV) and acquired immunodeficiency syndrome (AIDS) education programs, and even safe driving classes. There is also help for people who are having difficulty dealing with their problems, either physical or emotional. These initiatives (except for the safe driving classes) fall within the scope of practice of a community health nurse.

CDC is an agency of the Public Health Service that provides health information and conducts research to track down the sources of epidemics.

Reports from the **Centers for Disease Control (CDC)** support the need for all of these programs. In 1994, the CDC estimated that nearly 47 percent of premature deaths among Americans could have been avoided by changes in individual behavior, and another 17 percent, by reducing environmental risks. In addition, an estimated 11 percent of premature deaths among Americans were deemed preventable through improvements in access to medical treatment (DHHS, 1995). Significantly, these are all programs that are usually administered by registered nurses. Premature death, serious illness, and chronic disability are costly. Improvements in health status, risk reduction, public and professional awareness of prevention, health services, protective measures, and surveillance and evaluation are the means by which to decrease health care expenditures.

While no one can put a dollar value on a life, it is important to remain aware of the costs related to keeping someone alive. For example, the CDC reported that physical injuries, both unintentional ("accidental") and violent, cost more than $150 billion a year. The financial burden of those suffering with heart disease and stroke amounts to about $135 billion a year. The annual health care and related costs attributable to alcohol abuse is $98.6 billion and to illicit drug use, $66.9 billion. The yearly costs of those suffering from tobacco use amount to about $65 billion (DHHS, 1995).

While Healthy People 2000 may not provide us with the means by which to cure all the ills of our health care system, it does provide a vision for achieving improved health for all Americans and provides an opportunity to collaborate with other providers to meet clients' needs. The objectives of Healthy People 2000 have been adopted in one form or another by most of the states under the general headings of preventive services, health protection, and health promotion.

$\mathcal{H}$OME CARE: WHY IS IT CONSIDERED BIG BUSINESS?

Since home care is the fastest growing segment of community health, it is important to look at the home care industry from a business perspective. Home care is the term given to a variety of health and social services that can be delivered at home where the person lives and in various settings. These services can be delivered to anyone, at any age, who requires care while recovering from an illness either physical or mental, who is disabled or chronically ill, or who is challenged by a variety of social problems (NAHC, *Home Care*, 1995). The basic concepts of home care are discussed in Chap. 1. The number of disciplines that deliver home care are as diverse as the population they service. This section focuses on home health

⬦

TABLE 18-3

NATIONAL HEALTH CARE EXPENDITURES, 1995

	Percent
Total personal health care	100
Hospital care	40.2
Physicians' services	21.6
Nursing home care	9.1
Drugs and other medical nondurables	9.7
Other professional services	6.9
Dentists' services	4.8
Home care	3.7
Other personal health care	2.3
Vision products and other medical durables	1.7

NOTE: Reproduced by permission of the National Association for Home Care from *Basic Statistics about Home Care* (p. 3), by National Association for Home Care, 1996, Washington, DC: Author. Not for further reproduction.

---

care nurses who have been recognized historically as the main components of the home care business. Home health care nursing is a subspecialty of community-based nursing practice that integrates public health principles and components of community care (ANA, *Standards*, 1995). The ANA's Standards of Care for Home Care Nursing are detailed in Chap. 1.

In 1996, expenditures in home care exceeded $27 billion. Yet, according to the CBO memorandum of October 1993, this represents only 3 percent of the national health care expenditures as shown in Table 18-3. Home care is a cost-effective service. The CBO reported that in 1995 the average cost for a 1-day stay in a hospital was $1810 and in a skilled nursing facility, $293, while the cost for one home care visit was $86 (NAHC, *Basic Statistics*, 1996). This cost saving along with the estimates that as many as 9 to 11 million Americans need home care services are two reasons why there is such a strong movement toward home care.

Nursing Opportunities in Home Care

It was reported in 1996 that employment opportunities in home care had almost doubled since 1988, while employment in hospitals and in the total industry increased by approximately 25 percent as demonstrated in Table 18-4 (NAHC, *Basic Statistics*, 1996).

The BLS estimates that almost 500,000 persons were employed in home health agencies. The largest number of professionals employed in home care is nurses (Fig. 18-2). Compensation for nurses employed by home care agencies varies according to the section of the country in which these agencies are located. The average salary for registered nurses employed in home care as field staff is $36,294. The average fee paid to a registered

◙

TABLE 18-4

Number of Home Health Care Workers (1993) and Certified Agency Full-Time Employees (1995)

Type of Employee	No. Employees	No. Full-Time Employees
Registered nurse	90,950	135,694
Licensed practical nurses	32,240	29,545
Physical therapists	7,600	12,470
Home care aides	215,220	120,994
Other	104,160	72,787
Totals	450,170	371,490

NOTE: Reproduced by permission of the National Association for Home Care from *Basic Statistics about Home Care* (p. 8), by National Association for Home Care, 1996, Washington, DC: Author. Not for further reproduction.

nurse contracted on a fee per home visit basis is $30.24 (NAHC, *Basic Statistics*, 1995).

The average salary for top administrative positions such as chief executive officer (CEO), chief operating officer (COO), administrator, or director is $71,742. The average reimbursed cost of a home care visit made by a registered nurse is $94, and the average fee paid by an agency to the registered nurse making the home care visit is $30.24. This represents less than one-third of the reimbursement, leaving more than two-thirds or 68 percent to cover overhead and be taken as profit. As mentioned above, it has been estimated that as many as 9 to 11 million Americans need home

FIGURE 18-2.

◙

Employment growth as a percent of 1988 levels in selected health agencies. [NOTE: Reproduced by permission of the National Association for Home Care from *Basic Statistics about Home Care* (p. 9), National Association for Home Care, 1996, Washington, DC: Author. Not for further reproduction.]

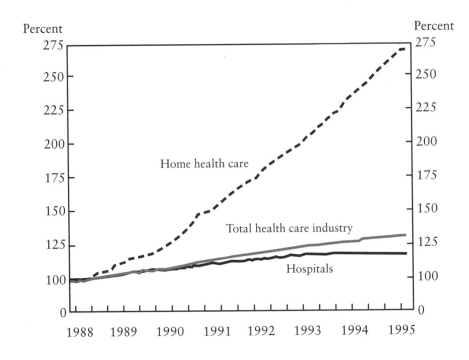

care services; thus, you can clearly see the potential for big business and handsome profits.

Being an independent contractor is another aspect of community health nursing that a nurse may want to consider. A nurse who is an independent contractor is paid on a per-visit basis. This type of an arrangement has many benefits. Nurses can set their own schedules and decide how many hours they wish to work. Nurses can determine the number of clients they wish to visit on any given day. This flexibility can also be very lucrative. For example, it is feasible that a nurse could visit as many as 12 clients in a day given the right geographical area and client case mix ($12 \times 30.24 = \$362.88$ average). This is the closest thing to having your own practice without the overhead and the responsibility of collecting fees or waiting for third-party reimbursement. However, there are downsides. Nurses must pay their own health insurance. There is no overtime for working on a holiday. If a nurse is sick or does not see clients for some other reason, she or he does not get paid. Nurses must also pay their own taxes, because as independent contractors they receive 1099 forms. And finally, nurses must consider whether there will be work when they want it.

Home Care Agencies

There are two types of home care agencies, licensed and certified. Both licensed home care agencies and certified home care agencies can be accredited. Accreditation signifies that the agency has met national industry standards. This is a voluntary process conducted by nonprofit professional organizations. Agencies may be accredited by the Community Health Accreditation Program (CHAP), the Joint Commission on Accreditation of Health Care Organizations (JCAHCO), or the National Home Caring Council, Division of the Foundation for Hospice and Home Care.

Licensed Home Care Agencies These agencies have been licensed by the state in which they do business. In most states, the agency must first apply for and receive a Certificate of Need (CON) from the State Department of Health. These agencies are not certified to receive reimbursement from the Health Care Finance Administration (HCFA). It should be noted that an agency's decision not to apply to the federal government for certification does not imply that it provides poor care or is financially insolvent. One of the primary reasons why an agency would not be certified is that it does not provide skilled nursing services.

Certified Home Care Agencies These agencies are licensed by the state in which they operate and have been certified by the federal government as having met minimum federal requirements for client care and financial management; therefore, they can provide home health services that are reimbursable from Medicare. To become certified, an agency must operate within the federal guidelines set by HCFA. To ensure that the federal government standards are upheld by an agency, the government contracts with a national accrediting body known as CHAP to conduct on-site reviews. This process is discussed in Chap. 16.

NAHC is the trade association that serves the nation's home care agencies, hospices, and home care aide agencies.

The **National Association for Home Care (NAHC)** reported that, as of June 1995, it had identified 18,874 home care agencies in the United States. Of this number, 9120 are Medicare-certified agencies, 1857 are Medicare-certified hospices, and 7897 home health agencies, home care organizations, and hospices that do not participate in Medicare (NAHC, *Basic Statistics*, 1996).

What Medicare certification means from a business point of view is that the certified agency is not closed off from receiving payment from the largest single payer of home care costs. Nearly 60 percent of the clients who receive home health care services have Medicare as their primary source of payment. In 1995, this represented 3,450,000 clients. Medicaid is the second largest payer source for home care at approximately 17 percent. And private insurance is the third largest payer source, representing approximately 8 percent of home health care costs incurred in the United States. To any agency, this means additional visits and additional revenue. According to HCFA, Medicare's home health expenditures for 1995 were over $14.5 billion. This represented over 228 million visits. There are a number of different types of Medicare-certified home care agencies, which are described below (NAHC, *Basic Statistics*, 1996).

Visiting Nurse Associations (VNAs)   VNAs are freestanding, voluntary, nonprofit organizations governed by a board of directors and usually financed by tax-deductible contributions as well as by earnings. The nation's largest certified voluntary home care agency is the Visiting Nurse Service of New York (VNS). In 1995, the VNS reported making 2,136,823 professional visits and logged 21,065,540 or 21.1 million hours of paraprofessional services.

Combination Agencies   These agencies are combined government and voluntary agencies; they are sometimes included among the counts for VNAs. Another example of a combination agency is the Veterans Administration Hospital system.

Public Agencies   These agencies are operated by a state, county, city, or other unit of local government having a major responsibility for preventing disease and for community health education. An example of this type of agency would be the Department of Health.

Proprietary Agencies   These agencies are freestanding, for-profit home care agencies. An example of this type of agency would be Staff Builders.

Private, Not-for-Profit (PNP) Agencies   These agencies are freestanding and privately developed, governed, and owned nonprofit home care agencies. VNAs are examples of this type of agency.

Hospital-Based Agencies   These are operating units or departments of a hospital. They may be agencies that have working arrangements with a hospital or perhaps are even owned by a hospital but operated as separate entities. They are classified as freestanding agencies under one of the categories listed above. The largest hospital-based home care agency in the nation is located in New York State. It is the Catholic Medical Center of Brooklyn and Queens-Home Care Division. This division is known as Mary Immaculate Home Care. In 1995, they reported making 379,610 professional visits and 497,248 paraprofessional visits. Some agencies are based in rehabilitation facilities, and some agencies are based in skilled nursing facilities (SNF).

Nurse as Entrepreneur

"Community health nursing had its origins in the late 19th century in the charitable bent of certain middle class women" (Brodie, 1994, p. 35). After all, it was not until the 19th century that women delivered nursing care outside of the home for financial reimbursement. Prior to this time, it was believed that obligation and duty bound the nurse to her client. Reverby, in her book *Ordered to Care*, quotes Dr. William Alcott who urges women to provide nursing care as a charitable duty. "If we do all the good we are able to do with our hands, we feel that we have better discharged our duties than if we first turned our labor into money" (1987, p. 13). Nurses have come a long way. Not only have nurses learned how to turn their labor into money, but they have become quite successful at doing so, especially in community health where nursing services have always been "costed out" and not lumped together with room and board as it is in hospitals. The first third-party arrangement for payment of nursing services for home care visits was made between the Metropolitan Life Insurance Company (MLI) and the Henry Street Settlement House. In 1910, the Welfare Division of MLI agreed to pay a 25-cent fee for each nursing visit made to a policy holder. Today, the average fee paid by a third party for a nursing visit is $94. No wonder there has been a proliferation of home care agencies (Brody, 1994)!

While entrepreneurship and private practice are terms that are often used interchangeably, they are not the same. A private practitioner can be an entrepreneur, but an entrepreneur is not always a private practitioner. *Webster's* defines an entrepreneur as "an organizer of an economic venture; that is, one who organizes, owns, manages, and assumes the risks of a business" (Gove, 1976, p. 759). The New York State Nurses Association (NYSNA) defines entrepreneurship in nursing as "a variety of business arrangements and practice/organizational models, owned and operated by a professional nurse or nurses, directed toward making nursing more directly accessible to the public" (1986, p. 2).

Do you have what it takes to be an entrepreneur? Are you a risk taker? More importantly, can you afford to be a risk taker? Are you innovative? Do you have the drive, foresight, and managerial skills it takes to be an entrepreneur? Are you creative, hard working, and willing to invest in yourself and your dreams to realize your goal? Do you have good interpersonal skills? Do you have a desire to achieve, control, and direct? Are you persevering? Positive responses to these questions may indicate your innate ability to create unique opportunities for your individual talents and skills that will enable you to transform your ideas into a marketable service or product.

After you have decided what service or product it is that you wish to sell, you must first determine whether or not there is a market for this service or product. This is referred to as a market/service analysis. This analysis is conducted by collecting data about the service or product you wish to sell. What type of service or product do you have the expertise to deliver? Would you be happy delivering this service or product? Are there any barriers to delivering this service or product? Are there any legal or regulatory constraints that you need to consider? Is there a need for this service or product? If so, where is the need? Is it in an area where people can afford to purchase your service or product to meet the need? Is this service or product offered in the same area by anyone else? If so, is the need great enough to allow both entities to survive and eventually flourish? Competition in an area can be positive, provided the nurse is able to command the needed share of the market. Thus, in doing a market/service analysis, it is not a bad idea to send up a *trial balloon*, that is, test your service or product in an area. Sources for data collection can be the literature, your own experiences, as well as colleagues, friends, family, or others who have had experience with this service or product.

When the data analysis is complete, it is extremely important to consider the advantages and disadvantages of being in business for yourself. Much of this information may have been gathered during your survey.

During the production of the video "Starting a Private Practice in Nursing" (Leonard, 1992), interviews were conducted with nurse entrepreneurs throughout New York State, and they were asked what they considered the advantages and disadvantages to being in private practice. The most prominent advantages were the: (1) autonomy, (2) personal satisfaction, (3) self-scheduling, which allows the nurse to work at home, and (4) pride in enhancing nursing by role modeling. The most prominent disadvantages were the: (1) isolation, (2) lack of cash flow, (3) number of hours necessary to get the practice off the ground, and (4) paperwork required by the insurance companies for payment.

Nurse entrepreneurs—that is, nurses who owned their own businesses (not practices)—who were interviewed had similar responses about the advantages and disadvantages. They spoke of the independence; the satisfaction of watching the business grow, knowing that it is yours; meeting new people; and the knowledge that they are showing people that nurses can do more than administer medication and change dressings. These nurses also mentioned similar disadvantages, such as the stress that comes from not knowing whether people will buy your service or product despite the market survey; the fear of failure after making a large financial investment; and the long hours.

Nurse entrepreneurs own and operate many different businesses. Some examples of nurse-owned businesses are licensed home care agencies, health care workers' employment agencies (head hunter agencies), educational seminar businesses, video production companies, publishing companies, nursing home placement counseling businesses, consulting businesses, durable medical equipment (DME) companies, health care supply companies, and nutrition companies. Consulting businesses have experienced a boom: it was reported that Empire Blue Cross and Blue Shield alone spent $55.8 million in 1995 in consulting fees (Lavan, 1996, p. 26).

Getting Started: Developing a Business Plan

A business plan is the vehicle by which dreams are transformed into reality. It should be carefully thought out because it could mean the difference between the success or failure of a venture. The planning stage could take as little as 6 months or as long as 12 months, but it is time well invested. This process forces the nurse to analyze thoroughly what it is she or he is proposing to do. The plan helps the nurse to focus on what is needed to be done and how, when, and where it should be done. Critical issues are brought to the forefront, and business decisions are made. A good business plan is not only a key tool for making sound business judgments, but it is also the comprehensive package that is presented to those who wish to invest time and capital into furthering your dreams. Developing a business plan is not very different from developing a nursing care plan for a community. Consider the similar factors listed below.

Need In a community nursing care plan, a *community assessment* is initiated to determine what is needed. Nurses collect objective and subjective data about the community, including the accessibility and availability of existing services; the demographics; statistics on mortality, morbidity, communicable diseases, and environmental hazards; and the community's resources and politics. In a business plan, this is called a *market/service analysis*.

Existing Barriers or Constraints In a community nursing care plan, community limitations, whether physical, geographical, or socioeconomic, that impede the health of the community and its ability to perform at its optimal level are identified. In a business plan, statutory limitations are identified, including the rules and regulations that will affect a business.

Community Resources In a community nursing care plan, it is important to know what the community is already doing to meet the identified need, such as with child care or day care centers, Meals on Wheels, senior citizen centers, clinics, urgent care centers, hospitals, churches, health department clinics, and outreach programs. In a business plan, this includes identifying the competition. For example, if a nurse wanted to set up a home care agency, she or he would want to know not only how many agencies are located in that community but also how many agencies outside the community service it. The nurse would also want to know the size of the employment pool.

Nursing Interventions In a community nursing care plan, the nurse evaluates the effectiveness of the treatments. If the nursing interventions are not successful, they are changed or adjusted. The same would hold true in a business plan. An evaluation of the service or product's effectiveness is done, and changes or adjustments are made as needed.

Resources The available resources that enable nurses to carry out their interventions must be identified. In a community nursing care plan, resources include the members of the interdisciplinary team who are available to lend their expertise and the supplies that are on hand (i.e., catheters, intravenous solutions, medications). In a business plan, resources include financial arrangements or supplies and equipment that are available.

Evaluation Taking the time to see how effective the business plan is and making adjustments to the plan as appropriate are imperative. These last steps—nursing interventions, resources, and evaluations—are the same for both a community nursing care plan and a business plan.

Elements of a Business Plan

Research has shown that there are many ways of developing a business plan but that most business plans contain essentially the same elements. Remember, presentation is everything. There is only one chance to make a good first impression. A typical business plan is shown in Table 18-5.

Introduction An introduction is usually in the form of a cover letter. This is where nurses introduce themselves and their ideas. In the introduction, nurses should tell the reader who they are, what their business entails, what product or services they can provide: "This is what I am asking from you" and "This is why you should invest in my business."

⊠

TABLE 18-5
ELEMENTS OF A BUSINESS PLAN

Introduction	Table of organization
Executive summary	Staffing analysis: management and support staff
Table of contents	
Mission statement	Plan of operations
Goals and objectives	Information systems analysis
Description of services or product	Projected operating budget
Company's legal structure and principals	Available resources
Industry survey	Risk analysis
Market analysis	Timeline projections
Marketing strategies	Supporting documents

Executive Summary While an executive summary appears at the beginning of the plan, it should not be written until the business plan has been completed. This is similar to an abstract; it should be brief and succinct.

Table of Contents The table of contents is a useful tool for the reader. In some instances, different parts of the business plan are reviewed by different people in the same agency, each person examining the portion of the plan in which she or he has expertise. For example, the marketing portion of the plan may be viewed by the vice president of marketing. The table of contents will direct that person to the appropriate section of your plan quickly and easily.

Mission Statement The mission statement tells the reader about the nurse and the company. This statement should reflect the business philosophy of the company.

Goals and Objectives This section of the plan delineates what the nurse expects the business to achieve and how. This is just an overview; a more detailed description is contained in the Plan of Operations.

Description of Services or Product In this section, a detailed description of the service or product is given. Here the nurse should describe the existing market and the knowledge of existing gaps that the company is prepared to fill. This section also explains why your services are better than those of the competition.

Legal Structure and Its Principals In this section, the nurse should describe the type of legal entity the company has formed (e.g., a corporation, a limited partnership). The names of the persons who serve as owners or officers of the corporation are included in this section.

Industry Survey Included in this section is a brief account of industry trends and projections of future industry growth. Also included is a description of what forces are driving the industry, both internally and externally. In this section, the nurse should explain the results of the research done regarding the industry of which she or he wants to be a part. Be sure to include information sources and to summarize and analyze your findings.

Market Analysis This part of the business plan was discussed earlier in this chapter. This analysis should be one of the first steps taken before investing your time, money, and energy on anything else because if there is no market for your services or product, a business plan will not be necessary.

Marketing Strategies This part of the plan is driven by the market analysis and is usually the second part of the plan to be addressed. Here ideas about how to market your services or product to your target audience are crystallized. Once the nurse determines to whom she or he will be marketing the product or services, a decision must be made as to the types of strategies that will be employed to reach that market. For example, will direct mailing be used? If so, what marketing materials will need to be designed and produced? Will telemarketers be used? How will advertising be handled? Will sales people be necessary? If so, then cost, availability, and effectiveness must be considered when making these decisions.

Table of Organization A table of organization will give the reader at a glance the hierarchy and the chain of command within the company. This chart should contain position titles only.

Plan of Operation In this section, an outline of how the company functions and who performs what function should be included. If a product is being produced, then the steps of production should be described.

Staffing Analysis: Management and Support Staff This section of the plan contains the names of the management team along with their curricula vitae or resumes and job descriptions. Support staff is listed by position only and includes the number of full-time and part-time employees. This section should also include a projection of the number of staff that is needed at different growth periods of the company.

Information Systems Analysis Increasingly, the need to collect and analyze data has become paramount. Therefore, it is important to identify the type of information management system that would best serve your needs. The nurse should also identify any software packages she or he may wish to purchase. The cost of hardware and software may be included in this section as well as in the operating budget.

It is important to analyze the kinds of data that the company should collect and how they should be collected. In this section, the different types of information systems that have been researched along with a cost analysis should be mentioned.

Projected Operating Budget The nurse may want to seek the advice of an accountant before projecting an operating budget. This is a line-item budget in which income, expenses, assets, and liabilities are projected. Figures must be realistic. A break-even analysis should also be included in this section.

Available Resources In this section, start-up capital and any additional financial resources available should be declared. Any equipment, information systems, databases, human resources, referral sources, real estate, office space, office furniture, and supplies already secured should be listed.

Risk Analysis In any comprehensive business plan, risks—actual and potential—must be addressed. The advice of an attorney and perhaps an insurance broker should be sought. When looking for these professionals, remember that many nurses today are also attorneys, accountants, insurance brokers, and financial advisers. Using qualified nurses for these services promotes entrepreneurism in nursing and helps to market your services to other nurses. Remember there are over 2.2 million nurses in the United States.

Insurance is another consideration when a risk analysis is done. For example, if the business is a partnership and one of the partners dies, it is important to determine if the remaining partner is covered in the contract or is the beneficiary of a life insurance policy. Is **malpractice insurance** needed? The cost of insurance along with the cost of workmen's compensation insurance must be researched.

Timeline Projections Time frames for beginning and completing each of the phases of the business plan are included in this section. Remember Murphy's Law "If something can go wrong, it will go wrong at the worst possible time." Thus, when these time frames are projected, it is important to allow for downtime due to weather, illness, equipment problems, learning curves, slow mail, and mistakes. It is always better to be ahead of schedule on any project.

Supporting Documents These documents are not included in the body of the business plan, but instead are submitted as attachments. Some examples would be resumés of key personnel, letters of commitment from a purchaser of your services or a bank, letters of support for work from community leaders or local politicians, letters of reference, and samples of marketing materials.

Malpractice Insurance. This is a policy that covers losses encountered as a result of a law suit for improper conduct of a professional in the performance of her or his duties, done either intentionally or through carelessness or ignorance.

Summary

An entrepreneurial explosion is underway in this nation, and it promises to continue for several decades. Nurses are part of this explosion. A significant number of these entrepreneurs are new entrepreneurs who were victims of recent corporate downsizing. Corporate downsizing and re-engineering are also affecting nurses and nursing positions across the nation. Many nurses have found themselves out of work, and many are being forced to work in areas of nursing for which they are not prepared. An increasingly large number of these displaced nurses are forming their own businesses or starting their own practices.

A significant number of these businesses or practices are being started right in these nurses' own homes. But nurses are not the only people starting home businesses. A large number of home-based businesses have appeared in recent years. This surprising increase has caused many economists to conclude that very small businesses (those with 20 or fewer employees) are increasingly becoming major players in the nation's economy. Therefore, it is probably wise to join one of the small business organizations listed in Appendix I, which would act as an advocate to ensure that your business interests are highlighted and not lost in the sea of regulations, mandates, and governmental requirements imposed upon them.

It is important to mention that many nurses who choose to become entrepreneurs do so on a part-time basis. This is done to accomplish three things:

(1) to determine whether or not they like being in private practice or owning their own business; (2) to see whether or not they can build up the practice or business to a level of financial solvency; and (3) to have the security of a guaranteed salary while the cash flow of the business increases.

If the reader has considered starting a practice or opening a business, I hope that the information contained in this chapter has been helpful. If entrepreneurship is not imminent at this time, keep this book as a reference guide when and if the opportunity for entrepreneurship presents itself. "Nurse entrepreneurship affects not only the destiny of certain individual nurses, but also the way in which nursing as a whole is practiced and viewed by the public. It expands the boundaries of nursing practice, and the results benefit patients, nurses and the profession itself" (Vogel & Doleysh, 1988, p. 259).

This journey through the business of community health was designed not only to give the nurse information but to explain the basic components of the business side of nursing. Whether the nurse is considering a career in community health or self-employment, the concepts explained in this chapter are important—the business of community health, factors that influence the rapid growth of community health business, the reasons for the shift from acute care to community care and home care, and the way to develop a business plan.

The concept of business and community health nursing merging has always been seen by nursings' visionaries who understood that caring alone was not enough to keep their clients well. Supplies, medication, healthy foods, housing, and clothing were also needed, and these things cost money. Therefore, a revenue stream must be created so that the delivery of care in the community to those in need of it can continue.

KEY WORDS

Business
Sole proprietorship
Corporation
Partnership
Home care

Certified agency
Healthy People 2000
Employment opportunities
Entrepreneur
Business plan

QUESTIONS

DIRECTIONS: Choose the one *best* response to each of the following questions.

1. The simplest form of organization for a business is
   A. nonprofit.
   B. limited.
   C. sole proprietorship.
   D. silent partnership.

2. The type of business where liability is unlimited is known as a

   A. for-profit corporation.
   B. not-for-profit corporation.
   C. sole proprietorship.
   D. general partnership.

3. A corporation is legally required to have

   A. shareholders' dividends.
   B. limited number of owners.
   C. a board of directors.
   D. capital gains.

4. The Healthy People 2000 consortium was composed of

   A. the President and his advisors.
   B. 300 organizations from across the United States.
   C. health care workers.
   D. a California-based research consulting firm.

5. The goals of Healthy People 2000 focus on all of the following *except*

   A. increased educational funding for nursing.
   B. risk behavior reduction.
   C. surveillance and evaluation.
   D. public and professional awareness of prevention.

6. Factors that have affected the shift from acute care settings to ambulatory and community settings include all of the following *except*

   A. Healthy People 2000 initiatives.
   B. an increased number of hospital beds.
   C. the inception of diagnosis related groups (DRGs), a system for reimbursement.
   D. the advances in health care technology that can be delivered in the home.

7. A licensed home care agency that is not certified cannot receive reimbursement from

   A. the clients.
   B. Medicaid.
   C. a commercial insurance company.
   D. Medicare.

8. All the following are examples of a nurse entrepreneur *except*

   A. a nurse who has begun a business venture.
   B. a registered nurse employed as the chief executive officer (CEO) of a certified home care agency.
   C. a nurse who owns her or his own practice.
   D. a nurse who operates her or his own business part-time while employed part-time elsewhere.

9. In a business plan, the business philosophy is included in which section?
   A. Mission statement
   B. Plan of operations
   C. Supporting document
   D. Company's legal structure and principals

ANSWERS

1. *The answer is C.* Sole proprietorship is the simplest form of organization for a business because it is owned and operated by one person. It is easy to form and easy to dissolve or sell. The business does not pay taxes. The business income is considered personal income. The sole proprietor has complete control over the business.

2. *The answer is D.* In a general partnership, the liability of a partner is unlimited. Each partner is liable for the business's debts and for the actions of the other partners. In this type of partnership, each partner is involved in and responsible for the day-to-day operations of the company.

3. *The answer is C.* A corporation is legally required to have a board of directors. It is not solely owned. Only a for-profit corporation may have shareholders and dividends; a not-for-profit corporation does not have shareholders.

4. *The answer is B.* A consortium of 300 organizations from across the United States composed the Healthy People 2000 consortium. While consultants and health care workers may have been a part of the consortium, it also consisted of people from multiple sectors of American communities. President and Mrs. Clinton and the President's advisors made health care reform the administration's priority, but they were not part of the Healthy People 2000 consortium.

5. *The answer is A.* The goals of Healthy People 2000 include health promotion, risk reduction, and public and professional awareness of prevention, health services, and protective measures, and surveillance and evaluation, but they do not address educational funding for nurses.

6. *The answer is B.* The shift from acute care settings to ambulatory and community settings can be attributed to the inception of diagnosis related groups (DRGs), a system of reimbursement. In this system, hospitals are reimbursed according to a rate assigned to each diagnosis. For example, if one is admitted to a hospital for a fractured hip, the hospital is paid one flat rate for the hospital stay whether it is for 3 days or 23 days. Therefore, it behooves the hospital to discharge the client as quickly as possible. Since the discharged clients still require skilled nursing care, a home care nurse follows the client. Advances in technology have also enabled the nurse to deliver highly technological care, such as peritoneal dialysis, in the client's home. Healthy People 2000 initiatives, which concern prevention, have decreased the number of hospital admissions, thereby decreasing the need for the present number of hospital beds.

7. *The answer is D.* Only a home care agency that has been licensed by the state in which it operates and is certified by the federal government is eligible to receive reimbursement from Medicare. A licensed agency can receive payment from Medicaid, commercial insurers, and from clients.

8. *The answer is B.* If a nurse is employed by a certified home care agency at any level, even as a CEO, and does not own another private practice or business, whether that business is a part-time or full-time practice or business, she or he is not considered an entrepreneur.

9. *The answer is A.* In a business plan, the mission statement tells the reader about the nurse and her or his company. This mission statement should also contain the business philosophy.

ANNOTATED REFERENCES

American Nurses Association. (1995). *Standards of community health nursing practice.* Washington, DC: Author.

This document is a revision of the Standards of Community Health Nursing Practice developed in 1973 by the Division on Community Health Nursing Practice (now the Council of Community Health Nursing). This document contains the standards that apply to community health nursing practiced in any community setting and the rationale for each standard. It is for the nurse generalist and the nurse specialist.

American Nurses Association. (1995). Today's registered nurse—numbers and demographics. *Nursing Facts*, Washington, DC: Author.

This publication contains statistics about the registered nurse population. It uses the U. S. Department of Health and Human Services, Public Health Services, Division of Nursing, Health Resources and Service Administration as its main source of information.

Brodie, B. (1994, November). From charity to business: Community health nursing, 1900–1926. *Nursing Connections 7*, 35–43.

This journal article talks about the establishment of Nurse's Settlement House in Richmond Virginia in 1900. It discusses how nurse Sadie Heath Cabaniss was inspired by the example of Lillian Wald who in 1893 established the Henry Street Settlement House and Visiting Nurse Association in New York City and turned the Settlement House into a thriving business.

Friedman, J. P., et al. (1987). *Barron's dictionary of business terms.* New York: Barron's Educational Services.

This dictionary contains 6000 clear definitions of key terms used throughout the business world. It is a pocket-sized paperback that is easy to use. All terms defined are short enough to be read in a few seconds but complete enough for the reader to grasp meanings and usage fully.

Gove, P. B. (Ed.). 1976. *Webster's third international dictionary of the English language.* Springfield, MA: G. C. Merriam.

Lavan, R. M. (1996, March 12). Outside work costs empire $67 million. *New York Daily News,* p. 26.

This is an article about Blue Cross and Blue Shield and how this insurance giant spent close to $67 million on outside consultants, attorneys, and accountants while struggling to improve finances and keep administrative costs in check.

Leonard, M. A. (1992). *Starting a private practice in nursing* [video tape]. New York: Rainbow Connections.

This 30-min video shows a series of interviews with some of nursings' leaders who own private practices in nursing. The questions asked revolve around the advantages and disadvantages of starting a private practice in nursing. It includes stories about why each of the nurses interviewed decided to start a private practice and how they did it. The video was produced and directed by a registered nurse, and the video company that produced the tape is owned and operated by a registered nurse.

Mershon, K., & Wesolowski, M. (1985, January). Strategic planning for the business of community health and home care. *Nursing and Health Care,* p. 33–35.

This article discusses the promising future for the business of community health and home care. The authors explain the importance of developing an action plan based on successful business practices to determine an appropriate and positive future for a nurse starting her or his own community or home care agency.

National Association for Home Care (NAHC). (1995). *Home care.* Washington, DC: Author.

This publication explains what the NAHC is and the benefits of membership. This is the largest organization representing home care and hospice in the world. Its mission is to promote quality care to home care and hospice clients; preserve the rights of caregivers; effectively represent all home care and hospice providers; and place home care in the center of health care delivery.

National Association for Home Care. (1996). *Basic statistics about home care.* Washington, DC: Author.

This publication contains statistics on many aspects of home care, including the different types of home care, the people who are serviced by home care, the types of services offered, and cost and reimbursement information.

New York State Nurses Association. (1986). *Nursing entrepreneurship in New York State.* Guilderland, NY: Author.

This booklet is designed to guide nurses who wish to explore professional autonomy as entrepreneurs. It defines a variety of business practices and gives examples of some of the different forms entrepreneurship can take.

Reverby, S. (1987). *Ordered to care*. Cambridge: Cambridge University Press.

In this book, Reverby presents a history of the development of nursing between 1850 and 1945 in the context of the changing health care system. It describes how nursing developed within the cultural expectation that caring would be a part of a woman's duty to family and community. Nursing is used as a case history of how the realities of the nursing work culture became politicized. The author also retells the political history of hospitals from the vantage point of nursing.

Rich, S. (1996, February 12–18). Saving Medicare for the boomers. *The Washington Post* (National Weekly Edition), p. 30.

This periodical is a special edition that is printed weekly. The format is designed to highlight major stories that have been reported in the course of the week.

United Hospital Fund (UHF). (1996). *Children and health: New York City and the nation*. New York: Author.

This book contains statistics on populations, socioeconomics, disease, deaths, health resources, and health services. It was used for the UHF conference "Child Health in a Managed Care Environment."

U. S. Department of Health and Human Services. (1995). *The health of the nation: Highlights of the Healthy People 2000 goals: The 1995 report on progress*. Washington, DC: Author.

This document is a report on the midcourse review of a national health promotion and disease prevention initiative called Healthy People 2000. This report details the preventive health objectives that have been set for the health of all Americans. It features the Centers for Disease Control and Prevention's statistical data on mortality and morbidity rates for the targeted disease states. It also contains the statistical data on how successful the United States has been in meeting targeted benchmarks for wellness and prevention measures set in 1990.

Visiting Nurse Service of New York. (1995). *Annual Report*. New York, N Y: Author.

This publication contains statistics and descriptions of the many services provided by this agency.

Vogel G., & Doleysh, N. (1988). *A nurse's guide to starting a business*. New York: National League for Nursing.

This book describes the authors' experiences of trial and error as they started their own business, Workstyles, a consulting business that offers workshops and seminars on a variety of management topics, plus career counseling to individuals. The authors also share their insights and knowledge about the process.

APPENDIX I: IMPORTANT RESOURCES AVAILABLE TO NURSE ENTREPRENEURS

1. American Nurses' Association (ANA), 600 Maryland Avenue, SW, Suite 11 West, Washington, DC 20024-2571; phone: 800-215-3727.
2. State nurses' association—a complete listing of each state's nurses' association can be obtained by contacting the ANA at the address or telephone number above.
3. Internal Revenue Service, 12th Street and Constitution Avenue, NW, Washington, DC; phone: 800-829-1040.
4. Small Business Administration, 144 L Street, NW, Washington, DC 20416; phone: 202-309-6565.
5. National Small Business Association 1604 K Street, NW, Washington, DC 20006; phone: 202-293-8830.
6. National Federation of Independent Business, 600 Maryland Avenue, SW, Washington, DC 20024; phone: 202-554-9000.
7. Service Corps of Retired Executives Association, 1129 20th Street, NW, Suite 410, Washington DC 20416; phone: 202-653-6279.
8. National Nurses in Business Association, 100 Burnett Avenue, Suite 250, Concord, CA 94520; phone: 510-356-2642.

THE POLITICS OF COMMUNITY HEALTH

National politics and the politics of workplaces, families, churches, social organizations, or communities touch the lives of everyone. Politics are sometimes referred to as an art, sometimes as a science, and sometimes as a game.

In this chapter, the structure of the U.S. government, as well as the legislative and political processes used by persons interested in achieving political changes, are described. The roles nurses play in these processes are also examined. Also, the power of the vote and the lobbying strategies that make the most of this power are discussed. It is hoped that by the time the reader finishes this chapter not only will she or he understand why nurses should be politically active but also will be interested in becoming politically active as well.

Politics, like nursing, is everywhere in the community, and it drives what is happening in health care today. In the Alliance Model for Community Health Assessment, the sphere that deals with politics is labeled influences on resource allocation decisions (see Chap. 5). This sphere has five components, one of which is the influence of special interest groups. Nurses are one of these special interest groups, their special interest being quality, cost-effective health care for all, delivered by qualified professionals. Since nurses are the largest group of professionals in our health care system, they have significant potential as a political driving force. Therefore, it is important that nurses understand how the political system works and how important it is to be politically active. A knowledge of the political system is necessary for nurses to maximize their role in shaping the health care delivery system.

Historically, nurses have been apolitical, largely because they believe that politics are something far removed from their agenda of caring. A number of other factors have contributed to nurses being apolitical, such as a predominance of women in nursing; a socialization of women and nurses into passive roles; a lack of preparation for political involvement; a fear of negativism about the political development of nurses; poor self- and occupational image; a lack of confidence, interest, and assertiveness; and fear of confronting other health professionals. Two other factors have kept nurses out of the political arena: the first is the fact that nurses tend to isolate themselves from policy-making groups and not assert their views, and the second is that nursing's internal strife has given it a conflictive image, which prevented it from making any serious impact on health policy decisions. Fortunately, several of nursing's leaders were visionaries; they saw politics as a vehicle for obtaining the funds needed to carry out their agenda of caring. Florence Nightingale (1820–1910) is an excellent example of the politically active nurse. She was politically influential because of her family's social status, and she used her political influence to solicit monies to fund projects important to nurses and to their patients. Her lobbying of the British War Office during the Crimean War about the unbearable conditions in the barracks used as hospitals resulted in reforms in the British Army Medical Service. These reforms were evident in improved dietary services, sanitation, and construction of new barracks for the soldiers and their families. Many similarly politically astute nursing leaders, such as Lilian Wald and Lavinia Dock, used their political influence to move nursing's agenda forward in the community. Individually, each of these women developed social and political clout. Together they were ardent crusaders for the indigent and for nursing.

Lillian Wald (1867–1940) was a brilliant nurse activist. She is best known as the founder of the Henry Street Visiting Nurse Association in New York City and the nurse who institutionalized the concept of public health nursing in the United States. As a suffragist, her feminist values were evident in her political activities, which were focused on the poor and on children. She was instrumental in the development of the Children's Bureau, which was begun as an effort to protect children against abuse.

Lavinia Dock (1858–1956) was a militant nursing leader in the feminist movement of the 19th century. Her main focus was on nursing education. She was also instrumental in the creation of the International Council of Nurses in 1901, the first international organization for professional women in history.

In politics, influence is measured by whom you know, how many votes you can deliver, and how much money you can contribute to political campaigns. Nursing organizations such as the American Nurses Association (ANA) have made great strides in the political arena for nurses. They have made our government's officials aware of nursing's power. They have done this through "grass roots" organizing of nurses: by letting the legislators know that 1 in every 44 registered voters is a nurse and by creating a political action committee (PAC). At present, the ANA is considered one of the ten most politically influential groups in our country. In the most recent election cycle (1992), the American Nurses Association Political Action Committee (ANA-PAC) ranked second nationwide in the increase of contributions to candidates for federal office. In the same year, ANA-PAC ranked 30th among the more than 4000 PACs in the United States, making it the third largest health care PAC.

$\mathcal{P}$RESENT POLITICAL CLIMATE

The term that is used to describe what is presently going on in the political arena is *political climate*, an appropriate name, since politics are as changeable as the weather. Indeed, it is virtually impossible for an author of a textbook to be as up-to-date about the current political climate as a political columnist or an author of a journal article. The political atmosphere at the time of this writing may be quite different from the political climate at the time this chapter is read.

Never before has the political climate been so challenging for nurses, and never before have so many nurses been politically active. The challenges have come in the form of changes: changes in where health care is delivered, how it is delivered, and by whom it is delivered. With the inception of diagnostic-related groups (DRGs) in 1983 (a payment reimbursement system whereby hospitals are reimbursed for services in predetermined amounts based on the client's principal diagnosis), the country began to witness these changes first-hand. Care delivery was shifted from acute care hospital settings to subacute (nursing homes) and in-home settings. Technological advances fostered the delivery of services such as intravenous therapy and peritoneal dialysis in the home. Another significant change was the change in the level of health care workers. On one end of the spectrum, care was delivered by family members or family designees, and at the other end of the spectrum care was delivered by advanced practice nurses (APNs) such as nurse practitioners, clinical nurse specialists, and certified nurse midwives. However, all of these changes had one common thread. Each change involved the cost of health care.

In recent years, nurses, along with most people in Congress and the general public, have been concerned about budget issues and the rising cost of health care. They have also been concerned about access to health care and the rising number of people in the United States who are uninsured or living in poverty (Tables 19-1 and 19-2).

Additionally, nurses have been alert to budget cuts that would affect nursing education monies, and they have been critical of a movement to use unlicensed assistant personnel (UAPs) to perform nursing tasks.

A unique feature of the current political climate is that, even as politicians have debated health care issues within established settings, the health care market has moved ahead with changes independent of the federal or state governments. There have been countless mergers and takeovers of major health care entities, and there has been rapid growth in the health care phenomenon called *managed care*. Since managed care remains a major issue, the entire next chapter of this book has been dedicated to the subject (see Chap. 20). The shift from tertiary (acute) care to preventive care (care delivered to people to prevent illness) contributed to the shift of nursing positions from acute care settings to community and ambulatory care settings. As part of this shift, health care facilities all over the country were downsized, and nursing positions that had existed in the health care field for decades were re-engineered. Many nurses were forced to work in

▩

TABLE 19-1

NUMBER OF POOR (IN THOUSANDS) IN THE UNITED STATES AND PERCENT OF FAMILIES IN POVERTY WITH RELATED CHILDREN UNDER 18 YEARS OF AGE BY FAMILY TYPE AND RACE (ETHNICITY)

Family Type	Total		White		Black		Hispanic Origin[a]	
	No.	Percent	No.	Percent	No.	Percent	No.	Percent
Female-Headed Household								
1980	2703	42.9	1433	35.9	1217	56.0	NA	NA
1985	3131	45.4	1730	38.7	1336	58.9	493	64.0
1990	3426	44.5	1814	37.9	1513	56.1	536	58.2
1993	4034	46.1	2123	39.6	1780	57.7	706	60.5
Percent change 1980–1993	49.2	7.5	48.2	10.3	46.3	3.0	NA	NA
Married-Couple and **Male-Headed Household**								
1980	2118	8.0	1644	7.0	367	16.0	NA	NA
1985	2455	9.2	1965	8.4	334	14.1	NA	NA
1990	2250	8.4	1739	7.5	374	15.8	549	21.3
1993	2717	9.8	2101	8.8	379	15.5	718	24.0
Percent change 1980–1993	28.3	22.5	27.8	25.7	3.3	–3.1	NA	NA

[a]In this table, persons of Hispanic origin may be of any race.

NOTE: From *Children and Health: New York City and the Nation* (Table 5), by United Hospital Fund, 1996, New York: Author. Adapted with permission.

areas in which they were unprepared; many lost their jobs, and many were forced to move from administrative positions back to staff positions. As a result, more nurses than ever before were either prepared or preparing to expand their scope of practice as APNs. In *ANA's 1995 Nursing Facts*, it was reported that there were 139,000 nurses prepared as APNs in the field: 58,185 clinical nurse specialists; 48,237 nurse practitioners; 25,238 nurse anesthetists; and 7400 nurse midwives (ANA, 1995).

These changes, both positive and negative, forced many nurses to take notice of what was happening to nursing and nurses, how it was happening, and why it was happening. As these nurses began to realize that politics were truly the driving force behind what was happening in health care, they came also to realize that *political clout* was a good thing. Through hard work, a unified voice, and dollars, nurses developed an unprecedented level of political clout. Nurses were learning how to play the game, and organized nursing was seen as one of the players.

In the 1990s, nursing made many political strides. The president of the United States invited the president of the ANA and presidents of several state nursing associations to the White House to share their views on health care issues. Throughout the states, nursing leaders have been appointed to

❈

TABLE 19-2

HEALTH INSURANCE COVERAGE STATUS (IN MILLIONS) IN THE UNITED STATES
AND PERCENT OF TOTAL POPULATION

	Total No. Persons	Private		Public		None	
		No.	Percent	No.	Percent	No.	Percent
Under 18	69.8	47.0	67.3	16.7	23.9	9.6	13.8
18–24	25.5	15.7	61.6	3.1	12.2	6.8	26.7
25 and Over	164.5	119.7	72.8	45.0	27.4	23.3	14.2
Total	259.8	182.4	70.2	64.8	24.9	39.7	15.3

NOTE: From *Children and Health: New York City and the Nation* (Table 20), by United Hospital Fund, 1996, New York: Author. Adapted with permission.

governor, assembly, and senate committee task forces on health care and related issues. The ANA's lobbying efforts were accelerated with the creation of its grass-roots network, Nurses Strategic Action Team (N-STAT). Nurses ran for political offices, and some were elected. In 1996, ANA-PAC contributions totaled approximately $1 million, and the success rate of its endorsed candidates was greater than 77 percent.

The political game has many rules, some of which are written or spoken, others unspoken, but one thing is certain, one of the most valuable chips in the political game is the health care chip. It is so valuable because it includes the rich and the poor, the well and the ill, the young and the old, the educated and the uneducated, and people of every race, creed, sex, color, and ethnic background. Everyone has a stake in health care.

To understand how the political game is played, one must first understand what the term "politics" means, who or what the government is, and how it works. One must also understand the legislative process and how to influence it.

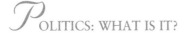 POLITICS: WHAT IS IT?

Webster's defines politics as "the art or science of political government; it is a science that deals with the regulation and control of [persons] living in society; a science concerned with the organization, direction, and administration of political units (as nations or states) in both internal and external affairs; the art of adjusting and ordering relationships between individuals and groups in a political community; the art or science concerned with guiding or influencing government policy; the art or science concerned with winning and holding control over a government (as by selection of government personnel) commonly known as the vote. Politics is a branch of ethics concerned with the state or social organism as a whole rather than as an individual person, a division of moral philosophy dealing with the ethical relations and duties of governments or other social organizations." In reading this extended definition, it is hard to miss the repeated use of two words also often used to describe nursing: "art" and "science" (1975, p. 1755).

On the other hand, Mason, Talbot, and Leavitt do not define politics as either an art or a science but as a process by which one influences the decisions of others and exerts control over situations and events (1993). Remember, another word for influence is power. Who is it that nurses are looking to influence? What is power? Who has the power? How do nurses get the power?

Power is the ability to command respect, influence people, and effect change. Nurses are in an ideal position to do all three of these things. Nurses in the workplace and in the community are in the unique position of being able to enter a person's life, home, and world probably more easily than any other professional. Nurses are there for people when people are at their worst and at their best. Nurses share in their clients' happiest and saddest moments. Nurses assist people in bringing new life into the world, and nurses comfort people as they die. Nurses assist clients with activities of daily living that clients find too embarrassing to ask of family members or their significant others. When people are ill, they not only see nurses as caregivers, confidants, and supporters but as skilled professionals who will assist and guide them back to their optimal level of functioning. Other professionals may do some of these things, but they are usually trained to assist in a specific area of the person's health care. For example, a physician assists a patient in diagnosing and curing a disease entity, the physical therapist works with restoring the functioning of an affected extremity, and a nutritionist works with a patient in designing and adhering to a specific dietary regime. However, the nurse deals with the whole person. People respect nurses for who they are and for what they do.

Most of the time, it is easier to influence people when they respect you than when they do not. Therefore, if patients, friends, peers, administrators, and community leaders respect nurses for what they stand for and what they have to say, they are more likely to be influenced by them. Conversely, if people perceive nurses as unresponsive, rude, unhelpful, unprofessional, or poorly informed, then nurses' ability to command respect or influence people positively will be greatly compromised.

In summary, respect can lead to influence, and influence is what nurses need to bring about change. This is politics, and nurses must be a part of it. Politics can no longer be looked upon as something about which the "other guy" has to worry. In a study conducted in 1991 that looked at the levels of political participation and the political expectations of nurses in New York State in nine defined roles—that is, voter, monitor, campaigner, player, lobbyist, negotiator, leader, spokesperson, and networker—it was found that, while nurses felt that it was important that nurses be involved in these nine different political roles, they themselves were not involved (Leonard, 1994) (Table 19-3). This study also showed that nurses who

▧

TABLE 19-3

COMPARISON OF MEAN POLITICAL PARTICIPATION SCORES BY ROLE FOR NURSES WHO ARE MEMBERS OF NEW YORK STATE NURSES ASSOCIATION (NYSNA) OR NURSES ASSOCIATION OF THE COUNTIES OF LONG ISLAND (NACLI) AND NURSES WHO ARE NOT MEMBERS

Role	Member Nurses		Nonmember Nurses		F	P
	Mean	(SD)	Mean	(SD)		
Voter	11.19	(3.83)	10.44	(3.08)	0.80	>.05
Campaigner	5.78	(3.28)	4.20	(2.42)	5.00	.02
Player	5.23	(2.83)	3.88	(2.01)	4.91	.03
Monitor	9.23	(3.66)	9.44	(2.42)	0.07	>.05
Networker	5.64	(3.01)	4.84	(2.48)	1.46	>.05
Spokesperson	5.17	(2.99)	4.48	(2.66)	1.06	>.05
Negotiator	6.02	(3.09)	4.68	(2.84)	3.75	>.05
Leader	5.56	(3.17)	4.24	(2.39)	4.29	.04
Lobbyist	5.30	(2.87)	4.52	(2.68)	1.47	>.05

NOTE: From "Levels of Political Participation and Political Expectation among Nurses in New York State" (p. 19), by M. Leonard, 1994, *Journal of the New York State Nurses Association*, 25(1). Reprinted with permission.

were members of professional organizations had significantly higher levels of political participation with respect to campaigner, player, and leader roles (Table 19-4). Therefore, it may be concluded that for nurses to continue to be players they should continue to be involved and encourage other nurses to be involved in their professional organizations.

▧

TABLE 19-4

COMPARISON OF LEVELS OF POLITICAL PARTICIPATION AND POLITICAL EXPECTATIONS IN NINE POLITICAL ROLES

Role	Actual Participation		Expected Participation		t^a
	Mean	(SD)	Mean	(SD)	
Voter	11.00	3.68	13.00	2.72	6.53
Monitor	9.26	3.42	12.76	2.37	10.65
Campaigner	5.42	3.17	11.20	3.35	13.93
Player	4.93	2.72	10.96	3.48	14.23
Lobbyist	5.12	2.83	11.01	3.61	14.39
Negotiator	5.45	3.08	11.64	3.35	14.53
Leader	5.31	3.06	11.35	3.47	15.25
Spokesperson	4.99	2.92	11.15	3.47	15.33
Networker	5.45	2.93	12.39	2.54	19.98

[a]All *t*-tests are significant at $P \geqslant .05$.

NOTE: From "Levels of Political Participation and Political Expectation among Nurses in New York State" (p. 20), by M. Leonard, 1994, *Journal of New York State Nurses Association*, 25(1). Reprinted with permission.

𝒢OVERNMENT: HOW DOES IT WORK?

Before nurses can influence government policies, they must first understand how the government operates. The government is that body of persons that constitutes the governing authority of a political unit or organization. It exists on many different levels. A community may have a local governing body and government system. While this local government entity may act independently in many areas, it is affected by the workings of the town, county, state, and federal governments. All of these governing bodies and systems are important for the community nurse to understand, and information about them can be obtained from the local governing boards or from the community library. This chapter offers a brief overview of how the federal and state governments function.

Federal Government

The government of the United States is founded on the Constitution. The Constitution of the United States was drafted by the Constitutional Convention at Philadelphia in 1787 and declared in effect on March 4, 1789. The Constitution established a republic with a federal system, in which extensive powers are granted to the states. Currently, there are 50 states that comprise the federal union.

The federal government has three distinct characteristics. First, powers are divided among three branches: the legislative, the executive, and the judicial. These three branches exist both in the federal government and in the state governments. Second, the power of each of the four elements of the federal government (the Senate, the House of Representatives, the president, and the federal courts) is limited by being shared with one or more of the other elements. Third, the different procedures by which the president, senators, and members of the House of Representatives are elected make each responsible to a different constituency.

Federal executive power is vested in the president, who serves a 4-year term and is limited by the twenty-second amendment to two consecutive terms of office. The president and the vice president are elected by an electoral college. Legislative power is vested in the United States Congress. The Congress is divided into two houses: the Senate and the House of Representatives. The Senate has two members from each state who are elected by popular vote for 6-year terms. Members of the House of Representatives are also elected by popular vote but for 2-year terms. At the time of this publication, there are no term limits for either senators or members of the House of Representatives. Each house is made up of many different committees, such as the Health Care Finance Committee, the Education Committee, and the Labor Committee.

Presently, there are two major parties in the United States: the Democratic party and the Republican party. The party with the greatest number of representatives in one or both of the houses is called the majority party. It does not necessarily follow that the president is of the same party. The party not in the majority is referred to as the minority party. There is a minority leader in both houses. The importance of which party is in power can be clearly seen in the composition of the different committees. For example, if the Democrats are in the majority in the Senate, each Senate committee is comprised of a majority of Democrats, and the committee chair is a Democrat. If the Republicans control the House of Representatives, each committee in the House will be chaired by a Republican and comprised of a majority of Republicans. Since most bills and actions are passed by a majority vote (one more than half of the total votes), the power of the party in the majority is quite significant.

State Government

The structure of each state government is similar to that of the federal government. There are three branches: (1) the executive branch, which consists of the governor, who carries out the laws; (2) the legislative branch, which consists of the Assembly and the Senate that make the laws; and (3) the judicial branch, which consists of the Supreme Court and the Court of Appeals, both of which interpret the laws.

The presiding officer of the Assembly is called the Speaker of the Assembly. The majority leader is a member of the party that has the most members in the Assembly. There is also a minority leader is who is a member of the party with the lesser number of members. There are many different committees in the Assembly, and each of these is chaired by a member of the majority party.

The presiding officer of the Senate is the president pro tem and the majority leader. In the Senate, as in the Assembly, there is a minority leader, and the committees are all chaired by a member of the majority party.

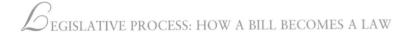

LEGISLATIVE PROCESS: HOW A BILL BECOMES A LAW

It is very important for nurses to understand how a bill becomes a law because it is during this process that nurses can exercise their influence over proposed legislation, which may affect their lives and the lives of their patients and loved ones.

Federal Legislative Process

Every bill starts with an idea. As can be seen in the example at the end of this segment, anyone can develop an idea for a bill; that is, nurses can generate ideas that eventually become bills and laws. An idea for a bill is given to a legislator who, it is believed, will support the idea. The legislator then discusses the idea and its rationale with one of his or her aides. This aide is usually the person on the legislator's staff who has the most expertise in the needed area. The aide researches the idea, gathers additional data, and

Presiding Officer. This is the leader in a specific House. The legislator is a member of the majority party.

writes a draft bill for the legislator to introduce. A bill is introduced either by handing it to the clerk of the House or by placing it in a box called the hopper. In order for the senator to announce the introduction of a bill, the legislator must first gain recognition from the **presiding officer** to do so. If there is any objection by any of the other senators, the bill's introduction is postponed until the next day.

After the bill is introduced, it is numbered. Each number is assigned a prefix which identifies it as either a House bill (H.R.) or a Senate bill (S.). The bill is then labeled with the sponsor's name and sent to the Government Printing Office. The bill is then referred to the appropriate committee. This referral is technically considered "read for the first time." Bills dealing with health care are referred to the House to the Committee on Energy and Commerce and its Subcommittee on Health and the Environment. Bills related to reimbursement or third-party insurance, such as Medicare and Medicaid, are referred to the House Ways and Means Committee and its Subcommittee on Health.

The bill is then placed on the committee's calendar for review, and its chances for passage are determined. This is where the majority of bills fall by the wayside because failure of a committee to move on a bill effectively kills it. Health care bills submitted to the Senate are reviewed by the Labor and Human Resources Committee. Legislation that deals with health programs under the Social Security Act is reviewed by the Senate Finance Committee's Subcommittee on Health. Usually, the committee's first action on the bill is a request for comment by any interested government agencies. The bill may also be assigned to a subcommittee to study or to hold hearings. A **hearing** can be public, closed (i.e., executive session), or both.

Hearing. This is a meeting that is called at a posted time for the purpose of presenting a bill either before the public or an executive committee for the purpose of hearing testimony and discussion on a proposed bill.

The bill is then brought back to the full committee for a vote. This is called "ordering a bill reported." A report is prepared that describes the purposes of the bill and any revisions that the committee has made. The report also indicates any proposed changes in existing law. Included in the report are any dissenting statements from the minority members of the committee. Amendments to the bill may be proposed, but the committee must approve, reject, or change the committee's amendments before voting on the bill

House Calendars. Once a House committee reports a measure to the floor, it is automatically referred to a Calendar where it awaits pending floor action.

A bill is placed on the appropriate **House Calendar** (Table 19-5). There are five House Calendars of the United States House of Representatives, each of which is designed to handle different types of bills. In the Senate, there is only one legislative calendar as well as a single executive calendar for treaties and nominations.

Bills are usually debated when they come to the floor. In the Senate, each senator is limited to 5 min of debate on each bill that is called on the Senate Calendar. In the House, the duration of debate is determined by a number of factors and can continue for varying periods of time. It is important to lobby a legislator before a bill is referred to a calendar so that the legislator has a person's input and is aware of that person's particular concerns.

In both the House and the Senate, bills may be voted on repeatedly before they are approved or rejected. Votes can be cast in one of three ways: (1) an untabulated voice vote, (2) a standing vote, or (3) an electronically recorded roll call, by which yeas and nays are recorded for each legislator. This third type of voting is the most enlightening to the public since

◙

TABLE 19-5

THE FIVE U.S. HOUSE OF REPRESENTATIVE CALENDARS

1. The **Union Calendar** to which are referred bills raising revenues, general appropriations bills, and any measures directly or indirectly appropriating money or property. It is the Calendar of the Committee of the Whole House on the state of the union.
2. The **House Calendar** to which are referred bills of public character not raising revenue or appropriating money or property.
3. The **Consent Calendar** to which are referred bills of noncontroversial nature that are passed without a debate when the Consent Calendar is called the first and third Monday of each month.
4. The **Private Calendar** to which are referred bills for relief in the nature of claims against the United States or private immigration bills that are passed without debate when the Private Calendar is called the first and third Tuesday of each month.
5. The **Discharge Calendar** to which are referred motions to discharge committees when the necessary signatures are signed to a discharge petition.

NOTE: From "House and Senate Rules of Procedure: A Brief Comparison" (p. 3), *Congressional Research Service Report for Congress*, 1990, Washington, DC: Author. Adapted with permission.

it is the only form of voting that records how each legislator has voted for a bill. There is also a *teller vote*, which is used only in the House. This system of voting only gives total votes; it does not identify how a particular legislator has voted.

Once a bill has passed one chamber, it is sent to the other. The second legislative body may choose one of several options. It may pass the bill as it has been received, retaining the other chamber's language; it may send the bill to committee for review and perhaps alteration; or it may reject the bill. Finally, if the second house is preparing its own version of the proposed bill, it may simply ignore the bill. This often happens when the majority in the Senate is of one party and the majority in the House is of the other party.

When the identical form of a bill has been passed by both the House and the Senate, it is forwarded to the White House, where it awaits action by the president. There are two ways by which the president can approve a bill, and there are two ways by which the president can veto a bill. To approve a bill, the president signs and dates it, sometimes writing "approved" across the document. A bill can also be approved if the president does not sign the bill within 10 days (not counting Sundays) of receipt of the bill and Congress is in session. The president vetoes a bill by refusing to sign it then returning it to Congress along with an explanation of his refusal within a 10-day period. The president can also use what is known as the *pocket veto*. This procedure is followed when the president has not signed a bill and Congress adjourns before the 10 days expire. Congress may override the president's veto and enact the bill if there is a two-thirds vote to do so in both houses wherein there is a quorum; this vote must be by roll call. When a bill finally passes, it is given a law number.

State Legislative Process

As is shown in Fig. 19-1, the state legislative process is similar to the federal legislative process; that is, an idea for a bill is developed, a bill is drafted and introduced in the Assembly or the Senate, and the bill is referred to the appropriate committee in each house. There it is debated and reported out to the legislative body and is either killed by vote or dies from lack of interest. The bill is then sent on for a second and a third reading calendar, and it is either recommitted to a committee or debated. If the bill passes, it is referred to the other House, where it is debated. If it passes the second House, it is sent to the governor for approval or veto. If it is approved, the bill becomes public law. If the governor vetoes the bill, it can still become law if it repasses both Houses with a two-thirds vote.

CASE STUDY: POLITICAL CASE STUDY

Virginia Murphy, a nurse in private practice in a rural county, recently considered inviting another nurse to join her, thus expanding her practice. Nurse Murphy's practice deals primarily with oncology patients. Nurse Murphy routinely sees her patients in her office but also visits them in their homes when necessary. Nurse Murphy generally practices traditional nursing, but she has incorporated some alternative healing modalities into her practice. Her excellent holistic nursing care and business acumen have produced a growing practice.

When Nurse Murphy first made the attempt to expand her practice by bringing in another nurse, she was told by the Home Care Association (HCA) that, since she and her partner would be making house calls, they must first become licensed as a home care agency. One of the steps towards licensure involves making application for a Certificate of Need (CON) from the Department of Health, which can be a lengthy process. Nurse Murphy was upset by the fact that nurses were the only health care professionals who had to go through this process. Neither the physicians in her area nor the physical therapists, chiropractors, and nutritionists needed to be licensed as home care agencies, despite the fact that they, too, made occasional house calls. The restriction upon nurses struck her as exclusionary and unfair.

Nurse Murphy decided that she was not going to take this lying down. She made sure that she knew the issues and that her information was correct, and then she went to her local legislator. She explained the issue to him and asked him for some assistance in changing this law. At the same time, realizing that there is power in numbers, she went to her State Nurses Association (SNA) for help.

The SNA drafted a letter describing the major elements that they would like to see in a bill and brought it to Nurse Murphy's

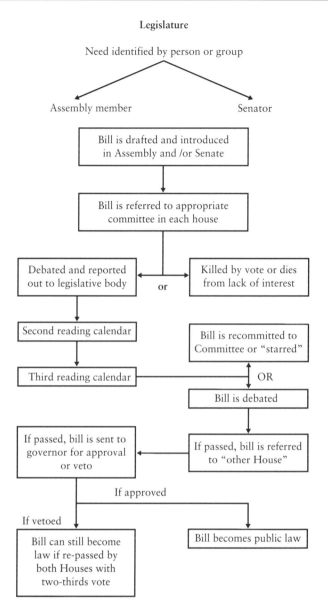

Legislature

Need identified by person or group

Assembly member   Senator

Bill is drafted and introduced
in Assembly and /or Senate

Bill is referred to appropriate
committee in each house

Debated and reported   Killed by vote or dies
out to legislative body   or   from lack of interest

Second reading calendar

Bill is recommitted to
Committee or "starred"

Third reading calendar   OR

Bill is debated

If passed, bill is sent to   If passed, bill is referred
governor for approval   to "other House"
or veto

If approved

If vetoed

Bill can still become   Bill becomes public law
law if re-passed by
both Houses with
two-thirds vote

FIGURE 19-1

⬔

How a bill becomes a law.
(NOTE: From *The Legislative
Process* [p. 3], by New York
State Nurses Association, 1993,
Guilderland, NY: Author.
Reprinted with permission.)

assemblyman, who was considered a **"friend of nursing."** The assemblyman agreed to sponsor such a bill and to bring it before the appropriate committee.

As a member of the majority party and a sincere believer in the
bill, the assemblyman was able to withstand the opposition to it. The
opposition came mainly from the HCA. The HCA lobbied strongly
against the bill, arguing that if nurses were able to have a practice
with more than one nurse and to make house calls to their clients,
they would be in direct competition with the licensed home care
agencies. This, of course, was not the intent of the bill.

To date, the HCA lobbying efforts have been successful in the
Senate but not in the Assembly. The bill has been around for several
years now. At one time, there was an Assembly bill and a companion
Senate bill. The Assembly passed it, but it never came out of committee in the Senate, which effectively killed it. This bill is then consid-

Friend of Nursing. This is a
name given to a legislator who
has proven to be accessible to
nurses, open to their views, and
whose voting record on issues
important to nurses is in line
with what nurses have lobbied
for or against.

Dead Bills. Any bill that does not get approved during a legislative session is considered dead. In order to keep the hope for legislation alive, a new bill with a new number and sometimes new sponsors must be introduced in the next session.

ered a **dead bill**. This year there is a new bill. Although it passed the Assembly, to date, it still lacks a sponsor in the Senate. Nonetheless, Nurse Murphy and the SNA have not given up hope.

ᒪOBBYING STRATEGIES: HOW TO GET YOUR MESSAGE ACROSS

Lobbying is a multibillion dollar industry in the United States. Some people see lobbying as a God-given right, while others see it as the devil's work. Whether you like it or hate it, approve of it or condemn it, you should know that it is considered the most effective way to achieve legislative change in this country. Lobbyists come in all shapes and sizes and all levels of sophistication, ranging from the occasional signer of a petition to the full-time paid lobbyist. While it is difficult to calculate how many lobbyists there are, the government office that maintains the files of active, registered lobbyists reports that there are about 6000 individuals or organizations, representing approximately 11,000,000 clients. It is estimated that the actual number may be as much as four times higher (Sachs, 1991).

Lobbying: What Is It?

According to Richard Sachs, an analyst for the United States government, *lobbying* is the process of achieving public policy goals, most often by private interest groups, through the selected application of political pressure (Sachs, 1991). In the United States, lobbying is a protected activity under the First Amendment, that part of the Constitution that guarantees the rights of free speech, assembly, and petition of government for redress of grievances.

Lobbying is actually a major form of the art of influencing people. Every minute of every day someone somewhere is lobbying someone for something. People lobby different people for a variety of reasons and causes, both formally and informally. For instance, a child may lobby a parent for permission to go on a special trip with her or his friends, a worker may lobby her or his boss for a raise, or a head nurse may lobby an administrator to protect a nursing position. For the purposes of this chapter, lobbying is considered on a grander scale; nurses can lobby policy makers so that the health care of the community can be preserved or improved. Therefore, how a lobbyist persuades public policy makers to adopt a certain course of action is examined.

There are many different lobbying strategies, including letter writing, telephoning, faxing, E-mailing, using the Internet, sending postcards, and making personal visits to your legislator. A few of those strategies along with how-to steps for each are discussed below.

Organizing a Grass-Roots Campaign One way to improve the effectiveness of your lobbying efforts is to organize a *grass-roots* network. Anyone can lobby on her or his own, but there is strength in numbers. First, the nurse must research the issue thoroughly; the nurse cannot pos-

sibly convince someone to lobby for a cause if she or he does not understand the issue. Moreover, it is always easier to get people involved if the
issue being addressed affects them directly.

Second, the nurse must identify people in her or his immediate circle of
friends who would like to be involved. If possible, a meeting can be held
to explain the issues, describe the lobbying strategies, and list the individuals targeted by the lobby.

Third, each person in the core group must be asked to identify five people she or he would be willing to contact to assist in this lobbying effort.

Fourth, all of the health care institutions and nursing schools in the area
must be listed and a key person in each of those institutions identified.
Then an individual in the core group must contact that key person. That
key person must then be asked whether she or he would be willing to act
as a liaison between the core group and the nurses in their institution. As
liaison, that person would be expected to distribute lobbying information
among his or her colleagues. Cooperation at this level is usually very high
because people do not see this role as burdensome.

Fifth, a list of telephone numbers, called a *telephone tree*, must be compiled so that the core group and the people identified as key contacts will
have this list from which to work when the time comes to take action on
a specific issue. The telephone tree is a very effective lobbying tool.

Please keep in mind that the people enlisted in the grass-roots network
do not have to be nurses. They can be family members, friends, or acquaintances. It also important to remember to treat all grass-roots workers with
respect. Keep the lines of communication open in both directions. Let people know that their input is valuable. Work projects should be well organized, so that there is always something for these workers to do when they
call to volunteer to help. Make working on campaign projects fun; serve
refreshments whenever possible. Most importantly, always thank your
workers for what they do and show appreciation. Remember, these people
are usually volunteering their time.

Postcard Campaign   To set into motion a successful postcard campaign,
it will be helpful if a grass-roots network has already been established.
A postcard campaign is simple: it is an organized effort to send as many
postcards as possible containing the lobbying message to targeted legislators. (Please remember that the people enlisted as grass-roots workers do
not have to be nurses; they can be family members, friends, or acquaintances). A postcard campaign can be conducted in a number of ways. For
instance, the members of the network can be asked to send their own postcards with their own messages, using their own stamps, to the targeted legislators. Alternatively, the nurse can supply the postcards with the message
printed on them with or without the postage already affixed.

Telecommunications Campaign   In this era of sophisticated telecommu-
nication systems, it is not unusual for nurses to use means other than the
telephone to contact their legislators, but for years the telephone has been
a quick and easy way to contact legislators or their aides to discuss issues
of concern. When using the telephone, make sure that your name and any
affiliation you wish to have acknowledged are stated. Ask for the name of

the person to whom you are speaking and her or his title. Be brief and to the point. Document your call for your records.

E-mail and Faxes In today's highly technological world of communications, most legislators can be contacted through these media. Again, either your grass-roots people can compose their own messages on the lobbying issue, or the nurse can supply a message. In either case, the nurse must supply the network with the contact information for the targeted legislators.

Internet and the World Wide Web Since participation on the information highway is increasing every day, it is important to determine how many people in the grass-roots network can employ these modes of communication in their lobbying efforts.

Letter Writing While letter writing is a skill that most nurses feel they already possess, letter writing as a lobbying strategy has a special set of guidelines.

1. Handwrite your letters whenever possible or at least address the envelope by hand. An envelope that is handwritten is more likely to be opened than one that has a label affixed or the information typed.
2. Make sure that the legislator's correct title is used and that the legislator's name is spelled correctly.
3. Write or type legibly; if the legislator or his or her aide cannot read the message, the purpose of the message has been defeated.
4. Make sure that your name and address are on the letter and on the envelope.
5. Sign the letter, including your degrees or title (e.g, R.N.) after your name.
6. Identify yourself as a registered voter, and, if applicable, make sure to mention that you are a constituent.
7. Identify yourself as a member of whatever groups with which you are associated (e.g., the ANA, the PTA, your local church group).
8. Identify the issue that concerns you.
9. Limit your letter to one subject and be concise.
10. Give the bill number and key provisions. (e.g., bill number S _____ , which states that _____).
11. State your relationship to the bill; for example, "This bill will have a direct negative effect on the clients for whom I care."
12. Support your position; for example, "This bill, which calls for a co-payment for health care services for people on Medicaid, will result in a decrease of available health care services. For many of my clients, passage of this legislation will mean choosing between getting needed health care or putting food on the table."
13. Clearly ask for action on the bill; for example, "I am asking you to vote against bill number S.___ or for bill number H.R.___." Sometimes, this is the only piece of information that is actually relayed to the legislator. Remember that most of the legislator's correspondence is not opened or read by the legislator.

14. Write clearly and concisely, using straightforward language.
15. Adopt a reasonable and respectful tone. Remember: "You catch more bees with honey."
16. Ask for a reply.

Face-to-Face Lobbying Visiting your legislator and discussing your issues face-to-face is a very effective way to lobby. If it is your good fortune to actually meet with your legislator that is wonderful, but alas, that is not always the case. Very few lobbying visits are conducted with the legislator actually in the room. Instead, it is more than likely that you will meet with the legislator's aide. Do not fret. Most of the time you are better served when you meet with the aide because the aide is usually the person who is handling the issue about which you are concerned anyway.

Anyone can lobby; but your lobbying efforts should have an impact. Here are some tips on how to get the most out of your lobbying visit.

1. Call your legislator's office and ask for an appointment. To increase your chances of seeing your legislator in person, you must always consider the legislative calendar. What days will your legislator be in session? This session calendar will also have a bearing on where you wish to visit your legislator. Do you want to meet at the legislator's local office or at the legislator's capital office?
2. Do your homework. Make sure that you understand the issue you wish to discuss. Also, try to find out where your legislator stands on the issue. A review of the legislator's voting record or news articles related to the issue will help to determine this.
3. Be on time for your appointment.
4. If there is a sign-in book, make sure you sign it.
5. Bring printed material that describes your position on the issue and any other information that you would like your legislator to have. You can hand this material to your legislator as soon as you walk in. You can then say, "Here is some information regarding _____, which I would like to discuss with you today." This allows the legislator to direct her or his attention to what you have to say without worrying about jotting down notes.
6. Address your legislator by her or his title, (e.g., Senator Brolly).
7. When you introduce yourself, give the legislator your card.
8. Clearly state the issue and your position. Allow the legislator to discuss her or his position. Allow time for dialogue.
9. Offer your expertise on health care issues to your legislator. Offer to be a resource person, to be a member of any task force she or he may create, or to attend any meeting that is convened.
10. Thank her or him for giving you time and repeat your request; for example, "Thank you for your time, Senator Brolly. It has been a pleasure meeting with you, and I hope you will support bill number S._____."
11. Send a follow-up letter thanking your legislator again for taking time out of her or his busy schedule to meet with you. Repeat your lobbying message.

All of these steps should be taken whether you meet with the legislator or with the legislative aide.

Lobbying Strategies: Some Added Advice   In regards to all of the strategies mentioned here, it is important to note that *timing is everything!* Contact your legislator either before the issue about which you are concerned is to be considered or while it is being considered. There is no real harm done if you begin to lobby your legislator too early on an issue, but you can lose any impact that you might have had if you lobby too late—that is, after the bill has passed a particular house, both houses, or the executive branch.

Something else nurses should keep in mind is that, although a legislator has the power to take action on the bill that may interest nurses, they have the power to vote that same legislator into or out of office. Remember: the power is in the vote, and you cast the vote.

Campaign Contributions and Political Action Committees (PACs)   One of the most powerful lobbying strategies involves making financial contributions to a politician's campaign. For many years, this part of the political game was played largely by a select group. These players represented business, commerce, labor, and agriculture. Recently, however, Washington has seen a diversification of special interest groups; lobbyists now represent the professions, education, welfare, science, the arts, public interest groups, and the consumer.

This form of lobbying has inspired a great deal of controversy. Those who see it as a positive force feel that it facilitates the flow of knowledge and understanding to and from the government. To these people, lobbying is seen as an activity that encourages the participation and involvement of citizens in the workings of the government. However, there are also many Americans who view lobbying as a harmful force. They see lobbyists and the special interest groups that they represent as exercising influence that is not in the best interest of the public; an example is the lobby for the tobacco industry. Critics also contend that many lobbying activities are conducted in secret, deliberately avoiding public scrutiny. Antilobbyists see campaign contributions and social relationships with elected or appointed officials as unsavory if not illegal or improper. These same people see lobbyists and lobbying as obstacles to the decision-making process of our government.

Many people feel that lobbyists are in a position to buy a legislator's vote through unreported campaign contributions, by giving legislators expensive trips and gifts, or through some misuse of PAC funds. Therefore, campaign reform has been a hot political football for several years.

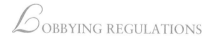

LOBBYING REGULATIONS

Lobbying is a very difficult industry to control because there are so many gray areas. The first major gray area is created by the difficulty in drawing a distinction between socializing and lobbying. How can you regulate with whom legislators can socialize in their own homes or on vacation? The second gray area arises from the difficulty in differentiating between lobbying and information exchange. It is very difficult to make this distinction when conversations about political issues have a tendency to be viewed as lobbying when a legislator is involved. Finally, it has been difficult to regulate lobbying because Congressional investigators of alleged improprieties or illegal activities often become the target of the lobbyists under investigation. This is almost a natural result of an investigation because lobbyist have friends everywhere. Friends are a by-product of a lobbyist's business.

Congress does, however, control lobbying in a limited way. Listed below are some of the laws of which nurses should be aware.

- **Treasury and Postal Services Appropriations for Fiscal Year 1996** [Public Law (P.L.) 104-52, H.R. 2020]. A Senate floor amendment sponsored by Senators Simpson and Craig prohibits lobbying by certain tax-exempt organizations who receive federal awards, including grants and loans. Signed into law on November 19, 1995.
- **Lobbying Disclosure Act of 1995** (P.L. 104-65, S. 1060). This act requires the disclosure of all lobbying intended to influence the federal government. It also prohibits gifts from lobbyists to members of Congress and for other purposes. Signed into law December 19, 1995.
- **Hatch Political Activities Act** limits the political activities of United States government employees. Congress passed the act in 1939 and a major amendment in 1940. The 1939 act prohibits most federal employees from taking an active part in political campaigns. The 1940 amendment extends these provisions to most state and local employees in federally funded projects. The 1940 amendment also set limits on campaign contributions by individuals, but the Federal Election Campaign Act of 1971 removed overall ceilings.

The Federal Election Campaign Act of 1971 required detailed reporting of both campaign contributions and expenses. In 1974, amendments to the Act established public financing of presidential campaigns and created an agency called the Federal Election Commission to enforce the rules. The amendments further limited the amount an individual or group could contribute to any one candidate. In 1976, the Supreme Court of the United States ruled that only presidential candidates who accept public financing must stay within the spending limits.

The United States Civil Service Commission administers provisions of the Hatch Political Activities Act. The act was named for its sponsor, Senator Carl Hatch of New Mexico.

Naturally, all of these laws affect how nurses and the ANA lobby. A PAC is limited by law as to the amount of cash and **in-kind services** it can contribute to a campaign. The ANA-PAC must also engage a qualified person to prepare the financial reports and filings for submission. However, it is also nice to know that all PACs must abide by these same laws and regulations.

In-Kind Services. This is a term used to describe political contributions that are not monetary such as manpower, printing services, phone calls, and so on.

‭N‬URSES AND POLITICS

The ANA is nursing's professional organization, representing approximately 2.2 million nurses. The purposes of the ANA are: (1) to work for the improvement of health standards and the availability of health care services for all people; (2) to foster high standards of nursing; and (3) to stimulate and promote the professional development of nurses and so advance their economic and general welfare. The ANA has several functions, three of which will be mentioned here: (1) to assume an active role as consumer advocate; (2) to represent and speak for the nursing profession with allied health groups, national and international organizations, governmental bodies, and the public; and (3) to protect and promote the advancement of human rights related to health care and nursing. These three functions are directly related to political activity. There can be no effective consumer advocacy without political activity; there can be no effective representation for the nursing professions if there is no political activity; and there can be no effective protection or advancement of human rights related to health care and nursing without political activity. Therefore, the ANA has worked hard to develop its governmental affairs department and to enhance its visibility in the political arena.

As was said earlier, politics is the art of influencing people, and if one expects to be an advocate for consumers, nurses, and human rights, one needs to be able to influence people. The ANA has evolved into a very influential force in the political arena through its grass-roots organizing and its PAC.

It is important that nurses understand how the ANA is organized, how their SNA is organized, and how the two organizations interact. This relationship between the ANA and the SNA is not unlike the relationship between the federal government and the individual state governments. The chart on the facing page (Fig. 19-2) is an illustration of the organizational structure of the ANA. It shows how the state organizations relate to the ANA and how the district constituencies relate to the state organizations. At the top of the chart is the voting body. Here, as in the federal and state governments, the most powerful voice is the voter.

One of the ways that the ANA carries out its commitment is through organized lobbying efforts. The N-STAT, a grass-roots network of nurses coordinated by the ANA in conjunction with the SNAs, is the power behind the ANA's lobbyists.

N-STAT nurses are all volunteers who understand the critical role they play in advancing nursing's political and legislative agenda. Certain N-STAT nurses are assigned to be liaisons between the ANA and a congressman or senator. N-STAT nurses are kept abreast of issues that are important to nursing through *Action Alerts and Legislative Updates*. In addition, all N-STAT nurses receive a letter outlining the legislative priorities, copies of *Capital Update* (ANA's legislative newsletter for nurses), and a *Congressional Directory*.

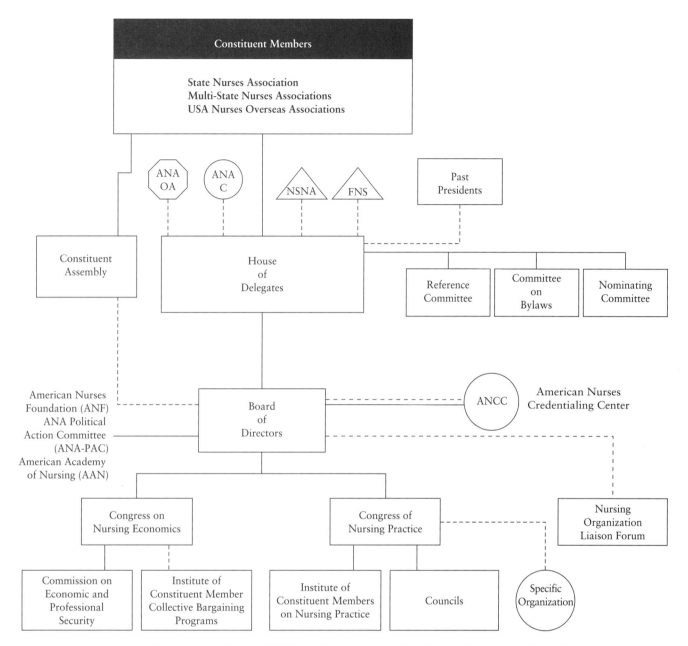

FIGURE 19-2. American Nurses Association (ANA) table of organization. [NOTE: From *American Nurses Association Bylaws as Amended July 2, 1995* (p. 45), by ANA, 1995, Washington, DC: Author. Reprinted with permission.]

At the SNA level, there are similar grass-roots networks in place. In New York, for example, there are nurses who act as liaisons between the New York State Nurses Association (NYSNA) and the state legislators. These nurse liaisons are called legislative district coordinators (LDCs). In their capacity as liaisons, these nurses contact their assigned legislators whenever there is an issue of concern to nurses.

The ANA reports that the N-STAT network is 40,000 nurses strong. Forty thousand nurses speaking in one voice can be heard "loud and clear" on Capitol Hill.

American Nurses Association Political Action Committee (ANA-PAC)

The ANA-PAC as we know it today has evolved over the last couple of decades. The first formal meeting of the group of nurses that would come to be known as Nurses for Political Action (NPA) was held at Adelphi University on July 10, 1971. This group of about ten nurses met "to determine how the nursing profession might exert greater influence over health care in this country" (Rothenberg, 1985, p. 133). These nurses were disturbed by the fact that "although nurses constituted the single largest group of providers and despite our vital contribution to health care, the profession continued to have little power or influence" (Rothenberg, 1985, p. 133). These nurses were aware of the power that the American Medical Association (AMA) had achieved through the American Medical Political Action Committee (AMPAC). These nurses decided that it was necessary for organized nursing to have its own political action arm. Since there was no movement at this time from their SNAs or the ANA to create such an organization, these ten nurses decided to move forward on their own, hoping that their new entity would eventually become the political action arm of the ANA. To do this, seed money was needed. These nurses raised this seed money by each pledging to lend NPA $1000, a great deal of money in 1972. NPA moved forward, developing a grass-roots campaign in which nurses spread the word about NPA to other nurses and nursing organizations. In January of 1973, a meeting was held between NPA and the ANA to discuss the feasibility of making the NPA the political arm of the ANA. Talks continued. The idea was becoming a reality. On September 20, 1973, the ANA Board of Directors voted to create a PAC. The new organization was named Nurses Coalition for Action in Politics (N-CAP). At the 1974 ANA Convention in San Francisco, the formation of N-CAP was announced. Today, the ANA-PAC, as it is now known, has experienced dramatic growth as a result of the commitment of thousands of nurses to political action. It is now the third largest health care PAC in the United States.

The ANA-PAC endorses candidates for federal office. The ANA-PAC endorsement process relies on both the SNAs and the N-STAT leadership team (i.e., SDCs, CDCs) for input on each candidate being considered for endorsement. Representatives from the SNA or the N-STAT team meet with candidates and review candidates' voting records to see where these candidates stand on issues important to nurses. Evaluations with recommendations are written and forwarded to the ANA-PAC Board for review. The ANA-PAC is governed by the ANA-PAC Board of Trustees. Presently, the Board is responsible for directing the fund-raising activities of the ANA-PAC as well as the candidate endorsement activities. The ANA-PAC Board of Trustees votes on candidates they want to support for election or reelection and the amount of monies or in-kind services that will be contributed. The amount of monies that a PAC may contribute to an individual is limited by federal law. A PAC may contribute up to $5000 per candidate per election. The PAC endorsement recommendations are sent to the SNAs for final approval. SNAs may veto the endorsement.

The ANA-PAC has also been very successful in getting its endorsed candidates elected to office. Approximately 77 percent of the candidates it supported in the 1996 election won their races.

SUMMARY

This chapter discusses the important part that politics play in shaping today's health care policies and explains how important it is for nurses to become politically active. It also describes how nurses can obtain and exercise political influence in their workplaces as well as in their lives. Many different lobbying strategies are detailed so that nurses can put them to use immediately. Laws regulating lobbying and lobbyist's activities are also described. Additionally, this chapter describes the federal and state governments of the United States and the legislative process of each. This chapter also describes the organization, purpose, and functions of the ANA as they relate to political activism, including the ANA's N-STAT program and its PAC. This chapter strongly emphasizes how important it is for nurses to belong to professional nursing organizations such as the ANA and to support the ANA-PAC.

KEY WORDS

American Nurses Association (ANA)
Federal government
Grass roots
Legislative process
Lobbying
Nurses Strategic Action
   Team (N-STAT)

Political Action
   Committee (PAC)
Political climate
Political clout
Politics
Power
State government

QUESTIONS

DIRECTIONS: Choose the one *best* response to each of the following questions.

1. Historically, nurses have been apolitical because
   A. most nurses do not understand politics.
   B. a nurse has never run for a major political office.
   C. nurses are too busy caring for patients to get involved in politics.
   D. most nurses feel that politics are far removed from their agenda of caring.

2. The issue of health care has been considered a politically "hot issue" for all the following reasons except

    A. health care affects every constituent of every politician.
    B. health care costs are a major budget issue.
    C. 1 in every 44 registered voters is a registered nurse.
    D. voters monitor their legislator's actions on health care issues when deciding how to cast their vote.

3. Which of the following actions relate most directly to the legislative process?

    A. Using the Alliance Model to assess the health of a community.
    B. Bringing an idea for a health-related bill to the local legislator.
    C. Administering immunization to the uninsured and underinsured.
    D. Writing a letter to the editor of the local paper regarding poor housing conditions.

4. An example of an action by the executive branch of the government is the

    A. ruling of a family court judge to issue an order of protection for an abused spouse.
    B. vote of a Senate committee on a bill to increase Medicare funding.
    C. decision of the Speaker of the House not to take action on a health care bill.
    D. president vetoing a bill that has been passed by both houses.

5. The most prudent course of action for nurses to take if they wish to influence health care policy and practice positively is to

    A. introduce as many ideas for "nurse friendly" bills as possible to as many legislators as possible.
    B. wait for a bill to be introduced by Congress that appears to be in line with nursing's agenda.
    C. bring an idea for a bill to a legislator in the majority party to sponsor.
    D. attend public hearings on all health-related bills.

6. One of the most effective lobbying strategies for nurses is

    A. speaking with clients to discover what political issues are of interest to them.
    B. organizing a grass-roots campaign.
    C. identifying the issues about which nurses are most concerned.
    D. calling a legislator in a neighboring district to ask her or him to vote yes on third-party reimbursement for nurses.

7. The factors that have contributed most to the success of the American Nurses Association Political Action Committee (ANA-PAC) include all of the following *except* the

    A. establishment of the Nurses Strategic Action Team (N-STAT).
    B. ability of the nursing profession to raise monies for the PAC.
    C. passage of the Lobbying Disclosure Act of 1995.
    D. ANA ability to become recognized as one of "the players."

8. When planning a face-to-face meeting with a legislator to lobby for passage of a particular bill, the nurse should do all of the following *except*
    A. cancel the meeting if the legislator is not available.
    B. bring a written position statement as well as be able to state her or his position clearly.
    C. identify her- or himself as a nurse and, if applicable, as a constituent.
    D. lobby the legislator on timely issues.

9. Nurses who are politically active in the community usually
    A. are not nurses who deliver "hands-on" care.
    B. work with the interdisciplinary team and the client to influence resource allocations.
    C. will not attend town meetings because it is not in their job description.
    D. realize that only issues that affect the delivery of health services to the community are the ones with which nurses should be involved.

10. In the Alliance Model, the community health nurse works with the interdisciplinary team to influence the inner circle, which deals with resource allocation decisions by
    A. becoming politically active in the local community.
    B. coordinating the care of the interdisciplinary team.
    C. identifying issues that may have a negative affect on the health of the community.
    D. telling clients to move from their community if it lacks needed services.

ANSWERS

1. *The answer is D.* Historically, nurses are known to be apolitical because they feel that politics are far removed from their agenda of caring.

2. *The answer is C.* Although it is true that 1 in every 44 registered voters is a nurse, the reason why health care is such a politically "hot" issue is that every voter wants to have a say in how the health care issue will be resolved. Accordingly, voters are monitoring their legislator's actions in regards to this issue to see whether or not that legislator deserves their vote. It is not just a nursing issue.

3. *The answer is B.* Bringing an idea for a health-related bill to a local legislator is the first step of the legislative process both on the state and federal level.

4. *The answer is D.* The federal executive power is vested in the president.

5. *The answer is C.* By bringing an idea for a bill to a legislator in the majority party to sponsor, the chances for passage in the House are increased. This is so because each committee is made up of a majority of members from the majority party and is chaired by a member of the majority party.

6. *The answer is B.* Organizing a grass-roots campaign is one of the most essential elements of a successful lobbying effort.

7. *The answer is C.* The passage of the Lobbying Disclosure Act of 1995 prohibited lobbyists from presenting gifts to members of Congress.

8. *The answer is A.* Most lobbying meetings are held with the legislator's aide because the legislator's calendar is so full. The legislator's absence is not a reason to cancel a meeting because a meeting with the aide can be effective.

9. *The answer is B.* A politically active nurse works with the interdisciplinary team and the client to influence resource allocations so that the health of a community remains stable or improves.

10. *The answer is A.* Becoming politically active in the local community can contribute significantly to the effectiveness of both the nurse and the interdisciplinary team.

ANNOTATED REFERENCES

American Nurses Association. (1995). Advanced practice nursing: A new age in health care. *Nursing Facts.* Washington, DC: Author.

This fact sheet contains statistics on advanced practice nurses (APNs), such as how many there are, who they are, and how they are prepared.

American Nurses Association (ANA). (1995). *Keeping nurses' issues alive.* Washington, DC: Author.

This brochure explains what the Nurses Strategic Action Team (N-STAT) is and what it does as the ANA rapid response team.

American Nurses Association (1995). *American Nurses Association Bylaws.* Washington, DC: Author.

This booklet contains information about the association's purpose, function, membership, and workings.

Congressional Research Service. (1992). *The legislative process in brief.* Washington, DC: Author.

This document contains a brief overview of the legislative process of the United States government.

Cove, P. B. (Ed.). (1975). *Webster's Third International Dictionary.* Springfield, MA: G.C. Merriam.

Kalisch, P. A., & Kalisch, B. J. (1987). *The changing image of the nurse.* Palo Alto, CA: Addison-Wesley.

This book discusses the changing health care delivery system and how nursing's image has changed.

Kelly, L. & Joel, L. (1996). *The nursing experience: Trends, challenges, and transitions* (3rd ed.). New York: McGraw-Hill.

This book contains a detailed compilation of facts about the practice of nursing. It contains charts chronicling nursing organizations and the accomplishments of nursing leaders.

Leonard, M. (1994). Levels of political participation and political expectation among nurses in New York State. Journal of the New York State Nurses Association, 25(1), 16–24.

This article describes a study that investigated the relationship of area of practice, educational level, and membership in a professional organization to political participation and political expectations among a group of nurses.

Mason, D., Talbot S., & Leavitt, J. (1993). *Policy and politics for nurses* (3rd ed.). Philadelphia: W. B. Saunders.

This book contains the information, the encouragement, and the how-tos to help nurses get involved in the political and policy-making processes.

New York State Nurses Association. (1993). *The Legislative Process.* Guilderland, NY: Author.

This pamphlet describes the legislative process on a state level.

Rothenberg, J. S. (1985, May/June). The growth of political activity in nursing. *Nursing Outlook*, p. 133–135.

This article traces the history and describes the formation of the Nurses Coalition for Action in Politics (N-CAP).

Reader's Digest Association. (1975). *Family encyclopedia of American history.* Pleasantville, NY: Author.

This book contains a compilation of facts and dates about American history.

Sachs, R. (1991, October 23). Lobbying in the United States. *Congressional Research Service Report for Congress.*

This report is developed by Congressional Research Service (CRS), the Library of Congress. It describes lobbying as a protected activity under the part of the Constitution that guarantees the rights of free speech, assembly, and petition of government for redress of grievances.

Sachs, R. (1996, February). Regulating interest groups and lobbyists: Issues in the 104th Congress. *CRS Issue Brief.*

This publication of the Congressional Research Service (CRS), Library of Congress contains recent developments on actions of the 104th Congress as they pertain to regulating lobbyists.

United Hospital Fund (UHF). (1996). *Children and health: New York City and the nation.* New York: Author.

This book was used for the UHF Conference "Child Health in a Managed Care Environment." It contains statistics on populations, socioeconomics, disease, deaths, health resources, and health services.

ℳANAGED CARE: FRIEND OR FOE

In discussing the Alliance Model for Community Health Assessment in Chap. 5, we noted three interrelated areas of concern, one of which was the influences affecting resource allocation decisions. A more in-depth look at this sphere showed five variables that influence how resource allocation decisions are made. The fifth variable had to do with patterns of insurance coverage, the most controversial of which today is managed care. This chapter defines managed care, explores its many facets, and describes how nurses acting as part of interdisciplinary teams can work to produce healthier communities by bringing this sphere of the Alliance Model into increased connection with community-based needs and systems of care management.

The impetus behind the managed care movement is cost containment. Since many believe that cost containment has led to unscrupulous and unethical practices by some managed care organizations (MCOs), nurses, who are both consumers and providers of health care, have banded together with consumer groups and other professional disciplines to voice their concerns about some controversial issues. While nursing agrees with the major concepts of managed care—prevention, wellness, client outreach, and education—the impetus behind nursing's involvement in the managed care movement is the need to ensure access for all to quality health care. This chapter discusses how the challenges and opportunities of managed care have been or will be met by nurses.

$\mathcal{M}$ANAGED CARE

Public Awareness of Managed Care

A great deal of the managed care controversy comes from a lack of understanding of the managed care industry itself. Managed care has spread across this nation like wildfire, advancing fastest in the west. It is an industry with a whole new vocabulary (e.g., enrollee, capitation, full-risk contracts, any willing provider, gag rules, **reinsurance**) and a whole new set of rules (e.g., preadmission authorization, concurrent reviews, prior approvals, in-plan and out-of-plan authorizations). As if all this were not confusing enough, many people also have difficulty making sense of managed care's many new acronyms [e.g., preferred provider organization (PPO), independent practice association (IPA), point of service (POS), health maintenance organization (HMO), physician-hospital organization (PHO), exclusive provider organization (EPO)] and the many news headlines [e.g., "Penny-pinching HMOs Showed Their Generosity in Executive Paychecks" (Freudenheim, 1995, p. D1), "Managed Care Contributed Significantly to Recent Declines in Health Inflation" (Fubini, 1995, p. 3)]. Moreover, many people do not know who the players are, and they are unaware of what legislation and regulations are in place or are being proposed for the managed care industry. Therefore, how can they possibly make an accurate assessment of the advantages and disadvantages of managed care?

Many people believe that managed care was created in response to public demands to control the chaos caused by the rapidly escalating costs of our fragmented *fee-for-service health care system*, a system that may reward providers for delivering too much care or ordering too many diagnostic tests for a client. There are also people, however, who hold the contrasting belief that managed care has compromised the quality of health care delivered to clients under the *capitated reimbursement system*, a system that may reward providers for limiting the services available to a client. What are the differences between fee-for-service reimbursement and capitated reimbursement? How do these differences affect the care delivered under each system? Most people just do not know.

Despite the widespread ignorance and confusion about managed care, more and more people are enrolling in managed care plans every day. Currently, there are approximately 53.3 million enrollees in the nation's 593 HMOs (Spragins, 1996, p. 58).

Reinsurance is sharing of risk among insurance companies. Part of the insurer's risk is assumed by other companies in return for a part of the premium fee paid by the insured. Reinsurance allows an individual company to take on clients whose coverage would be too great a burden for one insurer to carry alone.

Economic Perspective on Managed Care

Managed care comes at a time when our country is experiencing a dramatic escalation of health expenditures; in 1995, health care cost $1.069 trillion, approximately one-seventh of the United States gross domestic product (GDP). Consumers, the business community, and the government

Indemnity Plan. This is an insurance plan whereby an individual pays a premium to secure against loss or damage that may occur in the future.

all have a vested interest in containing the cost of health care. Each of these groups is concerned with rising health care costs and the negative impact that these costs are having on the overall inflation rate.

Many reports have touted managed care as the vehicle that can both contain health costs and lower insurance premiums. The average cost of health care per employee across the nation was significantly less when the employee was covered by an HMO than if the employee was covered by an **indemnity plan**, and the average premium costs for both individual and family coverage were less when provided by an HMO.

The two most notable sources of federal governmental, third-party reimbursement are Medicare, which has 35 million participants at a cost of $135 billion, and Medicaid, which has 30 million participants at a cost of $80 billion. Therefore, it is no wonder that the government jumped on the managed care bandwagon after seeing that corporations providing HMO coverage for their beneficiaries experienced significant savings.

Managed care has emerged as a very powerful and lucrative industry. While there are a number of government initiatives in the works to bring both Medicaid and Medicare recipients into the managed care arena, the number of beneficiaries opting into HMOs without any government mandates or incentives is astounding. For example, the Health Care Financing Administration (HCFA) recently reported that 70,000 Medicare beneficiaries opt into Medicare HMOs every month.

Managed Care: A Definition

Managed care has been defined as a health care system that combines cost-effectiveness with quality care. The American Nurses Association (ANA) Task Force on Standards and Regulation of Managed Care defines managed care as a system for delivering a prepaid health-centered benefits package to a defined population or membership. Managed care covers the full continuum of health care, integrates the services of various providers, seeks appropriateness in the type and intensity of care, and requires collaboration among a variety of providers or provider groups. Managed care members (i.e., clients) are involved in making decisions within the system, and the system attempts to balance the assignment of risk between clients, providers, and the administration and to provide an ethical framework for the resolution of disputes (ANA, 1996).

This definition was developed as part of a report to the Congress on nursing practice in April, 1996. This definition contains elements that nurses see as important safety nets for consumers: full continuum of care, collaboration, client involvement in decision making, balance of risk assignment, and an ethical framework component. These elements will be discussed in greater detail later in this chapter.

Types of Managed Care

MCOs are legal entities licensed by the state and regulated by state departments of insurance or health. There are many types of MCOs, each of which represents a sector of health insurance in which health care providers are not independent businesses (e.g., physicians in private practice) but administrative firms (e.g., HMOs, PPOs) that manage the allocation of health care benefits. MCOs use various financial incentives and management controls to direct clients to efficient providers responsible for giving appropriate medical care in cost-effective treatment settings. These providers participate in HMOs, PPOs, EPOs, and other POS arrangements.

Health Maintenance Organization (HMO) An HMO is a comprehensive health care financing and delivery organization that provides or arranges for provision of covered health care services to a specified group of enrollees at a fixed periodic payment through a panel of providers. Historically, four types of HMO models have been common: (1) the *staff model*, in which physicians are salaried employees of the HMO; (2) the *group model*, which contracts with multispecialty physician group practices; (3) the *IPA model*, which contracts with IPAs, which, in turn, contract with independent physicians who practice in their own offices; and (4) the *network model*, which contracts with two or more independent group practices or IPAs. HMOs can be sponsored by the government, medical schools, hospitals, labor unions, consumer groups, insurance companies, or hospital medical plans.

Preferred Provider Organization (PPO) A PPO is an arrangement whereby a third-party payer contracts with a group of preferred medical care providers who furnish services at lower-than-usual fees in return for prompt payment and access to a certain volume of clients.

Exclusive Provider Organization (EPO) An EPO is a more rigid type of PPO that requires the insured either to use only designated providers or to sacrifice reimbursement altogether.

Physician-Hospital Organization (PHO) A PHO is an organization of physicians and hospitals that—at a minimum—is responsible for negotiating with third-party payers.

Point of Service (POS) A POS is also referred to as an open-ended HMO-PPO. In a POS plan, each time the **enrollee** seeks care she or he is given a choice of receiving health services either from an in-plan network provider or an out-of-plan provider. This option to receive services from an out-of-plan provider usually entails higher costs to the enrollee in the form of higher premiums, deductibles, and copayments (Fig. 20-1).

Enrollee is one who has signed on to be a member of a managed care plan.

How Does Managed Care Work?

Managed care operates by balancing three essential components of health care: utilization, cost, and outcomes. Utilization is monitored closely by the MCOs to protect against both under- and over-utilization of services by either providers or the enrollees. Costs are monitored to ensure savings,

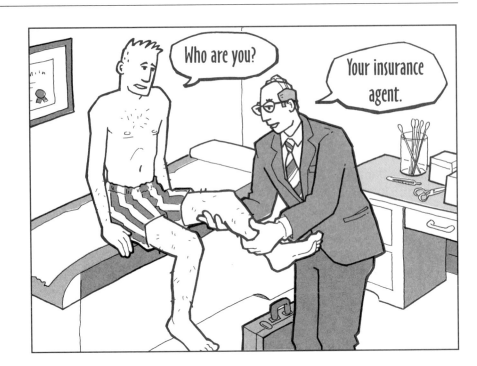

FIGURE 20-1

and outcomes are monitored to ensure that appropriate quality care is delivered. All three of these components are controlled through capitated reimbursement, case management, authorization/certification, and precise contractual language.

Capitated Reimbursement System or Capitation Capitation is a method of payment for health services in which a practitioner or hospital is prepaid a fixed per-capita amount to cover a specific period of time for each person served, regardless of the actual number of services provided to each person. Most plans arrange their capitation rates according to **actuarial classes**. In this type of managed care arrangement, the MCO does the marketing of the PCP, usually establishing a large **panel** for MCO network providers.

Actuarial Class. This is a classification of enrollees that is arrived at by using the mathematics of insurance, including probabilities. It is used in ensuring that risks are carefully evaluated, that adequate premiums are charged for risks underwritten, and that adequate provision is made for future payments.

Panel is the term used to describe the number of enrollees assigned to a provider who acts as the PCP for those enrollees.

CASE STUDY: THE CASE OF DR. MCGRAW

Dr. McGraw, an internist, has applied to and been accepted as a part of Lionheart HMO. Dr. McGraw's name will now be offered to the enrollees of Lionheart HMO for selection as their primary care provider (PCP). When an enrollee chooses Dr. McGraw as her or his PCP, the enrollee's name is added to Dr. McGraw's monthly enrollee roster. This roster is used to track the number of enrollees on Dr. McGraw's panel for whom he receives a monthly capitation payment. This payment is inclusive for any and all services delivered to these enrollees.

Each month, Dr. McGraw receives an updated roster listing the names of the enrollees on his panel. Dr. McGraw has already agreed to the capitation rate of $30 a month; accordingly, Dr. McGraw receives $30 per month per enrollee. If Dr. McGraw's panel grows to 500 or 1000 enrollees (the average enrollee capacity threshold prescribed by MCOs is between 1000 and 1500), he would then receive a monthly payment (assuming all enrollees fall into the same actuarial class) of $30,000 ($30 $\times$ 1000). Dr. McGraw will receive this same payment whether he sees every client ten times that month or only one client one time that month. It should also be noted that presently there are no restrictions on the number of MCO plan networks to which a PCP can belong. Therefore, it is feasible that a PCP can belong to many MCO networks and receive similar monthly payments from each. Hence, managed care capitated agreements can be very lucrative for Dr. McGraw.

Provider Incentive Programs Many managed care plans have provider incentive programs. These plans usually offer financial incentives for PCPs who deliver care in a cost-effective manner.

In order for a PCP to be considered eligible for an incentive program, a provider profile is compiled. The profile looks at: (1) quality outcomes; (2) number of **enrollee months**; (3) utilization patterns of services (both over- and under-utilization), including laboratory tests, durable medical equipment, supplies, and pharmaceuticals; and (4) enrollee satisfaction.

Enrollee Month. This is the number of months a member is enrolled in a plan.

A review of quality of care issues usually includes looking at a PCP's file to see if there have been any complaints lodged; the PCP is submitting encounter data on a timely basis; the PCP has remained accessible to the enrollees; and the PCP is adhering to the quality standards set by the plan. If the PCP is deemed eligible for the incentive, a check is issued.

The two most widely employed forms of incentive programs are *bonuses* and *withholds*. Bonuses are monies paid in addition to the agreed-upon capitation fees. A withhold is the HMO practice of holding back a portion of a physician's annual pay until the end of the year as an incentive to keep costs below certain targets. If the physician is able to achieve this goal, the money is paid.

Complaints have been lodged by consumers and providers against MCOs in the areas of capitation and incentives because it has been reported that many plans exclude or expel physicians who order tests or consultations deemed unnecessary by the health plans. It has also been charged that these plans punish physicians who either fail or refuse to inform clients and regulators of financial incentives that networks offer to practitioners. Some MCOs have also been found to have "gag rules" in place under which HMOs threaten to dismiss physicians if they inform clients about alternative care that might add to the costs.

As a result of a deluge of these complaints, state legislators and regulators around the country are moving to outlaw or restrict these controversial practices. More than half a dozen states, including Illinois and Georgia, have required MCOs to include any physician who has the appropriate credentials in their network. This is known as the Any Willing Provider Bill.

Maryland, which has been one of the most active states in regulating managed care, has prohibited withholds. Moreover, a few states have passed legislation stating that clients and state regulators must be informed of financial incentives offered to practitioners by networks, and at least six states have outlawed gag rules.

Clinical Pathway. This is a comprehensive algorithm designed to manage the care of clients from the time they enter the system until they are returned to their optimal level of functioning.

Case Management   Case management is a service implemented by MCOs to coordinate care and manage the cost of expensive, resource-intensive cases, such as AIDS, cancer, and major traumas. The term case management first appeared in social welfare literature during the 1970s, but the concept evolved from community service coordination, which began at the turn of the century. Today, **clinical pathways** are being developed as one methodology to incorporate and implement case management. Case management can be likened to the systems of care management sphere of the Alliance Model for Community Health Assessment (see Chap. 5); in both, the variables considered include client mix, expectations of the public for care, the competence of the professionals, accepted standards of care, and the use of interdisciplinary care plans.

To illustrate care management by an MCO, the problem of acquired immunodeficiency syndrome (AIDS) is considered. Many MCOs have found that care for enrollees with AIDS is extremely expensive. Therefore, they have decided that it is in the best interest of their clients and themselves to employ someone to oversee the coordination of the care of these clients. This case manager is usually a clinical nurse specialist (CNS) in the field of infectious disease, who functions as an integral part of the interdisciplinary team caring for the client. The case manager monitors the client's hospital stay to see that no unnecessary days are spent waiting for certain tests or procedures. The case manager then works with the hospital discharge planner to coordinate any services that the client may require, such as transportation, home care, durable medical equipment (DME), supplies, or pharmaceuticals. This case manager works with the client and the provider to coordinate the services required to assist the client to return to her or his optimal level of functioning. Case management is probably the one area of managed care that has received the least amount of resistance, simply because the concept makes clinical and fiscal sense to everyone involved, including the client, the provider, and the MCO.

CASE STUDY: THE CASE OF ALICE BEAR

Alice Bear is a client who has been newly diagnosed with human immunodeficiency virus (HIV). Alice is enrolled in Lionheart HMO. She recently experienced an exacerbation of her disease, and her provider admitted her to St. Joseph's Hospital. After giving authorization for the hospitalization, the utilization review agent (URA) at Lionheart HMO referred the case to the utilization management department of the HMO, where a case manager was assigned. The case manager assigned to Ms. Bear's case was Kathleen Boggan, a CNS with 7 years of experience working with infectious diseases and who had most recently worked at an acquired immunodeficiency syndrome (AIDS)–designated facility in Denver.

Nurse Boggan called Ms. Bear's PCP to discuss the case. Ms. Bear's PCP, a general internist, asked Nurse Boggan if he could transfer the medical coordination of Ms. Bear's case to Dr. Jack, a physician who was board certified in infectious disease medicine. Nurse Boggan, agreeing with the PCP's decision, coordinated the transfer. She then contacted Dr. Jack after the PCP had spoken to him. Dr. Jack also felt that it would be very beneficial to Ms. Bear to be transferred from St. Joseph's Hospital to Colorado Hope Hospital, where there was a designated AIDS center. Nurse Boggan informed Dr. Jack that Colorado Hope Hospital was not part of the Lionheart network and suggested the AIDS-designated center at St. Mary's Hospital, which was part of the Lionheart network. Since Dr. Jack had admitting privileges at both hospitals, it was agreed that Ms. Bear would be transferred to St. Mary's.

Once Ms. Bear was transferred, Nurse Boggan contacted the nurse in charge of Ms. Bear's care and set a date to be called back with an update on her condition and progress. During each subsequent call received from the nurse or Dr. Jack, Nurse Boggan would discuss Ms. Bear's condition, give further authorization for needed care, and set a date for the next follow-up call. During the third call, the hospital nurse reported that Ms. Bear was still waiting to have a series of diagnostic tests performed that had been rescheduled due to the overbooking of appointments. Nurse Boggan informed the hospital nurse that the hospital would not be paid for any additional hospital days that were the direct result of a failure on the part of the hospital to keep assigned appointments for scheduled testing. The hospital nurse said she would relay this information to the billing department.

Throughout the following month, Nurse Boggan continued to coordinate Ms. Bear's care with all the different members of the interdisciplinary team, arranging for transportation, home care, prescribed medications, DME, respite care for Ms. Bear's family, and home visits by a nutritionist, a physical therapist, and a social worker. Through effective case management, Nurse Boggan was able to ensure continuity of care for Ms. Bear and peace of mind for Ms. Bear's family. After Alice Bear's death, the family sent Nurse Boggan a very touching letter thanking her for all that she had done for Alice and for them.

The case management approach to this client's care produced the desired results of client satisfaction, provider satisfaction, and plan satisfaction because the client received quality, cost-effective care. In this case study, the value of appropriate case management can be seen (see Fig. 20-2).

Authorization or Certification Authorization is a form of utilization review employed by MCOs. Through this system, an assessment is made of the medical necessity of a client's admission to a hospital, some other inpatient institution and emergency department, an ambulatory care site,

FIGURE 20-2

FIGURE 20-2

Illustration of the value of case management. [NOTE: From "Critical Challenges for Nursing at the Millennium" (p. 6), by A. M. Zuckerman, 1996, paper presented at the National League for Nursing Annual Meeting, Philadelphia, PA. Reprinted with permission.]

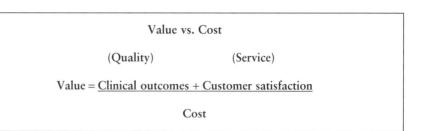

Value vs. Cost

(Quality)   (Service)

Value = $\dfrac{\text{Clinical outcomes} + \text{Customer satisfaction}}{\text{Cost}}$

or a home care service. These assessments are performed to assure that only clients requiring these levels of care receive them. Lengths of stay deemed appropriate for the client's admitting diagnosis are usually assigned and certified, and payment is supposed to be assured. These authorizations and certifications can be done before admission (preadmission), shortly after admission (concurrent), or after discharge (retrospective).

Thus, if a provider deems it necessary that a client be admitted to the hospital for a surgical procedure, the provider calls the client's MCO and requests authorization. A URA for the MCO speaks with the provider, and after obtaining the necessary demographic data, asks the provider a number of questions, such as: What is the client's diagnosis? What type of surgery will be performed? Where will the surgery be performed? The URA then determines if the requested surgery can be performed in an ambulatory surgery setting or if it requires hospitalization. The URA also determines whether or not the facility requested is a participating provider with the plan before an authorization is given. If an authorization is not given, a provider can ask to speak to the director of the utilization review department or the plan's medical director.

Utilization review has been an area of great concern and controversy among health care professionals and MCOs. Currently, URAs function without regulatory oversight, and many health care professionals feel that URAs create unnecessary barriers to needed health care services for the consumer and the provider. Another area of concern involves the qualifications of URAs. Providers feel that denials of service must be made by a licensed health professional whose qualifications, experience, and specialty have prepared them to assess effectively the service under review. Legislation to address this issue is being considered.

Another authorization and utilization review issue that has both consumers and providers up in arms is the MCO practice of withholding payment for certain types of care. At least 27 states have recently enacted laws limiting these practices by MCOs. At least 18 states have banned so-called drive-through maternity care, the hospital practice of sending mothers home less than 48 h after they give birth. Meanwhile, at least 14 states have barred insurers from refusing to pay for what turn out to be unnecessary emergency room visits such as when chest pains are traced to heartburn rather than to a life-threatening heart attack. More than 12 states guarantee a client's right to go directly to certain types of specialists (e.g., obstetrician, gynecologists) without first getting approval from a primary care physician who is called the gatekeeper by insurers.

Contracts Contracts are the life blood of a successful MCO. To stay financially solvent, a MCO must know what elements are essential for inclusion in their contracts with providers and vendors. A contract is an agreement that gives rise to an enforceable legal obligation or duty (Northrop & Kelly, 1987). The three most common contract models are: (1) the full-risk/comprehensive benefit model; (2) the partial-risk/limited benefit model; and (3) enhanced fee-for-service.

In a full-risk/comprehensive benefit model, the provider assumes financial risk for all covered services and is responsible for controlling the use of unnecessary or duplicative services. Under this arrangement, a managed care provider receives a monthly capitation rate per enrollee to cover a wide range of services, including hospital inpatient services. The provider may furnish services directly or under a subcontractual arrangement; in either case, the provider is responsible for both the quality and the cost of services reimbursed within the capitation payments. This type of contract is likely to define the relationship between an HMO and governmental agency.

In a partial-risk/limited benefit model, the provider's financial responsibility is for a limited benefit package, usually limited to the services provided directly (e.g., primary care services) and would typically exclude inpatient and other specialized services. This type of agreement is likely to be found between an HMO and a primary care practitioner or community health center.

An enhanced fee-for-service model is most likely to be employed in conjunction with a less-than-comprehensive service package. It uses as its base the existing fee-for-service **reimbursement structure** adapted to a managed care delivery system, and it may include enhanced fees. Such enhanced fees may include fee increase or case management fees. This type of agreement might be found between an HMO and a provider, clinic, or outpatient department.

All contracts should explicitly state the standards to which the MCO will hold its providers. Standards pertaining to access, quality, credentialing, confidentiality, utilization, coordination of care, and submission of encounter data all need to be spelled out in a well-written contract.

> **Reimbursement Structure.** This is a name given to a system in which a payment source is identified for services rendered.

Medicaid Managed Care

One of the most costly government programs is Medicaid, a program whose annual expenditures exceed $80 billion. The Medicaid program is a public assistance program administered and operated by participating state and territorial governments. It provides medical benefits to eligible low-income persons needing health care, regardless of age. Given the reported success that managed care had in controlling health care costs for big businesses, it was not surprising that the government, too, would consider adopting the managed care option. Figure 20-3 is a graph that shows a national comparison of Medicaid costs per recipient per year in selected states.

In 1991, the governor of a state with major Medicaid expenditures signed into law the Statewide Managed Care Program Act, Chapter 165 of the Laws of 1991. It was one of the state's most significant health care initiatives in a decade, and it was designed to result in major improve-

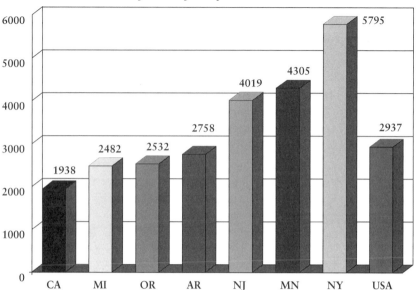

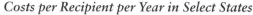

Costs per Recipient per Year in Select States

FIGURE 20-3

☒

National comparison of Medicaid costs. [NOTE: From "Critical Challenges for Nursing at the Millennium" (p. 9), by A. M. Zuckerman, 1996, paper presented at the National League for Nursing Annual Meeting, Philadelphia, PA. Reprinted with permission.]

ments in the delivery of services to Medicaid recipients. The act called for the creation of a comprehensive and coordinated system of medical and health care delivery that would encompass preventive, primary and specialty, ancillary, and acute care services.

In passing this act, legislators expected that each Medicaid recipient would be linked in a formal relationship to a primary care practitioner. The practitioner could be a private physician in solo or group practice, on staff in a community health center or outpatient department, associated with an HMO, or a nurse practitioner. The concept was that, regardless of the setting, the practitioner would be the focal point of the managed care system. This practitioner would be responsible for both the delivery of primary care and for the coordination and case management of most other services. The recipient would have access to primary care and continuity of care 24 h a day, 7 days a week. More specifically, this first state plan had the following policy objectives for managed care.

1. Enhance access to and availability of mainstream medical care and services for Medicaid recipients.
2. Ensure that managed care programs offer Medicaid recipients as wide a choice of primary care and other medical service providers as possible.
3. Promote more rational patterns of medical and health service utilization by Medicaid recipients.
4. Ensure quality of care within managed care programs.
5. Establish cost-effective managed care programs.

State and local districts were encouraged to begin new managed care programs on a voluntary basis. Once medical service providers became involved in managed care, they were obliged to work with the districts to develop and establish new strategies for quality assurance and monitoring of quality of care. In the meantime, the state was seriously considering accelerating into mandatory managed care, a process that would require waivers by the HCFA under Section 1915 of Title XIX of the Social Security Act.

Mandated Managed Care As a result of the Statewide Managed Care Program Act of 1991, many HMOs and **Prepaid Health Service Plans** (PHSPs) were developed. By 1995, there were approximately 30 HMOs and 11 PHSPs operating in this state. In 1995, the governor sponsored 1115 waivers from the HCFA for counties within the state, an action that could result in 100 percent mandatory enrollment of Medicaid recipients in managed care plans by 1998. Eventually, mandatory enrollment is expected to include special needs populations, child care, and home care.

The intent of the Statewide Managed Care Program Act was to create a coordinated care system that would provide increased access to primary care, facilitate the development of the client/provider relationship, and avoid indiscriminate and costly use of services. While this intent was excellent, a number of problems arose. Commercial HMOs, originally not interested, soon found Medicaid to be a profitable line of business. There was a shift to for-profit ownership fueled by the nationwide shift in the number of people enrolling in for-profit HMOs (Fig. 20-4). However, for some the shift was too quick. This course of action led to very heated debates between consumer groups, provider groups, and the state legislators. There were many areas of concern, the most significant of which was the marketing strategies employed by some of the HMOs and the PHSPs. It was felt that many Medicaid recipients did not understand managed care. Some recipients even claimed that they did not realize that they had "signed up for any-

Prepaid Health Services Plan (PHSP). This is a managed care plan that services Medicaid clients only.

Percentage of U.S. employees enrolled

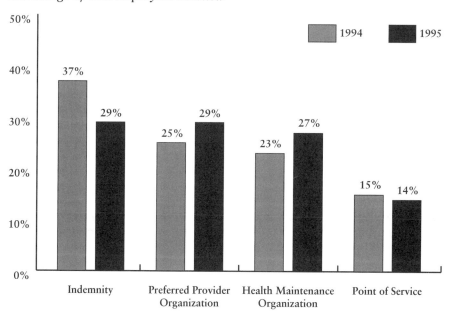

FIGURE 20-4

▧

The 1995 health maintenance organization/preferred provider organization (HMO/PPO) membership grows while indemnity falls. [NOTE: From "Medicaid Managed Care: A Challenge to the Health Care Ministry of the Catholic Church" (p. 5), by Department of Health and Hospitals, Archdiocese of New York, 1995, paper presented at the New York State Catholic Healthcare Council Annual Meeting, New York, NY. Reprinted with permission.]

thing." The questions raised about the marketing practices of some of the plans resulted in a freeze by the state's Department of Health, Office of Managed Care on all direct plan enrollments on August 1, 1995.

For some of the plans (PHSPs) with only Medicaid enrollees, this dramatic move by the state was devastating. It meant that there would be no direct enrollment of members for the plans. This extreme measure punished all of the plans, including the legitimate ones, for the misdeeds of a few. For the larger commercial plans, where Medicaid was just one of many products, this freeze on enrollments was not as difficult; after all, the Medicaid managed care population generally comprised only 25 percent of their total enrollee membership.

Managed care was also hit hard by the state's media that suggested that what you do not know about HMOs can kill you and that managed care casualties are enough to make you sick. Talk shows featured stories deploring the poor health care provided by HMOs. One of these stories was about a man who suffered a heart attack when an HMO delayed surgical treatment for an obvious cardiac condition. Another story told of a newborn baby boy who died after being sent home from the hospital after an HMO-mandated one-day maximum stay, even though his mother expressed concern about his health.

In spite of the terribly bad press received by the state's governor, the commissioner of health, and the state, support of mandatory Medicaid managed care continued. It continued because the managed care industry discounted the flurry of grass-roots protests, arguing that they were products of individuals who had a vested interest in maintaining the old style of health care, that few members had been dissatisfied enough to leave the plans, and that a number of independent studies found that HMOs matched or exceeded traditional fee-for-service medicine in the quality of several kinds of care.

The state's continued commitment to mandatory enrollment was expressed through forward-looking administrative action. HMOs and PHSPs wishing to be considered for selection as partners in the state plan when and if mandatory enrollment came into being submitted responses to state **requests for proposals (RFPs)** and participated in state readiness reviews. During these processes, plans were required to submit concrete examples of how their monitoring of quality, access and availability, and client satisfaction had resulted in improved service and care for their enrollees. The managed care plans were also asked to describe their client outreach and educational programs, any clinical pathways that had been developed, and what outcomes they had achieved or wished to achieve.

Requests for Proposals. This is a solicitation by a group, company, or government agency to interested parties for a submission of a proposal to become a participating entity in a project, to receive grant money, or to win a contract.

There are two schools of thought in the state regarding mandatory Medicaid managed care. The critics believe that this system will dissatisfy many Medicaid recipients because they will neither be able to obtain health care the way they did in the past nor utilize providers with whom they have already developed relationships. However, the system's proponents claim that the Medicaid population has not usually accessed care in a cost-effective manner, in particular citing the large percentage of Medicaid recipients who use the emergency departments of local hospitals as their major source of health care services. Proponents believe that MCOs will do extensive outreach to these enrollees to educate them to the proper use of emergency departments and encourage them to use preventive health services, which will be located at family health centers, PCP offices, and other sites conveniently located right in their own communities. It is believed that any provider now accepting Medicaid clients will probably be a member of the provider network of one or more of the MCOs, thereby allowing enrollees to maintain their existing provider relationships.

Managed care plans in the state are regulated by the Department of Health, Office of Managed Care. The Department of Health has very stringent and comprehensive standards, including quality assurance reporting requirements with which plans must comply. In 1996, the state's Department of Health contracted with the National Committee for Quality Assurance (NCQA) to assist with the monitoring of plan compliance.

Nurses and Mandated Medicaid Managed Care

During the early 1990s, many nursing associations became very concerned about the quality-of-care issues raised within the context of the managed care debate. After all, the number one item on the legislative agenda of the State Nursing Associations (SNAs) was consumer advocacy and health promotion. While nurses "believed that the conceptual framework for managed care was a good one and that, in fact, the basic concepts of prevention, maintenance of wellness, and patient education were consistent with nursing's model for an effective health care system," the growing number of concerns voiced by consumers caused some consternation (Myers, 1996, p. 1).

One SNA devoted much of its energies to the issues of managed care, working to develop a Health Care Bill of Rights—that is, legislation that required managed care plans to meet specific standards of operation in order to do business in the state. The bill contained essential consumer protections that ensured access to care and confidentiality of medical records; it also contained provisions for client outreach, continuity of care, choice of provider, and for a system that called for reporting pertinent data collected by the plan. Further, the bill urged provisions that assure that consumers are informed of their options prior to enrolling in a managed care plan. Of course, the SNA was instrumental in bringing about the provision that managed care plans were not allowed to deny privileges to health professionals solely based on the type of professional license held by a provider, thereby granting privileges and reimbursement for advanced practice nurses (APNs) as well as physicians for services rendered.

This SNA remains active in the managed care debate, supporting full choice of plans and access to care for all clients in the changing health care environment. The SNA's policies are as follows:

- Oppose improper and illegal recruitment of Medicaid clients into managed care.
- Support the Medicaid client's right to information that is presented in clearly understandable, culturally appropriate language; descrip-

tive of plan services; provided prior to enrollment in any managed care plan; and periodically updated.

- Advocate that Medicaid managed care maintains at least the basic set of benefits now available in the state's Medicaid program, that managed care also stresses prevention, offers access to a full range of health care providers (including registered nurses), provides services in geographically convenient settings, and supports traditional, community-based providers.

Nurses in this state have given testimony on managed care to a number of Legislative Task Forces on Health Care and at several town hall meetings called by area politicians. They have also worked on the governor's task force.

Next on this state's managed care agenda is the special needs population. Planning grants have been awarded from federal and state funds to MCOs interested in designing a proposal that will outline what a managed care plan for a special needs population should look like. You can bet that nurses will be involved in this phase of Medicaid managed care as well. While managed care pushes on, nurses, consumer groups, and state and federal government agencies will continue to monitor MCO activities and provide safeguards for enrollees.

𝓜ANAGED CARE ETHICS: AN OXYMORON OR DOES IT EXIST?

In a surprisingly short span of years, managed care has transformed from a cottage industry to big business. Some evidence of this change can be seen in the fact that the cash and stock awards to the chiefs of seven of the biggest for-profit HMOs averaged $7 million in 1994, the highest seen in any industry. The biggest pay package went to the chief executive officer of Healthsource, a medium-sized HMO in Hooksett, New Hampshire. The total value of the package was $15.5 million, which included a cash payment of $387,604 and stock options with a value of $15.1 million (Freudenheim, 1995, p. D1). Further evidence of managed care as big business can be seen in the rash of mergers that have taken place as health care companies have attempted to establish dominance in a lucrative, but changing, field. Recent examples include the merger of Aetna and US Healthcare, the merger of Kaiser and Community Health Plan, and the merger of two big California HMOs, Wellpoint Health Networks and Health Systems International. This last merger, a $1.8 billion stock swap, created one of the biggest stockholder-owned HMOs in the lucrative California market. Figure 20-5 lists the largest HMOs in the United States in 1995.

The acceleration of managed care penetration poses new challenges for nurses and other health care professionals, many of whom believe that human dignity and social justice are often incompatible with the business imperatives of for-profit initiatives, initiatives that have resulted in record-breaking profits.

As the government turns to managed care companies in a effort to keep down costs, the public, too, is rightfully questioning the ethics of the cost-containing strategies the managed care industry employs. No forecast is reliable, but some trends are clear. The number of uninsured, now almost 40 million, will grow. Private employers, who provide insurance for most workers and their families, are curtailing coverage in part by buying services from outside suppliers instead of retaining a regular work force. The public is nervous about who will control their futures. As cost-cutting intensifies, it seems unlikely that people will be willing to cede such sensitive authority to well-paid managed care executives who make larger profits every time they decide some procedure is not worth what it costs them. This shift in attitude is especially likely after people realize that managed care has achieved its profits in part by spending 15 to 20 percent of the premium dollar on mar-

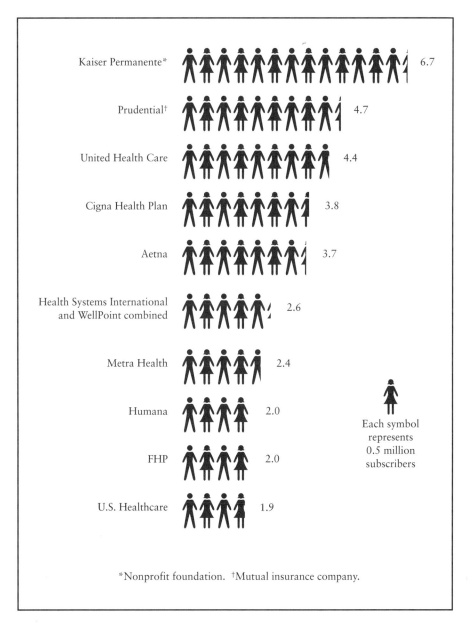

*Nonprofit foundation. †Mutual insurance company.

FIGURE 20-5

◎

The HMOs with the most subscribers in the United States in 1995. Figures are 1995 estimates in millions; they exclude people enrolled in preferred provider plans. [NOTE: From "Two California Health Care Providers Agree to an $1.8 Billion Merger" (p. B1), by M. Freudenheim, *The New York Times*, March 28, 1995. Reprinted with permission.]

Cottage Industry. This is an industry in which the production of goods takes place at the home of the producer rather than in a factory or other organized environment.

keting, administration, and profits, thereby diminishing the medical risk ratios to the residual 80 to 85 percent now being allocated to client care.

One of the concerns raised by this shifting of health care from a not-for-profit to a for-profit mode is where for-profit organizations' allegiance lies. As we discussed in Chap. 18, for-profit organizations or corporations have responsibilities to their shareholders; and, in most instances, the monies allocated to the shareholders represent a loss of the funding of care to the medically needy and underserved. Health care is no longer a **cottage industry**.

Although the stated goal of MCOs is quality client care at a low cost, allegations that this is not what the client necessarily gets are rampant. Horror stories of how clients are being denied care by their MCO or how providers have been denied payment have flooded the airways. And stories of how MCOs' cost-cutting strategies, which include denying authorization of services and payments, delays of as long as 2 years in payment of claims, and the overriding of physicians' medical decisions, are all reasons for the public to distrust MCOs.

One way to build trust is by adhering to ethical standards, but what are the ethical standards for managed care or what should the standards for managed care be? Consumers, providers, and MCOs all agree on certain basic health care rights: namely, the availability of accessible quality care delivered by a qualified provider in a confidential manner. However, a dilemma arises with regard to rationing that care. The Robert Wood Johnson Foundation has underwritten a grant for a study on the ethical dimensions of rationing decisions. The study will concentrate on five central issues: (1) physician incentives; (2) legal implications; (3) quality care assessment; (4) role of technology management; and (5) the relationship between administrators and physicians. Each of these issues is deserving of serious consideration. Currently, however, decisions on cases involving these issues are made by people who usually do not have all the facts or who do not know the client involved. Therefore, it is important that nurses take their role as client advocate seriously.

Three steps that MCOs can take to show the public that they are concerned about ethical practices are: (1) publish their clients' bill of rights; (2) acknowledge providers' rights; and (3) establish an ethics committee charged with identifying and reviewing problematic cases and policies. These steps would show the public that, although an MCO's goal is to contain costs, it does not intend to achieve that goal by sacrificing quality in the care that is delivered.

𝒜CCREDITATION OF MANAGED CARE ORGANIZATIONS

Accreditation is a process whereby a health care organization is evaluated by an objective body that has established standards to ensure that a specific level of quality is being met. There are four accreditation bodies of note in the managed care and community health field: (1) The Community Health Accreditation Program (CHAP) (see Chap. 16); (2) the Joint Commission on Accreditation of Health Care Organizations (JCAHO), an agency familiar to many in acute care settings that began a voluntary private accreditation program in 1994 for health care networks; (3) the Utilization Review Accreditation Commission (URAC), a private organization formed in 1990 by the American Managed Care and Review Association (AMCRA), a trade organization for utilization review firms, PPOs, and HMOs committed to improving the quality and efficiency of the interactions between the utilization review industry and the providers, payers, and purchasers of health care; and (4) the National Committee for Quality Assurance (NCQA), the accrediting body that has been recognized as the leader in the managed care field.

The NCQA is an independent, nonprofit HMO accrediting organization that has worked with independent health care quality experts, health care purchasers, state regulators, employers, labor union officials, and consumer representatives to develop standards that effectively evaluate quality management systems in managed care organizations. NCQA accreditation is mandated in several states but is voluntary in most. "Of the 222 plans in the country that have been reviewed by the NCQA, only 37 percent won full accreditation. An additional 39 percent got partial accreditation, 11 percent received provisional accreditation, and 12 percent were denied accreditation" (Spragins, 1996, p. 58). NCQA accreditation standards examine structure, process, and outcomes to ensure key rights of access, choice, quality, and confidentiality. Its accreditation eligibility criteria are based on meeting certain standards in quality improvement, utilization management, credentialing, members' rights and responsibilities, preventive health services, and medical records.

Regulatory Bodies with Oversight of the Managed Care Industry

Department of Health and Human Services (DHHS) is a federal cabinet-level agency, which oversees government health care programs and activities, including Social Security, Medicare, and Medicaid. The HCFA, the Health Resources and Services Administration (HRSA), and the Office of Prepaid Health Care Operations and Oversight (OPHOO) are all parts of the DHHS. HCFA is the federal agency responsible for administering Medicare, overseeing states' administration of Medicaid, and managing the Utilization and Quality Control Peer Review Program. HRSA is a federal agency of the United States Public Health Service within the DHHS responsible for developing primary health care services and resources, protecting and improving the health of mothers, infants, and children, improving the health of the medically underserved and those with special needs, and maintaining a high quality of health care nationally.

National Practitioners Data Bank (NPDB) was established through the Health Care Quality Improvement Act of 1986 (Title IV of Public Law 99-660). Responsibility for NPDB implementation resides in the Bureau of Health Professions, HRSA, DHHS. NPDB is an alert or flagging system used to facilitate a comprehensive review of health care practitioners' professional credentials.

NURSES AND MANAGED CARE

While nurses have many concerns regarding managed care, most believe that the conceptual framework for it is a good one. A philosophy of health maintenance and access to quality primary care in a cost-effective way is one that nurses can agree with as both consumers and providers. In fact, a seamless system of care that ensures continuity of care and promotes prevention, wellness, and client education are all consistent with nursing's model for an effective health care delivery system.

Issues and Concerns

Nationally, the ANA and other nursing organizations have been examining what effects managed care has had and will continue to have on health care and nursing. These organizations have been working together in an effort to educate nurses on evolving managed care markets. Nurses from all areas of the country and from every specialty agree that all consumers should have equal access to quality care delivered by quality providers, and they support most legislation that favors these issues.

At the ANA's Centennial Convention, resolutions that dealt with advocating for the rights of individuals enrolled in health plans were passed by the House of Delegates. The House of Delegates asked that the ANA: (1) seek, through federal legislation and rule-making, to have health plans operate in the best interests of plan participants and beneficiaries; (2) support full disclosure of contract provisions or other arrangements between purchasers, plan sponsors, and providers that could have the effect of dictating treatment decisions or care options to the detriment of the enrollee; and (3) seek state and federal regulation to grant participant access to information within the health plans, to increase and standardize the information reported and disclosed, and to provide for independent review and appeal of denied claims or services.

Nursing's Role in Managed Care

Nurses today are in a unique position. Not only do they possess the many skills and talents needed by the emerging managed care industry, but they are politically positioned to contribute significantly to the development of corporate and legislative policies that will guide the managed care industry in the future.

Currently, there is a myriad of roles available to nurses in the managed care arena. Depending on their level of expertise, nurses can fill positions on the entry, managerial, and executive levels. And, of course, for the nurse entrepreneur there is also the president's position. At whatever level nurses enter the managed care field, they can make a difference in how health care is delivered.

The nursing roles now associated with managed care are primary care provider, case manager, quality assurance nurse, triage nurse, client advocate, utilization review coordinator, risk manager, marketer, provider liaison, regulatory reviewer, reimbursement specialist, benefits interpreter, and information systems manager. Chapter 21 gives descriptions of some of these roles and the skills required to be hired for them.

Thomas Wolfe once said, "If a man has talent and cannot use it, he has failed. If he has a talent and only uses half of it he has partly failed. If he has talent and learns somehow to use the whole of it, he has gloriously succeeded, and won a satisfaction and a triumph few men will ever know" (Forbes Leadership Library, 1995, p. 58). By effectively utilizing their roles, nurses in the managed care arena can experience the satisfaction of which Thomas Wolfe speaks.

Role Settings

Although some roles in managed care call for nurses to work in the field (e.g., in a health care center, clinic, or traveling from hospital to hospital), most positions are office based. Because the only client or provider contact in these positions is by telephone, E-mail, or mail, a nurse who has become accustomed to personal contact and to the hustle and bustle of an institution may not be happy working with paper rather than clients. However, for the nurse who can reap satisfaction from knowing that this work is as important as direct hands-on care, it can be very rewarding.

Preparation for Nurses

Recognizing both the opportunities the field of managed care presents to nurses and the need for nurses to be prepared to assume diverse roles, the American Nurses Foundation (ANF) and the ANA developed a managed care curriculum for baccalaureate nursing graduates. The course was designed to benefit any professional nurse who lacks formal preparation in managed care delivery or whose prior experience has exclusively been in traditional health care settings (e.g., hospital, nursing home). The course is designed as a six-credit-hour course with three credits (45 h) allocated to didactic or theoretical content and three credits (135 h) allocated to clinical or practical experience. The course curriculum has eight major foci:

1. A shift in emphasis from illness care to prevention and health promotion
2. Community-based practice
3. Technological/electronic proficiency
4. Interdisciplinary collaboration
5. Quality improvement and risk management in a cost-sensitive environment
6. The philosophy of managed care
7. Ethics in managed care
8. Accountability

If you are considering a position in managed care, it would be beneficial to inquire where this course is being offered in your area. You can do this by contacting your local state nursing association, the National Student Nurses' Association, or the ANA.

$\mathcal{S}$UMMARY

Managed care is here to stay, for a while at least, and it is to every nurse's benefit to learn whatever she or he can about this rapidly growing phenomenon. This chapter has attempted to bring you a clearer understanding of what managed care is, how it works, who the players are, what Medicaid managed care is, and how mandated Medicaid managed care works, and what effect managed care has had and will continue to have on nurses, both as consumers and providers. The advantages and the disadvantages of managed care and the ethical conflicts that managed care has created are explored. Some of the many controversies surrounding managed care and the steps that are being taken to regulate, legislate, and accredit the managed care industry are discussed. Finally, the opportunities that managed care has created for nurses and how nurses are preparing to take advantage of these opportunities are considered. Managed care is a whole new world, a world in which nurses are playing a significant role.

KEY WORDS

Capitation
Case management
Exclusive provider organization
  (EPO)
Health maintenance organization
  (HMO)
Managed care
Managed care curriculum
Managed care organization (MCO)

Physician-hospital organization
  (PHO)
Point of service (POS)
Pre-authorization
Preferred provider organization
  (PPO)
National Committee for Quality
  Assurance (NCQA)
Utilization review

QUESTIONS

DIRECTIONS: Choose the one *best* response to each of the following questions.

1. The impetus behind the managed care movement has been the need

    A. for physicians to form independent practice associations (IPAs).
    B. to create positions for advanced practice nurses (APNs).
    C. to insure the uninsured.
    D. to control the rapidly escalating costs of health care.

2. The concepts of managed care that are most aligned with nursing's agenda include
   A. limiting the types of licensed professionals who may deliver care.
   B. refusal of care for nonmembers.
   C. determining the clinical appropriateness of care by nonclinical representatives.
   D. the delivery of quality, cost-effective care.

3. There are many types of managed care organizations (MCOs). All of the following organizations are considered MCOs except
   A. a preferred provider organization (PPO).
   B. a staff model health maintenance organization (HMO).
   C. emergency department of a local hospital.
   D. point of service.

4. In a capitated reimbursement system, a nurse would expect to find that
   A. no referral forms are necessary if a client needs to see a specialist.
   B. a provider is reimbursed the same dollar figure for every client, regardless of age.
   C. a provider is not paid on a fee-for-service basis.
   D. physicians may not participate in an incentive program.

5. The community health nurse using the Alliance Model would liken the care management inner circle to the managed care role of
   A. utilization management nurse.
   B. home care nurse.
   C. clinical nurse specialist.
   D. case manager.

6. Managed care organizations (MCOs) are licensed by
   A. the federal government.
   B. state licensing departments.
   C. the state.
   D. Department of Health.

7. In some states, the practices of some managed care organizations (MCOs) have led to the imposition of legislative minimums on
   A. the number of cases a nurse case manager can coordinate.
   B. the number of postpartum in-hospital days to which a woman is entitled.
   C. chief executive officers' pay levels.
   D. the number of MCOs a provider may join.

8. The National Committee for Quality Assurance (NCQA) has set accreditation standards for managed care organizations (MCOs) in the areas of
   A. quality improvement, utilization management, credentialing, preventive health services, and medical records.
   B. access, physician incentive programs, and primary care health maintenance standards.
   C. quality of care, "gag rules," physician "withholds," cost-effectiveness, and access to care.
   D. quality assessment and improvement, outcome studies, and emergency room triage service.

9. The community health nurse who is acting as a client advocate with a managed care company is working within which circle of the Alliance Model?

   A. The outer circle
   B. The focus on community-based needs circle
   C. The systems of care circle
   D. Influences on resource allocation decisions circle

10. The major foci of the managed care curriculum for baccalaureate nursing graduates designed by the American Nurses Foundation (ANF) and the American Nurses Association (ANA) include

   A. interdisciplinary collaboration.
   B. a shift from health promotion to illness care.
   C. the Alliance Model for Community Health Assessment.
   D. how to interpret coronary output.

ANSWERS

1. *The answer is D.* The impetus behind the managed care movement was cost containment.

2. *The answer is D.* The concept of delivery of quality cost-effective care is a managed care concept that is closely aligned to nursing's agenda.

3. *The answer is C.* The emergency department of a local hospital is not considered an MCO.

4. *The answer is C.* In a capitated system, a provider is usually not paid on a fee-for-service basis.

5. *The answer is D.* A managed care case manager and the Alliance Model care manager have many similar job responsibilities.

6. *The answer is C.* Managed care organizations (MCOs) are legal entities licensed by the state.

7. *The answer is B.* At least 18 states have banned so-called drive-through maternity care in which hospitals send mothers home less than 48 h after they give birth.

8. *The answer is A.* The NCQA has set accreditation standards for MCOs in the areas of quality improvement, utilization management, credentialing, preventive health services, and medical records.

9. *The answer is D.* The community health nurse who is acting as a client advocate with a managed care company is working within the influences on resource allocation decisions circle of the Alliance Model.

10. *The answer is A.* Interdisciplinary collaboration is one of the major foci of the managed care curriculum for baccalaureate nursing graduates designed by the ANF and the ANA.

ANNOTATED REFERENCES

American Academy of Nursing. (1993). *Managed care and national health care reform: Nursing can make it work.* Washington, DC: Author.

This publication defines managed care and explains the different types of managed care and what role nursing plays in it.

American Nurses Association. (1996, Winter). Understanding the moral life. ANA Center for Ethics and Human Rights Communique, 4(3).

This communiqué is published quarterly and contains articles on issues relevant to nursing.

American Nurses Association. (1995). Managed care: Challenges and opportunities for nursing. *Nursing Facts.* Washington, DC: Author.

This publication contains statistics on managed care including types of managed care organizations (MCOs), accreditation of MCOs, managed care settings, and nursing roles.

Forbes Leadership Library. (1995). *Thoughts on success.* Chicago: Triumph Books.

This book contains a selection of thoughts from leaders in industry, heads of state, philosophers, educators, authors, and military leaders. All focus on the meaning of success.

Freudenheim, M. (1995, April 11). Penny-pinching H.M.O.'s showed their generosity in executive paychecks. *The New York Times,* p. D1.

This article explores how HMOs put pressure on health care providers to cut costs, while they reward their chief executives with sizable pay packages.

Fubini, S. (1995). National health expenditures forecast 1994–1996. *Healthcare Trends Report, 9*(5), 3.

This monthly newsletter updates its readers on trends in the health services industry.

Hart, S. (1995). *Managed care curriculum for baccalaureate nursing program.* Washington, DC: American Nurses Association.

This publication contains the course overview, description, and objectives, and the outline of the curriculum. It also contains definition of terms, references, and bibliographies.

Kellet, A., Leonard, M., Craig, G., et al. (1996). *Report of the task force on standards and regulation of managed care to the congress on nursing practice.* Washington, DC: American Nurses Association. Unpublished paper.

This report contains an analysis of nine different regulatory bodies involved with managed care. The analysis looks at structure, process, and outcomes.

Kogan, R. (1996). *A closer look at federal caps and state matching requirements. Inside Medicaid managed care.* Gaithersberg, MD: Aspen Publications.

This publication contains articles on different aspects of managed care. The author is a senior policy analyst for the Washington, D.C.–based Center on Budget and Policy Priorities.

Leonard, M. (1996, May). Testimony to the New York State democratic task force on health care in New York State. Unpublished data.

This testimony pertains to managed care. It describes nursing's philosophy of health maintenance and access to quality, cost-effective care. It addresses nursing's concerns with issues such as access, patients' rights, and confidentiality. It also discusses the issue of nurses serving as primary care providers in the managed care arena.

Meyers, G. (1996). *Memorandum from the New York State Nurses Association (NYSNA) legislative program regarding managed care.* Guiderland, NY: NYSNA Legislative Department.

This document contains a compilation of information on federal budget cuts and the impact on New York State. Ms. Meyers is a lobbyist for NYSNA.

Department of Health and Hospitals, Archdiocese of New York. (1995). *Managed care: A challenge to the healthcare ministry of the Catholic Church.* Paper presented at the New York State Catholic Healthcare Council Annual Meeting, New York, NY.

This conference delved into how managed care is affecting the Healthcare Ministry and the projected effects.

New York State Department of Social Services and the Department of Health. (1991). *New York State managed care plan.* New York: Author.

This document was submitted to the governor and the legislature pursuant to Chapter 165 of the Laws of 1991 and contains the details of this managed care plan. It contains the objectives, key policy issues, types of reimbursement, and guidelines.

Northrop, C., & Kelly, M. (1987). *Legal issues in nursing.* St. Louis, MO: C. V. Mosby.

The authors of this book are nurse attorneys who want to educate nurses about the law. Each chapter gives an overview of a particular practice setting, identifies legal issues in that area of practice, applies specific case law and legislation, discusses standards, gives recommendations, and identifies trends.

Spragins, E. (1996, June 24). Does your HMO stack up? *Newsweek,* pp. 56–63.

This article contains the results of a survey rating 43 of America's largest HMOs.

Stiller, A., & Brown, H. (1996). Case management: Implementing the vision. *Nursing Economics, 14*(1), 9–20.

This article discusses case management as a strategy for restructuring the health care delivery system. It describes the planning steps for case management programs and how to educate agency personnel.

Wooster, D., & Fortham, T. (1996, March/April). Clinical pathways before implementing a clinical improvement program. *Best Practices and Benchmarking in Health Care,* p. 84.

This article objectively analyzes the clinical pathway phenomenon. It looks at the origins, elements, and purpose of this clinical improvement technique and critiques pathway outcomes.

FUTURE CHALLENGES AND OPPORTUNITIES FOR NURSES

Advance Practice Nurse (APN). This is the umbrella term used for some nurses who receive degrees or certification beyond the baccalaureate level such as nurse practitioners, certified nurse midwives, clinical nurse specialists, and certified registered nurse anesthetists.

"There is no security on this earth, only opportunity" (Douglas MacArthur). Never before have so few words had such great meaning for nurses. Nurses who have enjoyed the luxury of job security for most of their professional lives are now threatened with job insecurity and loss. Headlines in major newspapers across this nation are replete with doomsday predictions for those individuals employed in the health care field. Large-scale mergers in combination with the shift to a managed care environment have seriously impacted the nursing profession.

On the negative side, hospitals are downsizing, reassigning staff, and letting nurses go. Schools of nursing are closing their generic programs because they are too costly to run and their doctoral programs because they do not have an adequate number of faculty. Admissions are limited for fear that there will be no positions available for graduates. Nurse administrators have lost their jobs as hospital boards close hospital wings and eliminate upper management positions.

On the positive side, the shift from acute care settings to community and ambulatory care settings is projected to increase dramatically the number of nursing positions in these settings. In addition, the focus on primary health care that managed care has created calls for a significant increase in the number of **advanced practice nurses (APNs)** that are needed. In response to these changes, schools of nursing have begun to redesign their generic programs with a greater emphasis on community health nursing, and many have begun nurse practitioner programs. Fast track programs that offer accelerated associate degree to master's degree programs have gained in popularity. More and more nurses are beginning to realize the need for additional education and are returning to school for advanced degrees in nursing, public health, community health, and business administration.

Many nurses view these changes as threats to a profession in which they are comfortable. Therefore, it is important for nurses to realize that the changes brought by the large-scale mergers and managed care are simply new challenges that must be faced and that change plus challenge equals opportunity.

In this chapter, the status of nursing in this nation is examined, and nursing's strengths and weaknesses are discussed. Some of the reasons why nursing is a career of choice at this time and why it is not are explored. The opportunities that the changing health care system is offering nurses are examined, and the skills that nurses need to take advantage of these opportunities are described.

As the challenges and the opportunities nurses now face are explored, the different paths that have been created by nursing's leaders to prepare nurses for the future, paths that will guide nurses through role transitions, work setting transitions, and the paradigm shift that managed care has introduced, are also discussed. "The term paradigm implies a generally accepted world view or philosophy, a structure within which the theories of the discipline are organized" (Chin & Jacobs, p. 85). The viability of career ladders and the skills needed to climb them are examined. Differentiated nursing practice and educational tracks designed to move the nurse from novice to expert are discussed. Lastly, the importance of professional involvement and how nurses can benefit from belonging to their professional and specialty organizations are examined.

CURRENT STATUS OF NURSING

This chapter was designed to share important information about the current status of the nursing profession and give statistics on nursing that can assist nurses to draw their own conclusions. Information and statistics include: How many nurses are there? How many nurses will be needed in the future? What does the profession look like? Who are the people entering the profession? How are nurses educated? Where are they employed? What are the salary ranges? It is believed that this information will assist students in answering the question: Is nursing still the career of choice for me?

How Many Nurses Are There? There are over 2.2 million nurses with approximately 50,000 new graduates joining the ranks every year since 1984. This means that there are over 2 million nurses "assisting the individual (sick or well) in the performance of those activities contributing to health, or its recovery (or to a peaceful death), that he [or she] would perform unaided if he [or she] had the necessary strength, will, or knowledge" (Harmer & Henderson, 1960, p. 4). These nurses come from diverse backgrounds and have been educated at different levels to meet the distinct health care needs of our population.

Sign-on Bonuses. These are usually bonuses in the form of money that are paid to entice nurses to apply for employment with an institution or encourage nurses presently working in an institution to act as recruiters for an institution.

Downsize is the term used to describe the reduction of a work force.

How Many Nurses Will Be Needed in the Future? It is important to remember that the supply, demand, and need for registered nurses have been cyclical. Not long ago our nation experienced a severe shortage of nurses, which resulted from a prediction that there was going to be a glut. This false prediction led to a curtailing of nursing school enrollments, which, in turn, led to a nursing shortage. This shortage resulted in unprecedented raises in nurses' salaries and **sign-on bonuses** paid to new employees and to the nurses who referred the new employees. It also led to the extensive international recruitment of nurses from other countries, especially Ireland and the Philippines.

The profession is now concerned that this latest attempt to **downsize** the nursing work force will result in a nursing shortage. In the latest employment projections of the Bureau of Labor Statistics (BLS) for the health services industry for the period 1994 to 2005, it was reported that the health services industry was among the top 10 industries with the fastest projected growth; the BLS also ranked registered nurses fifth among occupations with the largest projected job growth. It has been projected that, in spite of the restructuring of the current health care industry, nursing will realize a 25 percent increase in the number of jobs by the year 2005.

What Does the Profession Look Like? Nurses come in all ages, colors, and sexes. Some are married, and some are single. Some have chosen nurs-

FIGURE 21-1

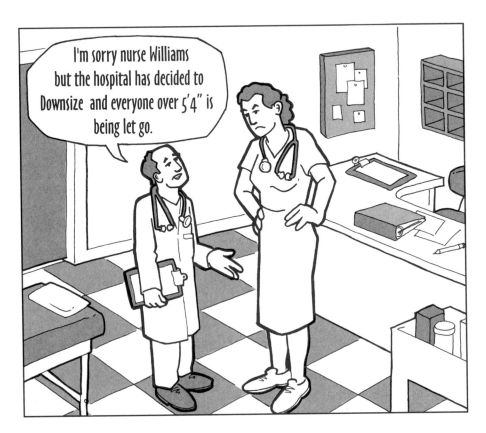

ing as their first career, while others have chosen nursing as a second career. The number of persons choosing nursing as a second career has increased in the last 10 years with many nurses possessing baccalaureate degrees in liberal arts or other fields of study. Nursing is also popular as a second career for policemen, fire fighters, and emergency medical technicians. According to *The Registered Nurse Population, Findings from the National Sample Survey of Registered Nurses* [U.S. Department of Health and Human Services (DHHS), 1992], the average age for registered nurses is 43 years. More than 60 percent of registered nurses are between the ages of 30 to 59, while only 11 percent are under 30.

Ninety percent of registered nurses are Caucasian, the remaining 10 percent are non-Caucasian including African Americans, 4 percent; Asian/Pacific Islanders, 3.4 percent, Hispanics, 1.4 percent; and American Indian and Alaskan Natives, 0.4 percent.

Approximately 95 percent of registered nurses are women, but more and more men are choosing nursing as a career. Between 1980 and 1992, there was a 97 percent increase in the number of men entering the profession.

Most nurses are employed full-time, and of all those nurses employed, approximately 33 percent have children. Approximately 72 percent of all nurses are married; 17 percent are widowed, divorced, or separated; and just over 1 percent have never married.

How Are Nurses Educated? In the past 5 years, it appears that the degree of choice was an associate degree with approximately 59 percent of nurses graduated from associate degree programs. Overall, 34 percent of nurses received their basic nursing education in diploma programs; 28 percent in associate degree programs; 27 percent in baccalaureate programs; and 3 percent are foreign educated. The trend, however, is moving toward higher education.

▧

TABLE 21-1
AVERAGE SALARIES OF REGISTERED NURSES

Hospital staff nurse	$36,618
Community/public health staff nurse	$32,621
Ambulatory care staff nurse	$27,949
Nursing home staff nurse	$31,298
Administrators	$45,071
Instructors	$36,896
Supervisors	$38,979
Clinical nurse specialists	$58,185
Nurse practitioner	$43,636
Nurse anesthetist	$76,053
Nurse midwives	$43,636

NOTE: Adapted from *Nursing Facts* (pp. 3–4), by American Nursing Association, 1995, Washington, DC: Author. Reprinted with permission.

Where Are Nurses and What Are They Paid? Approximately 67 percent of all employed registered nurses work in hospital settings; 10 percent in community and public health; 8 percent in ambulatory care; 7 percent in nursing homes and extended care facilities; 2 percent in nursing education; 2 percent in student health; 1 percent in occupational health; 3 percent in state boards of nursing, health planning agencies, and correctional facilities; and 2 percent are self-employed. The BLS projects a 127 percent increase in the number of nurses employed in home health for the period 1994 to 2005, and a 77 percent increase in the number of nurses employed in nursing home settings. Table 21-1 shows the national average of salaries for nurses in different settings and in different roles.

OPPORTUNITIES FOR NURSES

Believe it or not, the dramatic transformation of the health care industry has resulted in a number of opportunities for nurses, from the new graduate to the seasoned professional. The new graduate, if adequately prepared, will only see these changes as challenges; however, the nurse who is already employed in the nursing profession may find it difficult to live with these changes. It is hoped that these seasoned professionals will identify the challenges and prepare him- or herself to meet them. This chapter has been designed as a resource for not only the student, but also the new graduate and the seasoned professional. To quote Edgar Watson Howe "Every successful (person) [of whom] I have ever heard has done the best he [or she] could with conditions as he or she found them and not waited until the next year for better" (Forbes Leadership Library, 1995, p. 106). Thus, nurses must do "the best they can with the conditions as they find them," as well as exert influence to inform and shape the health care delivery system.

What are the conditions? Actually, the conditions are good. There are predictions of a 25 percent increase in registered nurse positions by the year 2005. Managed care has opened the door much wider for APNs. Nurses' salaries are at a record high, and most nurses have excellent health benefits packages. Tuition reimbursement still exists for many nurses, and many educational tracks are designed to fit the life style of the part-time adult student who works full-time and has many other responsibilities. Nurses have united, and nursing's voice has been heard by the legislature; nurses have been invited to discuss health care policies and have been recognized as one of the major players in the health care system.

Where Are the Opportunities for Nurses? The opportunities for nurses are in: (1) acute care, (2) community health, (3) long-term care, and (4) managed care.

Acute Care There will always be a need for acute care nursing, but many hospital-based nurses fear that the days of bedside nursing are coming to an end. They fear that the current trend to use certified technicians and unlicensed assistive personnel (UAP) to deliver patient care at the bedside is seriously jeopardizing patient care, patient safety, and nursing positions. This increased use of UAPs to staff hospitals is consistent with the projections released by the BLS, which show that while there will be an increase of 12.5 percent in registered nurse hospital positions, there will be a decline of 6.3 percent in the number of registered nurses employed in hospitals due to downsizing and layoffs. Therefore, the American Nurses Association (ANA) has launched a campaign to ensure that patients receive quality care delivered by qualified licensed nurses. This *multimedia campaign* is designed to heighten the awareness of the public as well as the legislators of this potentially dangerous practice. Simply put, an unlicensed health care worker who receives 6 to 12 weeks of training cannot possibly have the scientific knowledge base upon which licensed nurses make care delivery decisions.

Most acute care nurses will remain working in hospital settings, but a large number will be employed in ambulatory care settings, such as ambulatory surgical centers and in urgent care centers. Acute care nurses may also find themselves working in high-technology divisions of home care agencies.

Nurses in acute care must take the steps necessary to keep their skills and knowledge base updated, since opportunities for advancement of the bedside acute care nurse in hospital settings are usually in the form of career ladders or predicated on advanced competency levels. Many of these skilled acute care positions are being filled by APNs, and the numbers will continue to grow.

Community and Public Health The community offers the greatest number of opportunities for nurses. It also offers a variety of settings—home care, family health care centers, public health agencies, community nursing organizations, ambulatory care centers, school-based clinics, hospice care, occupational health sites, and the military. Another very interesting area in the public health arena is the Indian Health Service (IHS), which employs more than 2500 nurses. The IHS is an agency of the U.S. Public Health Service, DHHS. It operates a comprehensive health service delivery system for approximately 1.3 million of the nation's 2 million American Indians and Alaskan Natives among the 540 federally recognized tribes in the United States.

Long-Term Care Long-term care facilities have experienced a great deal of growth over the last decade. The BLS projects that growth will continue in this area, resulting in a 77 percent increase in registered nurse positions between 1994 and 2005. These projections are consistent with the expected increase in the number of persons over 65 by 2005 and the explosion expected in this age group in the year 2010 when the "baby boomers" begin to turn 65 (the graying of America).

There has also been an increase in the number of chronically ill patients who require care in extended care facilities and at home. This increase is the result of advances in the treatment for the chronically ill, which has extended the life expectancy for persons with chronic illness such as multiple sclerosis.

Long-term nursing care can be delivered in nursing homes, extended care facilities, assisted living facilities, health-related facilities, or in the patient's home. Nurses with expertise in geriatrics will fare well in this field.

Managed Care   A myriad of opportunities has been presented to nurses with the advent of managed care. The emphasis on primary care has dramatically increased the demand for APNs. Health maintenance organizations (HMOs) have created a whole flurry of new positions, such as utilization review nurses, benefits analysts, and reimbursement specialists, just to name a few. Many HMOs have taken existing positions and expanded them by adding responsibilities; for example, quality assurance nurses now must consider cost and utilization when they are assessing quality; case managers now manage the entire care of the patient (not just a segment of it) as well as aggregates of patients; and the triage nurse in the emergency room no longer simply assesses a patient's need to be seen by the physician but now also determines whether the patient should be triaged out of the emergency room to an urgent care center, a health center, or a primary care provider's office. While these new responsibilities can present new and important opportunities to nurses, they may also confuse some nurses who are trying to decide what career path to follow.

CAREER PATHS

It is important to realize that there is a significant difference between a career and a job. *Webster's* defines a job as "a piece of work; a regular renumerative employment," (1976, p. 1217) and defines career as "a course of continued progress; a profession for which one undergoes special education and which is undertaken as a permanent calling" (1976, p. 338). The decision to choose a nursing job or a career in nursing is a personal one but one that should be made early. If nursing is a career choice, then familiarity with the available career paths is essential. If your goal is to work in direct patient care, administration, academia, or research, it may be a good idea to speak with people who are already working in the field and ask them why they chose this field. How long they have been in the field? Are they happy with their chosen field? What are the downsides of the field? Are there opportunities for advancement? If so, what skills are needed, and what educational credentials are essential? This type of one-on-one discussion is invaluable when trying to choose among the available nursing fields. For each of the career paths discussed above, nursing offers a variety of specialty areas, areas such as acute care, primary care, community care, home care, ambulatory care, managed care, substance abuse treatment, education both in academia and in staff development, school health, occupational health, **nursing informatics**, public health policy, regulation and accreditation, and independent practice.

It is important to understand that all career paths follow the pyramid theory. There are many people with entry level skills who comprise the large number of nurses at the base of the pyramid. As one rises in the hierarchy of the pyramid, there are fewer nurses qualified to be at the next level where there is less room. This rise in the hierarchy is accomplished in different ways and through different career paths—for example, in a hospital system, it is usually accomplished through a mechanism of career ladders. In academia, becoming tenured is considered a giant step up the pyramid. Remember "the ladder of success doesn't care who climbs it" (Forbes Leadership Library, 1995, p. 108). Figure 21-2 shows various career paths. While there are hierarchies in different areas of nursing as well as different ways of rising in these hierarchies, there should be a mutual understanding and valuing of the different roles and capacities of all nurses in our health care system.

It has been stated in *A Model for Differentiated Nursing Practice* that "Mutual valuing and awareness by those practicing in the different roles is critical. . . . Collaborative relationships among nurses practicing in the

Nursing Informatics. This is a fairly new specialty area for nurses. There is an emphasis on computer expertise, data analysis, and information systems management.

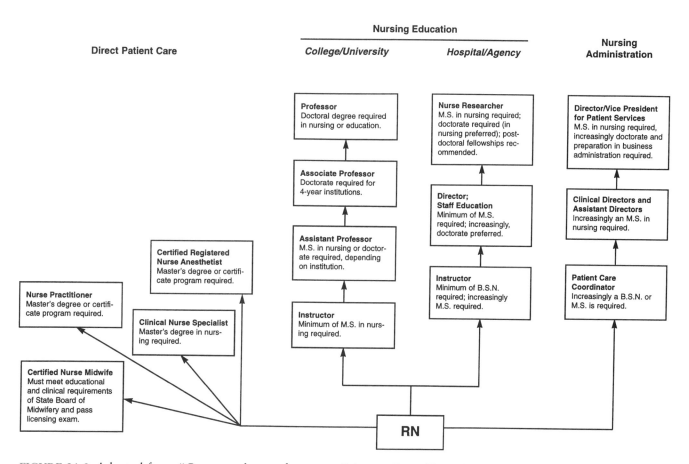

FIGURE 21-2. Adapted from "Career pathways for nurses." (NOTE: From *Your Future in Nursing: A Career Planning Guidebook for RNs* (pp. 8–9), by New York State Nurses Association, 1996, Latham, NY: Author. Reprinted with permission.

various nursing roles must be based on mutuality; each person's expertise is recognized as necessary for the provision of the highest quality care. Mutual valuing leads to growth, discovery, and insight into one's self and respect for the other practice roles. Relationship is the foundation for nursing practice; relationships with the client and family, as well as relationships among the various nursing roles within a differentiated professional community replaces the old paradigm 'a nurse is a nurse is a nurse'" (American Association of Colleges of Nursing, 1995, p. 13). This model may serve nurses well as the need for cross-training and the need for mutual understanding of what it is that nurses do comes to the forefront of nursing's thinking and the public's perception.

No matter which nursing career path is chosen, there is a pyramid approach to expertise, and there is room for only a few at the top of the pyramid. Those few who have made it to the top have been successful through hard work, experience, networking, and education.

Skills Needed to Survive and to Succeed

In this rapidly changing health care environment, one thing has become perfectly clear. Today's nurse must be flexible, resilient, informed, and involved. Some nurses have difficulty with change because they feel they are not prepared to handle the challenges that change presents. One way to avoid becoming a rigid, outdated, and unmarketable commodity is to consider individual growth a must. Benjamin Disraeli said "The great secret of success in life is for a man [woman] to be ready when his [or her] opportunity comes" (Forbes Leadership Library, 1995, p. 106).

Nurses can prepare for opportunity through self-empowerment, which can be acquired through self-accountability for life-long learning. To be effective leaders in the health care industry, nurses must possess many skills. Some of these skills should serve as a foundation for all nurses in today's health care environment as they follow their dreams and realize their career goals.

Knowledge Brokers

Nurses should be health care knowledge brokers and ambassadors of good health. This can be accomplished by gaining as much knowledge as possible through a variety of sources, using a number of tools. Once this knowledge is assimilated, nurses should then share the knowledge with their colleagues, patients, consumers, and legislators. Knowledge is power, and nurses need power to remain leaders in the health care industry.

Knowledge brokers are those nurses who are involved in the cutting edge of health care, that is, nurses who are part of the inner circle of "leaders and shakers" and who have first-hand knowledge of upcoming changes in health care. These are the nurses who sit on national health policy task forces and state committees on health care and state nursing boards. The knowledge these nurses possess must be shared (brokered) wisely so that the greatest benefits are realized.

To be knowledge brokers, nurses must learn how to collect and analyze data. They must have an understanding of how information systems work, and they should have input into how a system will be designed so that the desired data are retrievable.

Computer Skills

A basic knowledge of computers is necessary, not just for success but for survival in the health care industry. "The use of computers in health care is skyrocketing" (Henderson & Deane, 1996, p. 188). Studies have shown that student nurses have more computer experience than registered nurses, which can be attributed to the increased use of computers in educational settings. However, there is a history of nonuse and resistance to computers among nurses. The causes for resistance range from technical factors, such as lack of hardware (the computer itself) or poor technical quality of the computer system, to psychological factors such as computer anxiety and computer dissatisfaction. Nurses can overcome this resistance by: (1) becoming familiar with computers and computer language and (2) joining their organizations' management information systems (MIS) task force so that they can influence decisions about what computer systems are purchased and what programs are needed to assist nursing in its functions.

Computer literacy can be accomplished by taking computer courses and learning about the many applications computers have for nursing. Computer classes are offered in many settings, including colleges, hospital staff development departments, computer stores, adult education classes in high schools and libraries, and in the home. Today, in most states, the registered nurse licensing examination is given on computer.

Electronic mail (E-mail) and the Internet are two other features that can be useful to nurses. Many information sources now available "on line" allow nurses to do extensive literature searches. The **American Nurses Association Web Page** provides up-to-date information on legislative issues that affect nursing.

ANA Web Page is the ANA information format on the Internet.

Information Management Skills

The current health care environment must support innovative information systems as essential management tools that provide fast, efficient access to patient information. Nurses, as the largest group of professionals in the health care field, must be involved in this information management process. Nurses must know how to track, trend, and analyze data. They also must be able to project statistical probabilities from their data analysis. Computers, of course, can make this process much easier.

It has always been difficult to collect data from nurses because they are "too busy" to fill out questionnaires or complete additional report forms, which they feel are superfluous to what they do. Therefore, it is very important to explain the purpose of the data collection and to share the results of surveys and studies with the nurses who participate. It is also important that the data collection is made as unobtrusive to a nurse's workday as possible. This is where computers have proven to be very effective. If data are being tracked on a computer, nurses are more apt to comply with survey requests if only a few simple, entry strokes are necessary. These data can then be tracked and analyzed to produce useful information. Information is what drives both the health care industry and the nursing profession. Thus, it is to every nurse's benefit to learn how to use a computer; without these skills, nurses will lag behind.

Media Skills

Today's nurse should be a master of the media. Nurses should not only be able to use different types of media as teaching and learning modalities, but they should be able to contribute to enhancing the image of nurses and to advancing nursing's agenda through the use of mass media.

The increased use of audio and visual media and interactive computer disks as teaching and learning aids are testimony to their effectiveness. Soon there may be as many videos for sale from nursing organizations and publishing houses as there are printed materials. More and more textbooks are being sold with computer disk versions of the text.

Printed Media Printed media is the most important source for dispensing information and will no doubt remain so. The number of professional journals, industry communiqués, and specialty organization newsletters are at an all-time high. In addition, many nurses are also writing articles in nonprofessional publications (e.g., *Business Week*, *Modern Woman*). Many important issues that involve nursing have been featured as high profile stories in some of the nation's leading daily newspapers such as *The Washington Post*, *The New York Times*, and *The Los Angeles Times*.

A good way to get started with writing for publications is through letters to the editor of a local newspaper or writing an article for a local nursing organization's newsletter. The editors are usually very happy to receive letters and articles.

Radio and Television Nurses have also realized the wide-reaching impact that radio and television have on the millions of people who listen or watch. Stories that have featured nursing's issues have been featured on major stations across the nation, as well as local radio and cable stations. Many nurses have also joined the ranks of radio and television talk show hosts to produce health information shows that inform the public about these issues (e.g., Sigma Theta Tau International's television show, and *Community Nurse: On-Call*, a prime time health information radio show).

Videos In the fast-paced world in which we live, there are many things that are vying for people's time and attention. Educators are beginning to realize that they must present information in quick, hard-hitting, and attention-commanding formats. Videos, therefore, are becoming the media of choice because they have the elements that command attention. They are visual, colorful, and often have music. They can also be used repeatedly to reach larger audiences. Therefore, all nurses should be comfortable handling video tapes and players. Many nurses today are producing, directing, and starring in videos.

Audio Tapes Tapes have also gained in popularity as a teaching and learning aid. Almost every class has at least one student who tapes every lecture for later listening and review. A number of texts come on audio tape, and many students listen to the tapes as they drive to and from school or work. Therefore, nurses should be familiar with the operation of audio tape equipment.

Case Management Skills

Important skills for a nurse to have today are case management skills. These skills are used in all areas of nursing—acute care, primary care, community/ambulatory/home care, and managed care. They are also incorporated into nursing education programs.

"Nursing and case management are complementary professions. . . . Opportunities previously unknown to the profession of nursing are available as a result of case management" (Williams, 1996, p. 53). Yet, nurses are at a crossroads. On the one hand, there is resistance to change, and on the other, there is an opportunity to enhance the profession. The move today is for case management to become a specialty all its own. Case managers will be nurses and non-nurses. Some see this as an opportunity to work collaboratively as an interdisciplinary team, and some see this as a turf battle. Regardless of how it is viewed, one thing is certain: The number of nurses seeking to be certified as case managers is increasing rapidly.

Since the major focus of case management is the delivery of quality care in a cost-efficient manner, case management nurses must have special assessment skills—skills that allow them to make judgments about care that is needed, sometimes without ever seeing the client. The case manager must understand the concepts of utilization management, that is, the concept of delivering the most appropriate care, by the most appropriate provider, in the most appropriate setting, over the most appropriate time frame, using the most appropriate technology and the most appropriate equipment and supplies. The case manager must possess networking skills and negotiating skills since she or he will expend much time negotiating with others for services needed for their clients. The case manager must be sensitive to cost and quality issues and use **benchmarking** to establish guidelines and parameters for care. Nurses must be familiar with nationally recognized standards of care.

Benchmarking is a system of comparison. A benchmark or standard unit is identified in sufficient detail so that other similar classifications can be compared as being above, below, or comparable to the benchmark standard.

The case manager is a consumer advocate and, therefore, should be culturally competent to understand the needs expressed or sometimes not expressed by the client. The case manager must also be knowledgeable about benefits packages and reimbursement sources.

If a case management program is designed properly, a case manager is involved with a client's care as soon as the client is identified as one with a high-risk diagnosis or a diagnosis that requires high use of services or prolonged care. The case manager then develops a rapport with the client and the interdisciplinary team working with this client.

Case managers will play a very significant role in the health care system over the next decade, and it is important that nurses begin to assume the roles of case managers. If they do not acquire the skills needed to assume these roles, others will be very happy to assume them.

Business Skills

Business skills can range from a basic understanding of health care as a business to the skills necessary to own and operate your own business. These skills are discussed in detail in Chap. 18.

Leadership Skills

There are many differences between leadership skills and management skills. These differences stem from the basic difference between managers and leaders. A simple but insightful difference noted by Bennis, between managers and leaders, is the manager does things right and the leader does the right things (Bennis, 1989). In other words, someone who manages will do what she or he is directed to do and will do it well. The leader makes a decision as to what needs to be done and either does it or delegates it to someone who will do it well. The health care industry is now dangerously overmanaged but underled by people who know little about delivering care to clients.

Determining the right things for the industry has become progressively more complex and ambitious. Furthermore, decisions are made today not by top executives but by consultants who are engaged to interview managers throughout the health care organization to determine strengths and weakness, to summarize their findings, and to make recommendation for change. Usually, the consultants are hired to help restructure an organization—downsize or rightsize—and are more concerned with the bottom line than quality of care.

Nurses must take a larger leadership role in the health care industry. Leadership is fast becoming a critical dimension of interpersonal influence that must permeate the thinking of nursing managers if nurses intend to remain a core component of the health care system. Consequently, nurse managers must embrace leadership as a central component of their lifelong learning and their self-empowerment roles.

Mentoring Skills

Nursing mentors are leaders who must have excellent communication skills, interpersonal skills, business skills, decision-making skills, negotiating skills, teaching skills, and basic skills in legal interpretations. They must also be able to develop and implement algorithms to assist nurses in the decision-making process. These nursing leaders must also present a positive professional image.

Nurses who possess essential leadership qualities, such as vision and focus, should be mentored by other nursing leaders; that is, nurse mentors must encourage other nurses to engage in activities and studies that will enhance their growth and advancement in the nursing profession. Mentors provide needed support and nurturance and also offer challenges. Nurses can also benefit when their mentors share their experiences and warn of pitfalls. Mentors are also skilled at identifying signs of impending challenges, can offer options and alternatives, and can impart wisdom to those they advise. Nurses with mentors usually seek, find, and take leadership roles.

While leadership styles may vary, nursing leaders should be grounded in a powerful personal vision of what they intend to accomplish and should manifest their visions through their nurses by being exemplary managers of: (1) attention—they draw people through their strength and passionate focus on their visions, which they live; (2) meaning—they have an ability to communicate their vision in a way that allows people to make it their own and give it personal meaning; (3) trust—they are totally reliable, and their actions have integrity and embody a consistent interpretation of their vision; (4) self—they have high personal self-regard (Bennis, 1983).

Nurses who possess these skills and the aforementioned qualities have the effect of empowering other nurses by: (1) making them feel significant and recognizing their contributions, (2) focusing on their developing competencies rather than their failures, (3) creating a shared sense of community, and (4) making projects exciting and worthy of dedicated commitment. When these things are accomplished, nursing's voice becomes stronger and nursing's agenda of quality, cost-efficient health care for all is moved forward.

$\mathcal{E}$DUCATION

Have you ever heard the expression "you can't get there from here"? This expression is especially true for nurses. Nurses usually cannot reach the top of their profession without advancing their education. Education is one of the keys to self-empowerment and success, and education is what is assisting nurses in their transition from acute care nursing to community nursing.

For years, nurses have been educated at different levels through a 3-year diploma program, a 2-year associate degree (A.D.) program, or a 4-year baccalaureate degree (B.S.N.) program in preparation for state registered nurse licensure. For decades, nurses have been debating the issue of entry into practice with many nurses feeling that a baccalaureate degree should be the basic educational preparation for the nursing profession, while others argue against this notion.

It has been projected that the need for registered nurses who are prepared by baccalaureate degrees, masters' degrees, and post–master's degree certificate programs will increase significantly in the coming years. "The American Nurses Credentialing Center, the credentialing center that certifies more nurses than any group in the country (over 114,000), will require the B.S.N. for all of its specialty certifications by 1998" (ANA, 1995, p. 26)

As nurses begin to consider returning to school to further their education, the following variables must be considered: cost, accessibility, time commitment, philosophical comparability (the individual's and the school's), specialty tracks available, transferability of previous college credits, and whether or not the school awards credits for "life experiences."

Admission requirements must also be considered. Students should research review programs and courses that are offered to prepare examinees for entrance examinations that are required by universities or colleges or to prepare for challenge examinations.

Associate Degree to Baccalaureate Degree

Associate degree (A.D.) programs were originated by Mildred Montag who believed that there were two basic premises on which the associate degree program was developed: (1) the functions of nursing can and should be differentiated, and (2) these functions lie along a continuum with the professional at one end and the technical person at the other. Associate degree programs are probably the most popular and fastest growing programs in nursing education. This may be true for a number of reasons. Associate degree programs are usually based in community colleges, are therefore less costly than other programs, and are abundantly available throughout the United States; they are the quickest track to registered nurse licensure (2 years); and there are many job opportunities for associate degree graduates because employers do not necessarily differentiate between degrees when hiring staff nurses since both are licensed registered nurses. If an associate degree program is chosen, it is hoped that it will be seen as a jumping off point for more education, not a final destination.

There are over 500 universities and colleges that offer programs for the "returning registered nurse" who wishes to pursue a baccalaureate degree (B.S.N.). Baccalaureate degrees may be obtained in nursing or another health-related field, such as health science. For many nurses, self-marketability is one of the reasons for pursuing a baccalaureate degree.

It should be noted that a baccalaureate degree can also be attained through a nontraditional program offered by the Regents College, The State University of New York. This program is designed for the independent learner and offers home-study courses, which allow students to work at their own pace. It is available worldwide, and no residential study is required. The testing sites, however, are limited, and travel distances may be long.

Fast Track

For many nurses, time commitment is a major factor when they consider returning to school. For this reason, a number of institutions of higher learning have instituted an accelerated program, which allows the returning registered nurse to advance through a baccalaureate and master's program in 3 years. If a master's degree is the ultimate goal, researching these programs will be advantageous.

Master's Degrees

It has been projected that nurses who possess a master's degree will be more in demand than ever before in all areas of nursing. Therefore, the time may be right to consider pursuing this graduate degree. To enter a master's program, certain admission requirements and fee schedules must be met. Most schools require a B.S. degree, an undergraduate grade point average (GPA) of about a 3.0 or better, and acceptable scores on either the **Graduate Record Examination (GRE)** or the **Miller Analogies Test (MAT)**.

There are a number of master's degrees offered for nurses: Master of Arts (M.A.), Master of Science (M.S.), Master of Education (M.Ed.), Master of Science in Nursing (M.S.N), Master of Public Health (M.P.H.), and Master in Business Administration (M.B.A.). Presently, there are approximately 20 programs in the United States that offer a 2-year program through which students earn both an M.B.A. and an M.S.N.

Graduate Record Examination (GRE) is an examination taken before entrance into a college program, usually a graduate program. It looks at different mathematical skills and reading comprehension skills.

Miller Analogies Test (MAT) is an examination used to evaluate a student's level of preparedness for entry into graduate school. It deals primarily with problems that require solving by the use of logic.

Post–Master's Certificate Programs

Most post–master's certificate programs graduate nurses who are then referred to as advance practice nurses (APNs)—an umbrella term for registered nurses who have met certain advanced educational and clinical practice requirements. These programs have gained tremendously in popularity over the past decade as almost 140,000 APNs carved out their new role in delivering quality, cost-effective care. (It should be noted that not all APNs have educated at the post–master's degree level; many are prepared at the master's degree level). There are four principle types of APNs: (1) nurse practitioner (NP), (2) certified nurse midwife (CNM), (3) clinical nurse specialist (CNS), and (4) certified registered nurse anesthetist (CRNA).

Nurse Practitioner Programs In the United States, there are approximately 150 nurse practitioner programs that confer master's degrees.

There are at least 36 states that require nurse practitioners to be certified by national organizations.

Certified Nurse Midwife Programs Nurse midwifery programs are usually 1½ years long, and most do not have a specific degree prerequisite but instead require only completion of a basic nursing education in any accredited program. These midwifery programs generally confer certificates, but many of these programs are incorporated into master's programs. In some states (e.g., New York), certified nurse midwives require a separate license.

Clinical Nurse Specialist Programs Unlike nurse practitioner and certified nurse midwife programs, clinical nurse specialist programs must either confer master's degrees or require that a nurse entering the program have a master's degree in nursing.

Certified Registered Nurse Anesthetist Programs These programs are usually 2 to 3 years long, have a prerequisite of a baccalaureate degree, and must meet national certification and recertification requirements.

Doctoral Programs

There are several different doctoral degrees that registered nurses can pursue, such as a Doctor of Nursing Science (D.S.N.), a curriculum that tends to emphasize clinical expertise; a Doctor of Public Health, which emphasizes epidemiology and public policy; and a Doctor of Philosophy (Ph.D.), which focuses on the biological or social sciences. There are approximately 50 D.N.S. and Ph.D. programs in the United States. For nurses interested in academia, a Doctor of Education (Ed.D.) may be the track to follow. A doctoral degree that has gained in popularity among nurses is a Doctor of Jurisprudence (J.D.), a nurse attorney. Most doctoral programs require 90 credits beyond a baccalaureate degree.

Certification

There are several nationally recognized certification organizations in nursing. Many of these are specialty organizations that certify nurses in that specific specialty. In addition, The American Nurses Credentialing Center offers certification in dozens of specialty areas. "Certification is reserved for those nurses who have met requirements for clinical or functional practice in a specialized field, pursued education beyond basic nursing preparation, and received the endorsement of their peers" (ANA, 1995, p. 3). These examinations are based on nationally recognized standards of nursing practice.

Continuing Education

Many nurses hone their skills by attending educational programs that confer continuing education units (CEUs) to the nurses who attend these sessions. These are not college credits and are not used toward attaining a degree. Again, there are a number of organizations that confer these CEUs, but the ANA is the largest. CEUs can be obtained by attending a seminar, watching an educational video as part of a staff development program, or by reading an article, as in the *American Journal of Nursing (AJN)*, and answering the questions at the end of the article and mailing them in.

PROFESSIONAL INVOLVEMENT

One of the most important things nurses can do to ensure their professionalism is to belong to their professional organization. Many nurses belong to several organizations. They may belong to a specialty organization (e.g., Critical Care Nurses, the Black Nurses Association, the Philippine Nurses Association, the Irish Nurses Association), the state nurses association, the league for nursing, or a nursing honor society (e.g., Sigma Theta Tau International). Professional involvement is important because it gives the nurse a feeling of belonging, a sense of being a part of the whole. Professional organizations offer fantastic networking opportunities and an opportunity to have input into decisions that affect nurses. Professional organizations are also a great source of up-to-date information about what is happening in nursing. Some organizations serve as watchdogs over pending information that can either help or hurt nursing and can be heard as a collective voice for nurses. Professional involvement is another way to foster self-empowerment for nurses and help strengthen their commitment to the profession because to advance, we must unite.

SUMMARY

In this chapter, the current status of nursing and the opportunities available in the profession are examined. Different career paths and the skills that nurses need to pursue these paths are explored. The skills that nurses need to survive and to succeed in the present health care industry are also examined.

The concept of knowledge being power is highlighted through a segment that discusses the importance of nurses being knowledge brokers for clients, consumers, and legislators. Different educational tracks are explored to identify where and how nurses can pursue knowledge. Finally, the importance for nurses to belong to their professional organizations and how professional membership strengthens the profession are discussed.

KEY WORDS

Case management
Computer skills
Education
Fast track
Informatics
Knowledge broker

Leadership
Media
Mentoring
Nursing opportunities
Professional involvement

QUESTIONS

DIRECTIONS: Choose the one *best* response to each of the following questions.

1. The greatest numbers of opportunities for nurses are projected in all the following fields *except*

    A. community health.
    B. home care.
    C. hospital-based custodial care.
    D. managed care.

2. A Model for Differentiated Nursing Practice emphasizes which type of relationship among nurses?

    A. Mutually exclusive
    B. Collaborative
    C. Interdisciplinary
    D. Political

3. To remain employable, nurses must update their skills in which of the following areas?

    A. Computer technology
    B. Case management
    C. Communications (verbal and written)
    D. All the above

4. Benchmarking is used in case management to assist nurses in doing all of the following *except*

    A. approving claims.
    B. determining payment.
    C. negotiating services.
    D. determining who the client is.

5. Professional involvement is important for all of the following nurses *except* those who

    A. wish to keep current in their area of practice.
    B. need the benefits of networking.
    C. wish to limit their information sources.
    D. desire to become politically active.

ANSWERS

1. *The answer is C.* In most hospitals, discharge planners work diligently to find placement for clients who require custodial care in different types of facilities. Therefore, the need for nurses in this area of an institution has significantly declined.

2. *The answer is B.* In a Model for Differentiated Nursing Practice, collaborative relationships among nurses practicing in various nursing roles must be based on mutuality.

3. *The answer is D.* In order to be competitive in today's job market, a nurse must possess skills in computer technology, communications, and case management.

4. *The answer is D.* Benchmarking is a system of comparison. A benchmark or standard unit is identified in sufficient detail so that other similar classifications can be compared as being above, below, or comparable to the benchmark standard.

5. *The answer is C.* Professional involvement offers state of the art practice information, networking opportunities, and political activism.

ANNOTATED REFERENCES

American Association of College of Nursing. (1995). *A model for differentiated nursing practice.* Washington, DC: Author.

This publication details the activities, findings, and recommendations of a task force charged with identifying current differentiated practice and education efforts; developing a model for differentiated education and practice inclusive of associate, baccalaureate, and master's level nursing education; identifying a value-neutral terminology that describes differentiated clinicians' roles; and developing a plan for dissemination of these findings.

American Nurses Association. (1996). Supply, demand, need—nursing's numbers revisited. *Backgrounder.* Washington, DC: Author.

This publication contains statistics on nursing numbers from the U.S. Department of Labor, Bureau of Labor Statistics (BLS).

American Nurses Credentialing Center (ANCC). (1995). *Credentialing catalog. American nurses.* Washington, DC: Author.

This publication describes the different areas in which nurses can be credentialed by the ANCC.

Bennis, W. (1983). *On becoming a leader.* Reading, MA: Addison-Wesley.

This book looks at the differences between management and leadership skills. It describes different leadership styles.

Chin, P. L., & Jacobs, M. K. (1987). *Theory and nursing: A systematic approach.* St. Louis, MO: C. V. Mosby.

This text addresses the limitations of basing nursing theory and research on traditional scientific knowledge. It recognizes that scientific knowledge alone is inadequate to solve problems that are intimately related to human values, attitudes, beliefs, and personal interactions and expressions.

Forbes Leadership Library. (1995). *Thoughts on leadership.* Chicago: Triumph Books.

This book is a compilation of thoughts and reflections from history's greatest thinkers.

Harmer, B., & Henderson, V. (1960). *Textbook of the principles and practice of nursing.* New York: Macmillan.

This book is intended as a guide to nursing instructors and students and as a reference for nurses practicing in all settings. It presents the scientific principles that underlie nursing practice and suggests the methods that embody these principles.

Henderson, R., & Deane, F. (1996). User expectations and perceptions of a patient management information system. *Computers in Nursing,* 14(3), 188–193.

This article discusses a study that looked at the notion of disconfirmed expectations and the possible impact disconfirmed expectations may have upon the perceptions of the system the user group may develop.

Mattera, M. (Ed.). (1996). Nursing opportunities. *RN,* pp. 13–53.

This publication offers an alphabetical list of employer profiles, job opportunities, articles offering advice on interviewing skills, how to get your license, and how to add to your credentials to give your career a boost.

New York State Nurses Association (NYSNA). (1996). *Your future in nursing: A career planning guidebook for RNs.* Latham, NY: Author.

This booklet was prepared with assistance from the members of the NYSNA Council on Nursing Education. It describes opportunities afforded to nurses with college degrees and explains credentials needed for different career advancement.

U. S. Department of Health and Human Services. (1996). *Opportunities for nurses in the Indian Health Service.* Washington, DC: Author.

This colorful brochure details the opportunities available to nurses who wish to work in one of the 12 Indian Health Service areas. The brochure also contains a map of the United States with these 12 sites pinpointed.

Williams, D. (1996). The road less traveled. *Nursing Case Management,* 1(2), 53.

This editorial looks at case management as a field in which nurses can specialize. It also discusses the growth of case management and the Case Management Society of America.

*A*PPENDICES

*A*PPENDIX A

The definition and role of public health nursing was redeveloped in October 1996 and adopted in March 1997 by the APHA Public Health Nursing Section. The new definition of the role of Public Health Nursing states that "Public Health Nursing is the practice of promoting and protecting the health of populations using knowledge from nursing, social, and public health sciences" (APHA Public Health Nursing Section, March 1997).

Despite the recent trend, during the past 15 years, of hiring non-baccalaureate prepared nurses, the policy statement includes and expresses a need for basic baccalaureate preparation for all public health nurses (APHA Public Health Nursing Section, March 1997). The policy statement further states that all public health nurses should have a background in social and behavioral sciences, epidemiology, environmental health, current treatment modalities, and health care delivery options in order to fully understand health policy and research and treatment choices and to translate this knowledge into the promotion of healthy populations.

$\mathcal{A}$PPENDIX B

AGENCIES OF THE DEPARTMENT OF HEALTH AND HUMAN SERVICES

Office of the Secretary (OS)
Administration for Children and Families (ACF)
Administration on Aging (AOA)
Agency for Health Care Policy and Research (AHCPR)
Agency for Toxic Substances and Disease Registry (ATSDR)
Centers for Disease Control and Prevention (CDC)
Food and Drug Administration (FDA)
Health Care Financing Administration (HCFA)
Indian Health Service (IHS)
National Institutes of Health (NIH)
Program Support Center (PSC)
Substance Abuse and Mental Health Services Administration (SAMHSA)

$\mathcal{A}$PPENDIX C

CENTERS FOR DISEASE CONTROL AND PREVENTION (CDC)

Office of the CDC Director
   Information Resources Management Office
   Office of Health and Safety (OhASIS)
National Center for Chronic Disease Prevention and Health Promotion
National Center for Environmental Health
National Center for Health Statistics
National Center for HIV, STD, and TB Prevention
National Center for Infectious Disease
National Center for Injury Prevention and Control
National Institute for Occupational Safety and Health
Epidemiology Program Office
International Health Program Office
Public Health Practice Program Office
National Immunization Program

NOTE: The CDC is located in Atlanta, Georgia, and is an agency of the Department of Health and Human Services.

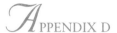

$\mathcal{A}$PPENDIX D

Organization of a Typical State Board of Health

State Health Officer
    Health Institutional Services
        Accrediting Bodies (Institutions and Professional Licensure)
    Research Services
        Vital Statistics
    Professional Education Services
    Public Health Education Services
    Health Care Services
        Dental Services
        Medical Services
        Nursing Services
        Medical Social Services
        Nutrition Services
    Environmental Health Services
    Legal Counsel

Organization of a Typical County Board of Health

District Health Officer
    Environmental Services
    Health Education Services
    Public Health Investigation Services
    Nursing Services
    Social Services
    Nutrition and Other Services
    Dental Services

INDEX

ISBN 0-07-105478-2

90000

9 780071 054782